D1310190

Cancer Chemotherapy and Biotherapy

A Reference Guide

Second Edition

Cancer Chemotherapy and Biotherapy

A Reference Guide

Linda Tenenbaum, R.N., M.S.N., O.C.N.
Professor, Nursing and Continuing Education
(Part Time)
Broward Community College
Ft. Lauderdale, Florida

W. B. SAUNDERS COMPANY
A Division of Harcourt Brace & Company
Philadelphia   London   Toronto
Montreal   Sydney   Tokyo

W.B. SAUNDERS COMPANY
A Division of Harcourt Brace & Company
The Curtis Center
Independence Square West
Philadelphia, PA 19106

RC271
.C5
T46
1994

Library of Congress Cataloging-in-Publication Data

Tenenbaum, Linda.
    Cancer chemotherapy : a reference guide / Linda Tenenbaum. — 2nd
ed.
        p. cm.
    Includes bibliographical references and index.
    ISBN 0–7216–6720–1
    1. Cancer—Chemotherapy.   2. Cancer—Nursing.   I. Title.
    [DNLM: 1. Neoplasms—nursing.   2. Antineoplastic Agents—therapeutic
use—nurses' instruction.   3. Neoplasms—drug therpay—nurses' instruction.   WY 156 T292c 1994]
    RC271.C5T46   1994
    616.99'4061—dc20
    DNLM/DLC   94–6844

CANCER CHEMOTHERAPY AND BIOTHERAPY:
A REFERENCE GUIDE   ISBN 0-7216-6720-1

Copyright © 1994, 1989 by W.B. Saunders Company

All rights reserved. No part of this publication may be reproduced or transmitted in any
form or by any means, electronic or mechanical, including photocopy, recording, or any
information storage and retrieval system, without permission in writing from the
publisher.

Printed in the United States of America

Last digit is the print number: 9   8   7   6   5   4   3   2   1

ABOUT THE AUTHOR

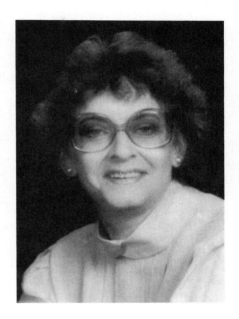

Linda Tenenbaum, R.N., M.S.N., O.C.N., received a B.S.N. from Adelphi University (Garden City, NY), an M.S.N. from Hunter College (New York, NY), and completed a National Cancer Institute Fellowship in Teaching Oncology Nursing at the University of Alabama (Birmingham). She has worked as a staff nurse at the Veterans Administration Hospital and as both a staff nurse and Nurse Clinician at Maimonides Medical Center in Brooklyn. She is currently a part-time Professor at Broward Community College in Ft. Lauderdale, Florida, where she teaches nursing and continuing education courses.

DBCN ACY-4165

MAR 28 1996

v

Notice

Extraordinary efforts have been made by the author to insure that dosage recommendations and all drug information are precise and in agreement with standards officially accepted at the time of publication.

It does happen, however, that dosage schedules and other drug data are changed from time to time in the light of accumulating clinical experience and continuing laboratory studies. This is most likely to occur with recently introduced products.

Uses for the medications include those officially designated by the manufacturers, and (in some cases) medications that show response in investigational studies.

It is urged, therefore, that you check the manufacturer's recommendations (the package insert) for dosages and other specifications and recommendations, *especially if the drug to be administered or prescribed is one that you use only infrequently or have not used for some time.*

PREFACE TO THE SECOND EDITION

A great deal of progress has been made in the field of cancer therapies since the first edition of *Cancer Chemotherapy: A Reference Guide* was prepared. This is partially reflected in the new title, with the words "and Biotherapy" added. Our understanding of neoplastic disease has expanded, and clinical investigations continue the search for new ways to halt tumor cell reproduction, with minimal effect to normal cells.

New agents have been added to those already in use. For example, luteinizing hormone releasing hormone (LHRH) agonists, such as luprolide (Lupron Depot) and goserlin (Zoladex), are developments of the late 1980s and early 1990s. Both have effects similar to diethylstilbestrol (DES) on prostate cancer, with fewer cardiovascular side effects. The nonsteroidal antiandrogen (flutamide, Eulexin) is now used in combination with LHRH agonists to suppress the associated "flare reaction," making the therapy more tolerable to the patient.

Through medical research, analogues of earlier medications, or "second generation" drugs, associated with fewer toxicities have been developed. Carboplatin, an analogue of cisplatin, is reported to be less emetogenic, neurotoxic, and nephrotoxic. Idarubicin, an anthracycline analogue, is reported to be less cardiotoxic than doxorubicin.

The fourth modality of therapy for cancers—biotherapy, or biological response modifiers (BRMs)—is addressed in Chapter 4. Some BRMs have demonstrated direct antitumor activity, while others can augment or moderate the immune system after myelosuppressive antininoplastic therapy.

The most common dose-limiting toxicity of antineoplastic therapy is myelosuppression. Colony-stimulating factors, such as filgrastim (Neupogen) and epoetin (Epogen) can ameliorate these effects by restoring circulating blood cells earlier and reducing complications such as infection.

Other pharmacologic agents have been developed that can prevent or alleviate some of the most undesirable and dose-limiting toxicities associated with cancer chemotherapy. Ondansetron (Zofran) and granisetron (Kytril) have made emetogenic therapy more tolerable and acceptable by minimizing the incidence and severity of nausea and vomiting. Mesna, a "uroprotective" agent, prevents hemorrhagic cystitis that may occur with ifosfamide or cyclophosphamide. Cardioprotective agents and other drugs that can reduce toxicities of chemotherapy are being studied in clinical trials.

A chapter on chemoprevention (Chapter 6) has been added, with information regarding medications such as Retin-A in clinical trials for prevention of skin cancers and tamoxifen as a preventive agent for persons at high risk for breast cancer.

As more persons are cured of cancer, we are more cognizant of long-term effects of chemotherapy, including second malignancies and organ alterations. Chapter 12 addresses the problem of second malignancies associated with chemotherapy. Another addition to the second edition, Chapter 15, presents information on the peripherally inserted central catheter (PIC or PICC line).

I hope that those of you who have the first edition found it helpful and that this edition will once again serve as your current resource on chemotherapy and biotherapy.

Linda Tenenbaum

ACKNOWLEDGMENTS

I would like to express thanks to those who offered suggestions, assistance, and support to make this book possible.

I am grateful to the many nurses and other health care personnel who prepare and administer chemotherapy and/or biotherapy and who care for persons receiving these medications. Many have given me suggestions to make this book accurate as well as practical. They include: reviewers for the second edition; Maria Buerga, R.Ph. Pharm. D., Director of Clinical Pharmacy, Florida Medical Center, Ft. Lauderdale, Florida; Linda Henke, M.S.L.S., Manager, Medical Library, Memorial Hospital, Hollywood, Florida; Mary Cochran, R.N., B.S.N., O.C.N., Nurse Manager; and Aleen Khan, R.N., O.C.N., staff nurse on the oncology unit, Memorial Hospital, Hollywood, Florida.

I owe thanks to the companies that market chemotherapy and biotherapy agents, chemotherapy safety equipment, vascular access devices, and nutritional supplements, and to many of the local Ft. Lauderdale representatives for valuable information they provided me as I revised and updated this book.

I appreciate Karon Titus, R.N., Ed.D., my friend and colleague, who provided the art for the original first edition cover. I am also grateful to a former student, Betty Scott, for her review and partial revision of the Plan of Care for the Patient with Alterations in Sexual Function, and to the library staff at Broward Community College, Central Campus, for their invaluable assistance.

Thanks are due to two oncologists: Dr. Abraham Rosenberg and Dr. Alan Kramer, for their review, suggestions, and answers to many questions I had in preparing the first and second editions of this book.

Special thanks to many at W.B. Saunders and P.M. Gordon Associates for the guidance and suggestions I received during the various stages of preparation; they truly added the "finishing touches" to the book. They are: Barbara Nelson Cullen, Editor, Nursing Books; Francine Rosenthal, Editorial Assistant; Cass Stamato, Staff Support Specialist; Peggy Gordon, Project Manager; and Joan Sinclair, Production Manager. Special thanks to Mary Finuoli, who answered W.B. Saunders' phone each time I called to speak to someone there. It was a pleasure to deal with persons who made a little extra effort to be as courteous and as helpful as possible.

Love to my Mom and members of my family for their understanding each time I said, "No—I can't" during the past three years of research and revision.

My final and greatest thanks, along with my never-ending love, go to my husband Arthur, for patience and love that has assisted me greatly during this time-consuming endeavor.

Linda Tenenbaum

CONTRIBUTORS

- **Cheryl A. Bean, D.S.N., R.N., C.S., O.C.N.**
Associate Professor and Project Director
Oncology Specialization in Primary Nursing
Indiana University School of Nursing
Indianapolis, IN

Nursing Management of the Client with Neuropsychological Alterations (Chapter 11)

- **Joseph Brown, R.N., B.S.N., C.R.N.I.**
Director of Education
Gesco International, Inc.
San Antonio, TX

Peripherally Inserted Central Catheters (Chapter 15)
Troubleshooting Vascular Access Devices (Chapter 18)

- **Jean Ellsworth-Wolk, R.N., M.S., O.C.N.**
Oncology Program Director/Oncology Clinical Nurse Specialist
Lakewood Hospital
Lakewood, OH
Clinical Faculty, Graduate Program
Case Western Reserve University
Cleveland, OH

Preparation/Administration/ Extravasation (Chapter 2)

- **Constance Engelking, R.N., M.S., O.C.N.**
Oncology Clinical Nurse Specialist
Westchester County Medical Center
Valhalla, NY
Adjunct Instructor of Medicine
New York Medical College
Valhalla, NY

Biologic Response Modifiers (Chapter 4)

- **Marianne Glasel, R.N., M.S., M.A.**
Director, Graduate Program in Oncology Nursing and Accelerated Masters Program
Columbia University School of Nursing
New York, NY
Consultant, Human Sexuality and Sexual Health Care
Memorial Sloan-Kettering Hospital
New York, NY

Effects on Reproduction/Sexual Function (Chapter 9)

- **Jody Gross, R.N., M.S.N., O.C.N.**
Director of Nursing
Hospice of the Florida Keys, Inc., and Visiting Nurse Association
Key West, FL

Cancer Drug Development (Chapter 5)

• **Jan Hawthorne, R.N., M.S.N., O.C.N.**
Clinical Nurse Specialist
Solid Tumor Unit
University Hospitals of Cleveland
Cleveland, OH
Clinical Faculty
Frances Payne Bolton School of Nursing
Case Western Reserve University
Cleveland, OH

*Preparation/Administration/
Extravasation (Chapter 2)*

• **Catherine A. Hydzik, R.N., M.S., O.C.N.**
Clinical Nurse Specialist–Oncology
Jack D. Weiler Hospital of the Albert Einstein College of Medicine
Bronx, NY

Second Malignancies (Chapter 12)

• **Patricia A. Kramer, R.N., M.S.N., O.C.N.**
Clinical Nurse Specialist–Oncology
St. Francis Memorial Hospital
San Francisco, CA

Chemoprevention (Chapter 6)

• **Debi Leshin, R.N., B.S.N., O.C.N.**
Clinical Manager, High Tech Division
Visiting Nurse Association of Dade
Miami, FL

Alterations in the Integumentary System (Chapter 10)

*Plans for the Client with: Alterations in the: Hematopoietic, Gastrointestinal, Renal, Cardiac, Respiratory, and Neurologic Systems
Fluid and Electrolyte Alterations
Allergic Responses*

• **Christine Miaskowski, R.N., Ph.D.**
Associate Professor
Department of Physiological Nursing
University of California, San Francisco
San Francisco, CA

Second Malignancies (Chapter 12)

• **Dixie Brennan Scelsi, R.N., M.S., M.S.N.**
Nursing Consultant
Port Charlotte, FL

*Vascular Access Catheters (Chapter 14)
Implanted Infusion Ports (Chapter 16)
Infusion Pumps (Chapter 17)
Troubleshooting Vascular Access Devices (Chapter 18)
Client Education (Chapter 19)*

• **Debra Wujcik, R.N., M.S.N., O.C.N.**
Clinical Nurse Specialist
Oncology/Hematology/BMT
Vanderbilt Medical Center
Nashville, TN

Biologic Response Modifiers (Chapter 4)

CONTENTS

LIST OF TABLES

General Information and Chemotherapeutic Agents

Chapter 1

The Cell Cycle and Cancer Chemotherapy

Linda Tenenbaum, R.N., M.S.N., O.C.N.

Goals of Chemotherapy

Cancer chemotherapy is the administration of antineoplastic medications alone or in combinations for treatment of malignant neoplasms. Tumors responsive to chemotherapy are listed in Table 1–1. The goals of chemotherapy include:

1. *Cure*—Eradication of all cancer, and the same life expectancy as an individual who does not have cancer. Cure is most often achieved for highly proliferative tumors, e.g., pediatric acute lymphocytic leukemia, Hodgkin's disease, neuroblastoma, testicular carcinoma, choriocarcinoma.

2. *Control*—Prolongation of survival by arresting or slowing growth of a metastatic tumor.

3. *Palliation*—Provision of relief of symptoms (e.g., pain, hypercalcemia) when it is no longer possible to achieve a remission.

4. *Adjuvant Therapy*—Administration of chemotherapy after removal of the primary tumor in an attempt to eradicate remaining tumor or micrometastases.

5. *Neoadjuvant Therapy* (primary chemotherapy, induction chemotherapy)—Administration of chemotherapy prior to other therapies (e.g., surgery, radiation therapy) in an attempt to decrease tumor size and bulk and make the tumor more responsive to the therapy.

3

Table 1–1   Tumors Responsive to Chemotherapy

Tumors Curable in Advanced Stages by Chemotherapy

Acute myelogenous leukemia	Hodgkin's disease
Burkitt's lymphoma	Lymphoblastic lymphoma (in children
Choriocarcinoma	and adults)
Acute lymphocytic leukemia (in chil-	Neuroblastoma
dren and adults)	Peripheral neuroepithelioma
Diffuse large cell lymphoma	Ovarian cancer
Embryonal rhabdomyosarcoma	Small cell cancer of the lung
Ewing's sarcoma	Testicular cancer
Follicular mixed lymphoma	Wilm's tumor

Tumors Curable in the Adjuvant Setting by Chemotherapy

Breast cancer	Osteogenic sarcoma
Colorectal cancer	Soft tissue sarcoma

Tumors Responsive in Advanced Stages But Not Yet Curable by Chemotherapy

Adrenocortical carcinoma	Gastric carcinoma
Bladder cancer	Glioblastoma multiforme
Breast cancer	Hairy cell leukemia
Carcinoid tumors	Head and neck cancer
Cervical carcinoma	Insulinoma
Chronic lymphocytic leukemia	Medulloblastoma
Chronic myelogenous leukemia	Multiple myeloma
Follicular small cleaved cell lymphoma	Prostate cancer
	Soft tissue sarcoma

Tumors Poorly Responsive in Advanced Stages to Chemotherapy

Carcinoma of the vulva or penis	Osteogenic sarcoma
Colorectal cancer	Pancreatic cancer
Hepatocellular carcinoma	Renal cancer
Non–small cell lung cancer	Thyroid cancer
Melanoma	

From DeVita, V.T., Jr., Hellman, S., and Rosenberg, S.A. (eds.): *Cancer: Principles and Practice of Oncology*, 3rd ed. (p. 297). Philadelphia, J.B. Lippincott, 1989. Reprinted with permission.

Cellular Kinetics

First order kinetics is a concept that refers to the destruction of a fixed percentage of tumor cells with each administration of antineoplastic chemotherapy. To eradicate all viable cells, the chemotherapeutic agent must be administered at repeated intervals over a period of time until the agents, along with the client's immune system, destroy all cancer cells. According to the *cell kill hypothesis* for tumor cells (Fig. 1–1), administration of a chemotherapeutic agent will kill a percentage of the total number of cells with each course of therapy. If, for example, a tumor body contains one million (1,000,000) cells and the treatment regimen

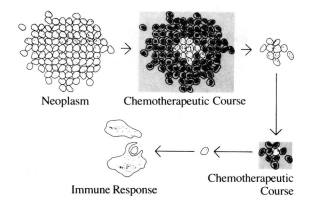

Neoplasm   Chemotherapeutic Course

Immune Response   Chemotherapeutic Course

Figure 1–1. Cell kill hypothesis. (From Goodman, M.: *Cancer: Chemotherapy and Care.* Princeton, NJ, Bristol-Myers Squibb Oncology Division, 1992, 22. Reprinted with permission.)

has a 90% cell kill rate, the first course of therapy would theoretically destroy 90% (900,000) of the one million cells, leaving 100,000 cells. The second dose would kill 90,000 cells, leaving 10,000 cells, and so on until one cell remained. Hopefully, the body's immune response would then destroy the final remaining cell. This theory explains why most chemotherapeutic regimens consist of medications administered at regular intervals over a period of months or years.

Phases of the Cell Cycle

The cell cycle (Fig. 1–2) is the pattern of cell growth and division for both normal cells and cancer cells. A concept of the cell cycle is necessary for better understanding of the way in which chemotherapeutic agents function.

During the cell cycle, all cell activities take place and each parent cell prepares for division into two identical daughter cells. One cell becomes two, two become four, four become eight, and so on.

Phases of the cell cycle include:

1. *Gap 1* (G-1)—The phase in which RNA, proteins, and enzymes necessary for synthesis of DNA are formed. This phase may last hours to days.

2. *Synthesis* (S)—The phase in which DNA is synthesized and chromosomes double in number within the cell nucleus in preparation for mitosis. DNA contains the genetic code information essential to the growth and reproduction of each cell. This phase may last 10–20 hours.

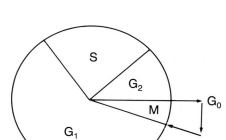

Figure 1–2. The cell cycle.

3. *Gap-2* (G-2)—The second period of RNA and protein synthesis. The mitotic spindle develops during this phase. This phase is also known as the *premitotic* phase and lasts from 2–10 hours.

4. *Mitosis* (M)—The phase in which one cell, known as the parent cell, divides into two new daughter cells. Each daughter cell contains the same number and kind of chromosomes as the parent cell. This phase is brief, lasting only 30–60 minutes.

5. *The resting stage* (G-0)—The phase in which all cell activity except cell division takes place.

The entire cell cycle (G-1, S, G-2, and M) is referred to as the *cell generation time.*

Most cells in the G-0 state can be activated to re-enter the G-1 phase when cell damage or destruction makes replication necessary. Some of the body's cells are always in the G-0 stage, such as the cells of the neurons, which are highly differentiated. Other cells do not normally reproduce after reaching maturity, but can do so to replace lost cells when necessary (e.g., hepatic cells can regenerate after hepatic damage or partial surgical resection of the liver).

The cell replication process is similar in normal cells and cancer cells. Normal cells replicate in response to the body's needs; initiation and termination of this process are controlled by biological feedback systems. Cancer cell replication occurs without control or response to biological feedback.

Actions of Chemotherapeutic Agents in Relation to the Cell Cycle

Chemotherapeutic agents vary in modes of action. They are classified as cell cycle phase–specific or cell cycle phase–nonspecific.

1. **Cell cycle phase–specific agents** exert their effect during a specific phase or phases of the cell cycle. These agents are most ef-

fective when used to treat tumors with rapidly dividing cells. This category includes:
   a. Mitotic inhibitors, which act by interfering with proper assembly of proteins necessary for formation of the mitotic spindle.
   b. Most subcategories of antimetabolites, which are specific to the S phase of the cell cycle.
2. **Cell cycle phase–nonspecific agents.**
   a. Act on cells that are actively dividing in any phase of the cell cycle or in the resting (nonreplicating) state. These include:
      (1) Alkylating agents.
      (2) Nitrosoureas.
      (3) Most antitumor antibiotics.
      (4) Purine analogs.
   b. Characteristics:
      (1) Dose dependent. The degree of cell kill is directly proportional to the dose administered.
      (2) Display no specificity for cells that are dividing.
      (3) Effects are directed toward the DNA molecule.
      (4) Effective when administered as a single bolus dose.

The phase or phases of the cell cycle in which chemotherapeutic medications act will be discussed throughout this book.

Categories of Chemotherapeutic Agents

1. **Alkylating agents.**
   a. Have the ability to bind or cross-link with the cell's DNA, interfering with DNA replication.
   b. Also interact with RNA and protein.
   c. Most kill dividing cells.
2. **Nitrosoureas.**
   a. Function in a manner similar to alkylating agents.
   b. Able to cross the blood–brain barrier.
   c. Myelosuppression is delayed, occurring 3 to 6 weeks after administration.
3. **Antimetabolites.**
   a. Structurally or functionally similar to normal essential metabolites, but with slight differences.
   b. Block or interfere with DNA synthesis when used by a rapidly dividing or slowly proliferating (tumor) cell.
   c. Most are cell cycle–specific to S phase of the cell cycle.
   d. Purine analogs are cell cycle–nonspecific.
   e. Subcategories include:

(1) Folate (folic acid) antagonists:
  (a) Methotrexate (MTX) (Mexate, Folex).
(2) Purine analogs:
  (a) Cladribine (Leustatin).
  (b) Fludarabine phosphate (Fludara).
  (c) Pentostatin (deoxycoformycin, Nipent).
(3) Purine antagonists:
  (a) 6-Mercaptopurine (6-MP) (Purinethol).
  (b) 6-Thioguanine (6-TG) (Thioguanine).
(4) Pyrimidine antagonists:
  (a) 5-Fluorouracil (5-FU) (Adrucil, Fluoroplex).
  (b) 5-Fluorodeoxyuridine (5-FUDR).
  (c) Cytarabine (Ara-C), cytosine arabinoside (Cytosar-U, Tarabine).
4. **Mitotic inhibitors.**
  a. Interfere with formation of the mitotic spindle.
  b. Most effective when administered:
    (1) In multiple, repeated fractions rather than one large dose.
    (2) When the cell mass is low and there is a large proportion of actively dividing tumor cells.
  c. Subcategories:
    (1) Vinca alkaloids (plant alkaloids):
      (a) Vinblastine (Velban, Velbe, Velsar).
      (b) Vincristine (Oncovin, Vincasar).
      (c) Vindesine (Eldisine).
    Vinblastine and vincristine are derived from the periwinkle (*Vinca rosea*) plant.
    (2) Podophyllum derivatives:
      (a) Etoposide (VePesid).
      (b) Teniposide (Vumon).
    Etoposide is derived from the American mandrake plant. Other podophyllum derivatives are currently under investigation.
    (3) Taxoids:
      (a) Paclitaxel (Taxol):
        (i) Originally isolated from the Western yew tree, *Taxus brevifolia*; synthetic form approved in 1993.
        (ii) Causes mitotic arrest by promoting formation of abnormal spindle fibers and mitotic asters (Rowinsky et al., 1990).
        (iii) Approved for use in the treatment of ovarian carcinomas unresponsive to first-line therapies.
      (b) Docetaxel (Taxotere, investigational):
        (i) Isolated from European yew tree, *Taxus baccata*.
        (ii) Mechanism of action similar to Taxol.

5. **Antitumor antibiotics.**
   a. Inhibit synthesis of RNA.
   b. React with or bind to DNA.
   c. Most are cell cycle phase–nonspecific.
6. **Miscellaneous cancer chemotherapeutic agents.** Some chemotherapeutic agents that have yet other modes of action or an unknown manner of action are classified in this category. As research identifies a specific mode of action, they may be placed in
   one of the preceding categories. These agents include:
   a. Hydroxyurea.
      (1) Interferes with DNA synthesis in a mode similar to the ac-
          tion of antimetabolites.
   b. Procarbazine.
      (1) Precise mechanism of action uncertain.
      (2) Effects resemble those of alkylating agents.
      (3) Cell cycle phase–nonspecific.
   c. Asparaginase.
      (1) An enzyme that inhibits protein synthesis of malignant
          cells by hydrolyzing asparagine, a required amino acid.
7. **Hormones and hormone antagonists.**
   a. Interfere with protein synthesis and alter cell metabolism by
      changing the cell's hormonal environment. Actions of all are
      not fully understood.
   b. Subcategories:
      (1) Adrenocorticoids (corticosteroids):
          (a) Prednisone.
              (i) Used as part of combination chemotherapy regi-
                  mens; used primarily for suppressant effect on
                  lymphocytes in leukemia and lymphomas.
              (ii) Administered for palliation of some solid
                   tumors.
          (b) Dexamethasone.
              (i) May inhibit induction of interleukin-2 and gamma
                  interferon in normal human lymphocytes (Arya et
                  al., 1984).
              (ii) Administered for treatment of cerebral edema
                   from primary or metaplastic neoplasms of the cen-
                   tral nervous system.
              (iii) Administered in antiemetic regimens (see Chap-
                    ter 8).
      (2) Estrogens.
          (a) Reduce secretion of testosterone from Leydig cells of
              the testes by blocking release of luteinizing hormone-
              releasing hormone (LHRH) and luteinizing hormone
              (LH) in the pituitary.

    (b) Examples:
        (i) Diethylstilbestrol (DES).
        (ii) Estradiol (Estinyl, Feminone).
        (iii) Chlorotianesene (Tace).

(3) Progestins.
    (a) Reduce LH secretion from the pituitary.
    (b) May have antiandrogenic properties.
    (c) Administered in treatment of carcinoma of the breast, endometrium, and prostate.
    (d) May be administered as an anabolic steroid with acquired immunodeficiency syndrome (AIDS) or cancer cachexia (see Chapter 8).
    (e) Examples:
        (i) Megestrol acetate (Megace).
        (ii) Medroxyprogesterone acetate (Provera).

(4) Antiestrogens.
    (a) Compete with estrogen for binding to receptors in breast cancer cells.
    (b) Inhibit action of estrogen at the cellular level.
    (c) Most effective against estrogen-receptor–positive breast cancer in the female (Aisner et al., 1992).
    (d) Examples:
        (i) Tamoxifen citrate (Nolvadex).
        (ii) Toremifene (investigational).

(5) Androgens.
    (a) Inhibit gonadotropin-releasing hormone (GnRH) and estrogen production (Aisner et al., 1992).
    (b) Examples:
        (i) Fluoxymesterone (Halotestin, Oratestryl).
        (ii) Methyltestosterone (Metandren, Oreton Methyl).
        (iii) Testolactone (Teslac).

(6) Antiandrogens (steroid type).
    (a) Compete with androgens for receptor sites in target cells at the cellular level.
    (b) Suppress gonadotropin and androgen production via negative feedback mechanisms.
    (c) Have no effect on circulating serum testosterone.
    (d) Used in combination with LHRH agonist to suppress androgen flare reaction.
    (e) Example:
        (i) Flutamide (Eulexin).

(7) Antiandrogens (progestational type).
    (a) Bind with and block dihydrotestosterone, the active metabolite of testosterone, to specific receptors in prostatic cancer cells.

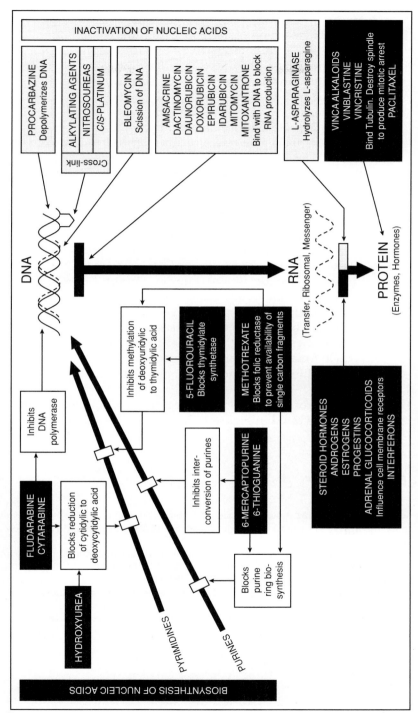

Figure 1-3. Mechanism of action of anticancer drugs. (From Krakoff, I.H.: Cancer chemotherapeutic and biologic agents. CA: A Cancer Journal for Clinicians. *41*:268, 1991. Copyright American Cancer Society, Inc. Reprinted with permission.)

      (b) Inhibit secretion of LH which, in turn, reduces production of testicular testosterone.

      (c) Do not cause a compensatory increase in androgen secretion and the "flare reaction" seen with conventional antiandrogens.

      (d) Example:

         (i) Cyproterone acetate (Androcur).*

(8) Luteinizing hormone-releasing hormone (LHRH) antagonists.

      (a) Suppress release of LHRH, with reduction of testicular and ovarian function.

      (b) Reduce circulating levels of testosterone, producing medical castration, which may be reversible if applied for a limited period of time (Eisenberger et al., 1986).

      (c) Indications: metastatic carcinoma of the prostate.

      (d) Examples:

         (i) Leuprolide acetate (Lupron, Lupron Depot).

         (ii) Goserlin acetate implant (Zoladex).

(9) Steroid blockers.

      (a) Block adrenal steroid synthesis.

      (b) Examples:

         (i) Aminoglutethamide (Cytadren).

         (ii) Mitotane (Lysodren).

The relationship of chemotherapy categories and specific agents to the cell cycle is illustrated in Figure 1–3.

References

Aisner, J., Eisenberger, M., and Fontana, J.A.: Hormonal agents for the treatment of cancer. In Perry, M.C. (ed.): *The Chemotherapy Source Book* (pp. 413–429). Baltimore, Williams & Wilkins, 1992.

Arya, S., Wong-Staal, F., and Gallo, R.C.: Dexamethasone-mediated inhibition of human T cell growth factor and α-interferon messenger RNA. J. Immunol. *133*:273–276, 1984.

Eisenberger, M., O'Dwyer, P.F., and Friedman, M.: Gonadotropin hormone releasing hormone: A new therapeutic approach for the treatment of prostate cancer. J. Clin. Oncol. *4*:414–424, 1986.

Rowinsky, E.K., Cazenave, L.A., and Donehower, L.A.: Taxol: A novel investigational microtubule agent. J. Natl. Cancer Inst. *82*:1247–1259, 1990.

*Available in Canada.

Recommended Readings

DeVita, V.T., Jr.: Principles of chemotherapy. In DeVita, V.T., Jr., Rosenberg, S.A., and Hellman, S. (eds.): *Cancer: Principles and Practice of Oncology*, 4th ed. (pp. 276–300). Philadelphia, J.B. Lippincott, 1993.

Goodman, M.: *Cancer: Chemotherapy and Care*, 3rd ed. Princeton, NJ, Bristol-Myers Squibb, 1992.

Guy, J.: Medical oncology—the agents. In Baird, S.B., et al. (eds.): *Cancer Nursing: A Comprehensive Textbook* (pp. 266–290). Philadelphia, W.B. Saunders, 1991.

Knobf, T., and Durivage, H.J.: Chemotherapy: principles of therapy. In Groenwald, S.L., et al. (eds.): *Cancer Nursing: Principles and Practice*, 3rd ed. (pp. 271–292). Boston, Jones and Bartlett, 1993.

Krakoff, I.: Cancer chemotherapeutic and biologic agents. CA: A Cancer Journal for Clinicians 41:264–277, 1991.

Quint-Kasner, S., Chisholm, L.S., de Carvahlo, M., et al.: Cancer chemotherapy: Basic principles (programmed instruction). Cancer Nurs. 16(1):145–160, 1993.

Yarbro, J.W.: The scientific basis of cancer chemotherapy. In Perry, M.C. (ed.): *The Chemotherapy Source Book* (pp. 2–14). Baltimore, Williams & Wilkins, 1992.

Chapter 2

Preparation, Administration, and Safe Disposal of Chemotherapeutic Agents

Linda Tenenbaum, R.N., M.S.N., O.C.N.
Jean Ellsworth-Wolk, R.N., M.S., O.C.N.
Jan L. Hawthorne, R.N., M.S.N., O.C.N.

Calculation of Chemotherapy Dosage

Chemotherapy doses are calculated according to (1) milligrams (or units) per kilogram of body weight, or (2) body surface area (BSA), which is based on height and weight. BSA is the more accurate way to compute doses for these medications and may be calculated by using a nomogram (Fig. 2–1). A straight edge (such as a ruler or index card) is placed with the left side at the patient's height (in centimeters or inches) and the right side at the patient's weight (in pounds or kilograms). A real or imaginary line is then drawn between the two points; the point at which the line crosses the center scale (BSA) is the m^2 (meters squared) used in calculating the dose. Children differ from adults in solid tissue and fluid proportions and a different nomogram (Fig. 2–2) must be used to determine a child's BSA.

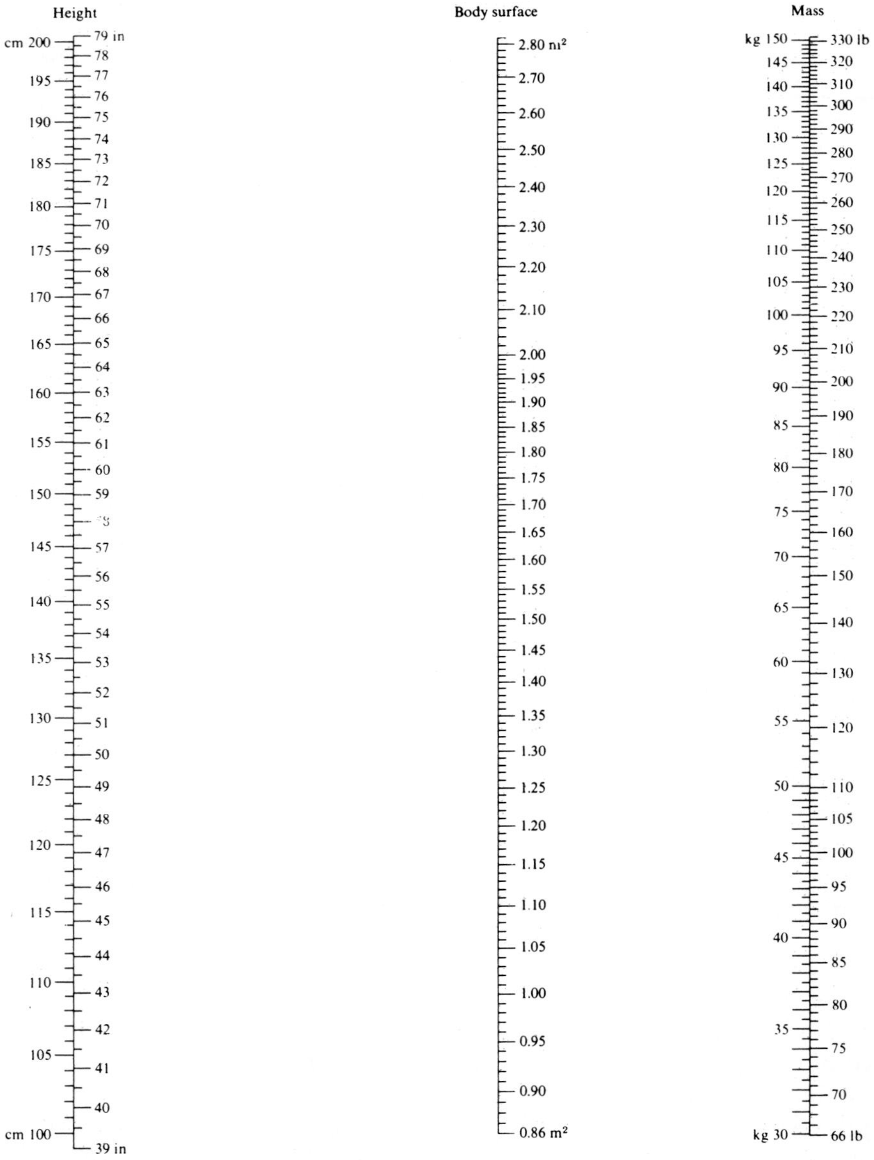

Height   Body surface   Mass

† From the formula of Du Bois and Du Bois, *Arch. intern. Med.*, **17**, 863 (1916): $S = M^{0.425} \times H^{0.725} \times 71.84$, or $\log S = \log M \times 0.425 + \log H \times 0.725 + 1.8564$ (S: body surface in cm^2, M: mass in kg, H: height in cm).

Figure 2–1. Adult nomogram. (From Letner, C. (ed.): *Geigy Scientific Tables*, 8th ed., Vol. 1. Basel, Ciba-Geigy, 1981, p. 226. Reprinted with permission.)

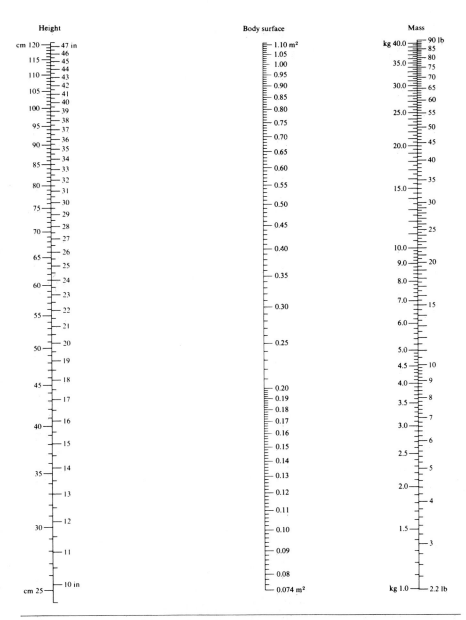

' From the formula of Du Bois and Du Bois, *Arch. intern. Med.*, **17**, 863 (1916): $S = M^{0.425} \times H^{0.725} \times 71.84$, or $\log S = \log M \times 0.425 + \log H \times 0.725 + 1.8564$ (S: body surface in cm²; M: mass in kg, H: height in cm).

Figure 2–2. Pediatric nomogram used for calculation of the BSA of a child. (From Letner, C. (ed.): *Geigy Scientific Tables*, 8th ed., Vol. 1. Basel, Ciba-Geigy, 1981, p. 227. Reprinted with permission.)

Modes of Administration of Chemotherapeutic Agents

Cancer chemotherapeutic agents may be administered in a variety of ways.

1. Oral route (P.O.).
   a. Tablet.
   b. Capsule.
   c. Liquid.
   d. Sublingual form (some hormonal agents).
2. Topical.
   a. Cream.
   b. Solution.
3. Parenteral routes, including:
   a. Subcutaneous.
   b. Intramuscular.
   c. Intravenous (I.V.) (most common parenteral route).
      (1) I.V. push (Fig. 2–3)—administration of the chemotherapeutic agent directly into a vein.
      (2) I.V. sidearm (I.V. sideport, I.V. Y-site) (Fig. 2–4)—administration of the chemotherapeutic agent from a syringe via a needle into the sideport or Y-site of a freely flowing I.V.
      (3) I.V. piggyback (Fig. 2–5)—administration of the chemotherapeutic agent diluted in a secondary I.V. bag, usually in 50–100 ml of diluent. The secondary line may be:

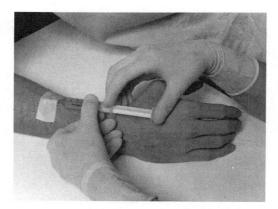

Figure 2–3. I.V. push—administration of medication from a syringe directly into a vein. Note: Extension I.V. tubing may be added between needle and syringe to allow for better visualization of blood return at intervals.

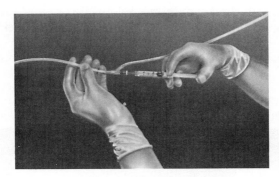

Figure 2–4. I.V. sidearm (sideport)—administration of a medication from the syringe via a protected needle or blunt cannula into the sideport of a freely flowing I.V. (Courtesy of Pharmacia Adria Laboratories, Columbus, OH.)

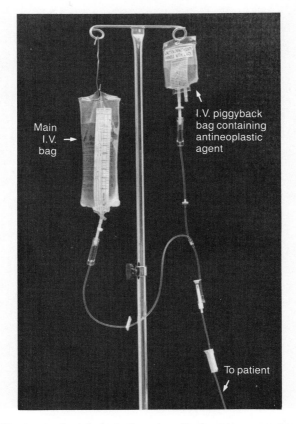

Figure 2–5. I.V. piggyback—adminstration of medication via a secondary I.V. bag and tubing, usually in 50 or 100 ml of diluent. Note: I.V. bag and tubing may need to be covered with aluminum foil or a light-resistant bag if medication is unstable when exposed to light.

> (a) Attached via a protected needle or blunt cannula to the primary line or to the I.V. or saline lock and removed when not in use, or
>
> (b) Part of a Y-set tubing that is clamped off but remains in place when not in use.
>
> (4) I.V. infusion (Fig. 2–6)—administration of the chemother-

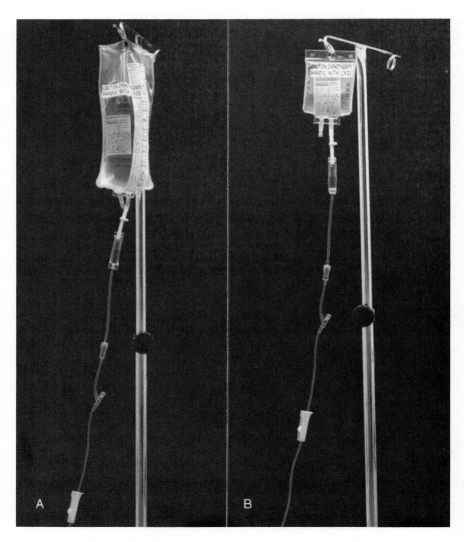

Figure 2–6. I.V. infusion. **A,** Administration of medication via the main I.V. bag, usually in 250–1000 ml of diluent. **B,** Primary medication bag may be 50 or 100 ml if a continuous I.V. is not necessary. Note: I.V. bag and tubing may need to be covered with aluminum foil or a light-resistant bag if medication is unstable when exposed to light.

apeutic agent diluted in the main I.V. bag, usually in 250–1000 ml of I.V. solution.

Some tumor types respond best when the chemotherapeutic agent or biologic response modifier is administered directly into the tumor area or into a body cavity. These modes of therapy include:

1. Intraperitoneal.
2. Intrahepatic.
3. Intravesical.
4. Intrapleural.
5. Intrapericardial.
6. Intrathecal.
7. Intracerebral.
8. Regional perfusion.

Further information on these modes of therapy can be found in Table 2–1.

Preparation and Safe Handling of Chemotherapeutic Agents

Chemotherapy is usually prepared in a pharmacy, using special equipment and procedures to ensure minimal exposure to and maximum protection from potentially dangerous agents. Occasionally, chemotherapy is reconstituted by a nurse in a hospital unit, in the physician's office, or in the home setting.

Oncology Nursing Society (ONS) Outcome Criteria

Outcome Criteria (ONS, 1988, modules 2, 3, p. 4; module 4, p. 5):

1. Health care personnel, the patient, and the environment will be protected from unnecessary exposure to potentially hazardous substances.
2. The sterility of the drug(s) being prepared for administration will be maintained.

Exposure to Antineoplastic Agents

Potential routes of exposure to chemotherapeutic agents and their components include direct skin or eye contact and aerosol inhalation. Effects of exposure may be short- or long-term. Short-term effects are usually seen at the time of exposure or within hours or days afterward. These include dermatitis and hyperpigmentation of exposed skin areas.

(*Text continued on page 29*)

Table 2–1 Alternative Routes for Administration of Cancer Chemotherapy

ANATOMIC REGION AND INDICATIONS	AGENT, DOSE, TOXICITY	NURSING INTERVENTIONS
Pleural Space		
Malignant effusion (usually secondary to lymphoma, sarcoma, and mesothelioma, and carcinoma of the stomach, ovary, or lung).	**Bleomycin** 15–240 U in 2 L. 0.9% sodium chloride solution (optimal dose 60 U). **Mechlorethamine** 0.2–0.4 mg/kg Toxicity—temperature elevation, nausea, vomiting, myelosuppression, local pain (rare). Vesicant if extravasation occurs. **Tetracycline*** 500 mg or 20 mg/kg Toxicity—local pain, temperature elevation, possible allergic reactions.	1. Orient client and answer any questions. 2. Assist in placement of thoracotomy tube or intrapleural needle. 3. Assess pleural drainage and maintain patency of tube. (When drainage is less than 100 ml in 24 hr.:) 4. Premedicate with systemic analgesic and/or narcotic (Demerol, Valium commonly used). 5. Administer antipyretic (acetaminophen commonly used) as ordered. 6. Administer antiemetic if ordered. 7. Assist physician in instillation of chemotherapy via chest tube or intrapleural needle. 8. Clamp chest tube. 9. Monitor vital signs and EKG. 10. Encourage client to change position while medication is in pleural cavity—every 5 min. for instillation time of 20 min. and every 15 min. for instillation time up to 2 hr. (When treatment is completed:) 11. Unclamp chest tube, resume water seal chest drainage with suction. 12. Assess respiratory status, temperature, blood pressure.

		13. Assess for and report severe chest pain or dyspnea.
		14. Administer analgesic p.r.n. as ordered for pain.
		15. Chest x-ray is usually taken at the end of the procedure and 24 hr. later. (When chest tube drainage is less than 100 ml in 24 hr.:)
		16. Administer analgesic (if ordered).
		17. Assist physician with removal of chest tube.
		18. Apply occlusive dressing (petroleum gauze dressing) to tube site.
		19. Continue to monitor client for stability of vital signs, respiratory distress.

Pericardial Space

	Intrapericardial	
Malignant effusion (usually the result of cancer of the breast or lung, leukemias, lymphomas).	**Mechlorethamine** 0.2 mg/kg (10–20 mg) in sterile water for injection or sodium chloride 0.9% for injection. **Thiotepa** 0.6–0.8 mg/kg	(Physician will administer medication via pericardiocentesis.) 1. Monitor client's vital signs and EKG for signs of arrhythmias or acute cardiac distress. 2. Encourage client to change position every 5–10 min. while medication is in place (usually 1–2 hr.).

Note: 2000–4000 rads of radiation is the treatment of choice for the client who has had no prior therapy to the cardiac region.

Peritoneum

	Intraperitoneal	
Malignant ascites (occurs with lymphomas, carcinoma of the ovary, colon, or stomach).	**Bleomycin** 60–150 U per day in 2 L normal saline solution.	1. Assist with paracentesis to drain most of fluid from peritoneum prior to instillation of medication.

(Continued)

Table 2–1 Alternative Routes for Administration of Cancer Chemotherapy (Continued)

ANATOMIC REGION AND INDICATIONS	AGENT, DOSE, TOXICITY	NURSING INTERVENTIONS
	Carboplatin 200–400 mg/m^2 in 1–2 L normal saline solution. Administer only if creatinine clearance is > 60 ml/min (Speyer, J.C. and Sorich, J., 1992). **Cisplatin** 90 mg/m^2 (may administer higher dose if sodium thiosulfate is administered to reduce renal toxicity). **Paclitaxel (Taxol)** 125 mg/m^2 in 1–2 L normal saline solution. See Table 2–4 for specific administration equipment specifications.	2. Peritoneal infusion may be administered via peritoneal trochar. Tenckhoff catheter or implanted port. When intraperitoneal trochar or catheter is in place, use sterile technique when assessing or dressing site. 3. Flush inlet to assure patency. 4. Administer chemotherapeutic agent(s) in 1–2 L of dialysate solution. 5. Allow solution to remain in peritoneal cavity for 2–6 hr. During this time, encourage and assist client to change position q 15–20 min. to allow solution to contact all surfaces of the peritoneal wall. 6. During infusion and retention period, monitor I & O, assess client for side effects (abdominal pain, cramping, anorexia, nausea, vomiting, diarrhea, fluid/electrolyte imbalances, toxicity of individual medications, dyspnea related to abdominal distention, low grade fever, peritonitis). (After designated dwell time:) 7. Allow chemotherapy solution to drain by gravity via paracentesis trochar or tube. Note: Nausea and vomiting may persist for 2–3 days after therapy. 8. Teach client to note and report side effects. (If Tenckhoff catheter is used:) 9. Teach client to care for site daily and to note and report signs of infection.

Liver

Hepatic metastases of colorectal carcinoma, carcinoma of stomach, esophagus, pancreas, breast, or lung, and malignant melanoma. Note: Tumor may be primary hepatic tumor.

Floxuridine (FUDR)

100 mg/m^2 daily for 5 days or 0.1–0.3 mg/kg for 24 days. Therapy may be administered until adverse reactions (nausea, vomiting, diarrhea, mucosal ulceration, myelosuppression) appear, and may be resumed when side effects have subsided.

Administered via intra-arterial catheter and pump into hepatic artery:

1. Ensure that catheter does not become dislodged.
2. Ensure that catheter is secured externally with Steri-Strips or other suitable dressing.

(On hospital unit or in the home setting:)

3. Educate client and elicit cooperation.
4. Monitor infusion, maintain regulation of rate by use of external pump.
5. Do not remove Steri-Strips.
6. Avoid pulling on catheter.
7. Prevent kinking of catheter.
8. Do not clamp catheter.
9. Use a stopcock or extension set.
10. Monitor liver function (AST [SGOT], ALT [SGPT], alkaline phosphatase). (Should stopcock or tubing separate from catheter in hepatic artery:)
11. Immediately connect a 10-ml syringe of heparinized saline solution to catheter and notify physician.

(Continued)

25

Table 2–1 Alternative Routes for Administration of Cancer Chemotherapy (Continued)

ANATOMIC REGION AND INDICATIONS	AGENT, DOSE, TOXICITY	NURSING INTERVENTIONS
Bladder	**Intravesical**	
Superficial papillary carcinoma of bladder wall.	**Thiotepa** Initiation: 30–60 mg in 30–60 ml sterile water for injection. May repeat once weekly for 4–8 weeks. After 4th week, may repeat monthly for up to 1 year. (Note: The need for additional courses of therapy will be determined by cystoscopic examination.) **Mitomycin-C** 20 mg in 20 ml sterile water instilled biweekly or 40–60 mg in 40–60 ml sterile water instilled weekly. May repeat monthly for up to 12 months. **Doxorubicin** 20–60 mg. Administer in sterile distilled water at concentration of 1–2 mg/ml.	1. Withhold fluids for 8–12 hr. prior to therapy. 2. Insert indwelling catheter, if it is not in place. 3. Administer chemotherapeutic agent in 60 ml distilled water for injection or sterile water for injection. 4. Clamp catheter. 5. Instruct client (assist if necessary) to change position q 10–15 min. to allow agent to contact all areas of superficial bladder. 6. Unclamp catheter and allow solution to drain. 7. Dispose of catheter, drainage bag, and other materials according to hospital or agency policy for chemotherapy waste. 8. Assess for signs of local irritation (frequent urination or pain when urinating). Systemic toxicities are not as common as with systemic administration of same medications.

Note: The following immunotherapy agent is currently under investigation for intravesical treatment of carcinoma of the bladder.

Bacille Calmette-Guérin (BCG)
120 mg weekly × 6 weeks.
Toxicity—transient hematuria, urinary frequency, dysuria, flulike syndrome.

9. Administer in 50 ml normal saline.
   Note: May be accompanied by simultaneous intradermal administration of BCG.
10. Assess for symptoms. Administer antipyretic as ordered for temperature elevation.

Central Nervous System

1. Intracerebral metastases

Intrathecal

Methotrexate†
6–12 mg/m²‡
(may be administered prophylactically in the child with leukemia).
Cytarabine†
30 mg/m² daily × 4 days, or once every 4 days until CSF is normal, followed by 1 additional treatment.

1. Assist physician with lumbar puncture if necessary, and with administration of chemotherapy.
2. Reassure client during procedure.
3. Monitor vital signs.
4. Assess for signs of neurotoxicity (headache, vomiting, fever, back pain, paresis, nuchal rigidity, confusion, irritability, somnolence, seizures).
(Note: Intrathecal medication may be administered via Ommaya reservoir or directly into cerebrospinal fluid every 2–5 days, or until the cell count of the CSF returns to normal.)
5. If chemotherapy is administered via spinal tap, instruct client to lie flat for 2–4 hr. after procedure to prevent headache.

(Continued)

27

Table 2-1 Alternative Routes for Administration of Cancer Chemotherapy (Continued)

ANATOMIC REGION AND INDICATIONS	AGENT, DOSE, TOXICITY	NURSING INTERVENTIONS
2. Leptomeninges (pia mater or arachnoid space)	Via lumbar injection or Ommaya reservoir: **Methotrexate**† 12 mg‡ or **Cytarabine**† 30 mg/m^2	See toxicity and nursing measures above.

Note: The usual therapy to reduce intracerebral edema and intracranial pressure with a tumor in this region is systemic administration of high doses of a glucocorticoid (dexamethasone or methylprednisolone). For additional information on these medications see Table 3-7. Osmotic agents such as mannitol may be administered as well.

Malignant Melanoma of Extremity	**Regional Perfusion of Extremity (Isolation Perfusion)**	
	Dactinomycin (alone or in combination with other antineoplastic agents) 50 μg (0.05 mg)/kg for lower extremity or pelvis, 35 μg (0.035 mg)/kg for upper extremity.	1. Assess extremity for signs of local edema, damage to soft tissue in area should extravasation occur. For other toxicities, see Table 3-4.

Note: The information in this table represents the most recent advances in regional administration of cancer chemotherapy. Some medications have not yet been approved for these specific modes of administration by the Food and Drug Administration (FDA); thus, these uses do not appear in the manufacturers' literature.

*Tetracycline is not an antineoplastic agent but is used for management of malignant pleural effusions.

†Medications and diluent for intrathecal administration should contain no preservatives. They may be diluted in Elliot's B solution, preservative-free saline, or the patient's own cerebrospinal fluid.

‡Dosage for intrathecal methotrexate is calculated based on the amount of cerebral extracellular fluid, which is less in children under age three years. This provides a more consistent concentration of methotrexate in the cerebrospinal fluid than when the methotrexate dose is based on body surface area, and may lead to a lower incidence of toxicity. (See Lasley, K., and Ignoffo, R.J.: *Manual of Oncology Therapeutics.* St. Louis, C.V. Mosby Co., 1981, p. 318.)

Long-term effects may develop months or years after exposure to chemotherapeutic agents. Although none has been conclusively associated with exposure to antineoplastic agents, there is concern about chromosomal abnormalities and carcinogenicity after long-term exposure to antineoplastic agents.

Procedure for safe handling:

1. Be familiar with the special nature of cytotoxic agents and the policies and procedures that govern their preparation. It is recommended that each hospital or agency maintain sufficient information on the safe use of cytotoxic drugs and procedures for their preparation and administration.
2. Adhere to sterile handling techniques and handwashing before and after mixing or administering antineoplastic agents.
3. Prepare chemotherapy in a Class II type B or Class III laminar flow biological safety cabinet (containment cabinet) to afford maximum protection. If this is not available, prepare chemotherapy in a quiet work space, away from heating or cooling vents and other personnel, and use a powered air-purifying respirator with high efficiency particulate air (HEPA) filter (OSHA, in press).
4. Check hospital or agency policy and use protective garments (gown, gloves, mask, and/or goggles) as indicated. If a gown is to be worn, the recommended type is one of a low-permeability, lint-free fabric that closes in back. Cuffs on the gown should be elastic or knit and long enough to tuck under the cuffs of gloves. If double gloves are worn, the outer glove should be over the gown cuff and the inner glove should be under the gown cuff. The gown should be removed before leaving the work area.
5. Protect the work area with a disposable plastic-backed absorbent pad to minimize contamination by droplet or spills. Change pad at the completion of each shift or after an accidental spill.
6. *Do not* eat, drink, smoke, or apply makeup in the area in which chemotherapy is prepared.
7. Review literature (hospital procedures, policies, package insert) before preparing or administering medication.
8. Wear gloves with the following specifications:
   a. Thick latex (0.007"–0.009") (Laidlaw, 1984).
   b. Talc-free.
   c. Disposable.
   d. Cuffs long enough to be tucked over the cuffs of the gown.
9. Change gloves regularly (hourly) or immediately after a puncture, tear, or medication spill.

10. When removing gloves, avoid skin contact and dispose of properly.
11. Wash hands before donning gloves and after removing gloves.
12. Use precautions to avoid skin contact when leakage of medication may occur, e.g.:
    a. Ejection of air from syringe or tubing containing a chemotherapeutic agent.
    b. Injection of chemotherapeutic agent into I.V. bag or tubing.
    c. Connection or disconnection of I.V. tubing with chemotherapy solution.
13. Syringes, tubings, and connectors used in chemotherapy preparation and administration should contain Luer-Loks at points of attachment.
14. Whenever possible, blunt cannulas or protected needles should be used to draw up medications or flush I.V. lines, to prevent accidental needle sticks.
15. When opening ampules:
    a. Clear all fluid from the neck of the ampule by "tapping down gently" before opening.
    b. Tilt the tip of the ampule away from yourself.
    c. Wrap a sterile gauze or alcohol pad around the neck of the ampule before breaking.
    d. Use a syringe that will be no more than ¾ full when desired amount is drawn up.
    e. Inject excess solution from the ampule into a sealed waste vial or dispose of according to agency policy.
16. To prevent aerosol generation from vials:
    a. Use an 18- or 19-gauge needle and a 0.2-μm hydrophobic filter, or dispensing pin.
    b. Create negative pressure in the vial when adding diluent by aspirating a volume of air slightly larger than the volume of diluent added.
    c. Add diluent slowly, allowing it to run down the inside wall of the vial.
    d. Perform final dose measurement before removing needle from stopper of vial.
    e. Clear drug from the needle and hub (neck) of syringe and allow air pressure to equalize from the vial back into the syringe before removing needle from vial.
17. Label all prepared solutions or syringes with:
    a. The client's name and I.D. number (if in hospital, include room and bed number).
    b. Medication—name, amount.
    c. Date and time of preparation.

d. Expiration date and time.
e. Name of person preparing medication.
18. When expelling air from a syringe or priming I.V. tubing with chemotherapy solution, do so *slowly* into a sterile gauze pad contained within a sealable 4-mil polyethylene bag.
19. Assess I.V. tubing and pumps for signs of leakage.

Management of Accidental Exposure

1. Should skin contact occur when preparing or administering chemotherapeutic agents, wash the involved area thoroughly with soap (not a germicidal agent) and water.
2. Should accidental contact with eyes occur when preparing or administering chemotherapeutic agents:
   a. Irrigate the involved eye(s) with water or an isotonic eye wash for at least 5 minutes while holding the eyelid open.
   b. Document the incident according to established institutional policies.
   c. Obtain a medical evaluation as soon as possible.
3. Obtain a medical evaluation after any accidental exposure to a cytotoxic agent.

Administration Procedure

1. Outcomes (ONS, 1988, modules 2,4, p. 5; module 3, p. 6):
   a. The patient will receive the prescribed chemotherapeutic agent(s) in a safe and appropriate manner.
   b. Health care personnel, the patient, and the environment will be protected from unnecessary exposure to potentially hazardous substances.
   c. The sterility of the drug(s) will be maintained.
   d. The patient should comprehend the consequences of treatment decisions.
2. Preliminary nursing measures:
   a. Verify medication and dose.
   b. Have knowledge of immediate and delayed side effects of the medication(s) being administered.
   c. Review client's history of past experience with chemotherapy administration.
   d. Review significant laboratory data (complete blood count, other laboratory values, electrocardiogram if indicated).
   e. Use proper procedure for identification of the client.
   f. Identify yourself to the client and family and answer questions that they may have concerning chemotherapy.

g. Verify that informed consent form (Fig. 2–7) has been completed if medication administered is an investigational agent or if otherwise required by institutional policy.

h. Explain procedure and any anticipated side effects of the medication(s) being administered and answer client's questions appropriately.

i. Inform client (or significant other) about procedure for reaching the nurse should this be necessary during or following treatment.

j. Wash hands and don gloves.

k. Administer antiemetics or other medications as ordered in preparation for chemotherapy (see Tables 8–2 and 8–3).

l. Administer medication observing the five rights:
   (1) The right medication.
   (2) The right time.
   (3) The right route.
   (4) The right dose.
   (5) The right patient.

m. Chart medication administration according to agency policy.

3. For intravenous medications:

a. Assemble equipment required to perform venipuncture if necessary.

b. Select site for venipuncture with regard to:
   (1) Location of proposed I.V. site. Use hand veins (Fig. 2–8) before using forearm sites (Fig. 2–9).
   (2) General condition of veins.
   (3) Previous trauma to proposed I.V. site.
   (4) Type of medication to be administered (e.g., vesicant and nonvesicant medications listed in Table 2–2). When vesicant medications are administered, avoid sites where damage to underlying tendons, nerves, or both is more likely to occur. These include:
      (a) Veins in the antecubital region.
      (b) Veins located near the wrist.
      (c) Veins on the dorsal surface of the hand.
      (d) Sclerosed veins.
      (e) Recent venipuncture sites.
      (f) Sites of recent I.V. infiltration.
      (g) Veins in or near which surgery has been performed (e.g., skin graft, mastectomy, or partial amputation).
   (5) Amount of medication to be administered.

c. Perform venipuncture using the most distal veins first, moving proximally with successive administrations.

d. Stabilize I.V. apparatus (winged needle Saf-T-Cath, or short-

Huntington Hospital

Huntington Memorial Hospital
100 W. California Blvd., P.O. Box 7013
Pasadena, CA 91109-7013

CONSENT FOR CHEMOTHERAPY OF MALIGNANT DISEASES

I understand that I am being offered this type of treatment for my disease. This treatment consists of one or more drugs.

I CONFIRM THAT I HAVE BEEN FULLY INFORMED ABOUT EACH OF THE FOLLOWING:

1. Therapeutic effects of the treatment: _____

_____

_____

2. The treatment will consist of the following drug(s): _____

_____

_____

_____

3. The method and frequency of drug administration has been described to me.

4. The drug(s) will be administered by the following routes: _____

_____

_____

_____

5. The treatment may have some unpleasant side effects. The expected ones have been read and explained to me. (See reverse).

6. Should I be pregnant or become pregnant during the course of therapy, the possibility of a miscarriage or damage to the unborn baby has been discussed.

7. I have been informed that frequent blood tests will be ordered to monitor the effects of therapy.

8. This treatment will be given in the hope of improving my condition, but I realize that no one can guarantee this will happen.

9. My doctors have discussed with me alternative methods in treating my disease. These include:

_____

_____

_____

10. My doctors have offered to answer any further questions I might have.

11. I understand that I may withdraw my consent and discontinue my participation in this treatment at any time. My doctors have pointed out that my consent is entirely voluntary.

12. I freely and voluntarily state that the risks and benefits of the use of the above medications have been explained to my satisfaction. I have read the above and give my consent to the use of the drug(s).

Date:_____   _____
                                   Patient Signature

Date:_____   _____
                                   Relative or Responsible Person

Witness_____   _____
                                   Physician

White — CHART   Canary — PATIENT   Pink — PHARMACY

Figure 2–7. Client consent form. (Courtesy of Huntington Memorial Hospital, Pasadena, CA.)

STATEMENT OF PREVIOUSLY DETECTED SIDE EFFECTS OF DRUGS LISTED BELOW:

(The physician will check the appropriate box, **read and clarify** for the patient, the drug and any possible side effects:)

☐ **AMINOGLUTETHIMIDE (Cytadren, Elipten):** Rash, lethargy, visual blurring, dizziness, nausea, anorexia, facial flushing, enlarged thyroid gland, low white and red cells, susceptibility to infection and bleeding, in women: facial hair growth and voice deepening. Extreme fatigue.

☐ **ASPARAGINASE (L-Asp; Elspar):** Nausea, vomiting, fever, lowered red white cell and platelet count, susceptibility to infection and bleeding, damage to liver and kidney, unconsciousness, inflammation of pancreas, low blood pressure, skin rash, asthma, mood changes.

☐ **BLEOMYCIN SULFATE (Blenoxane, Bleo):** Fever and chills, blisters and numbness of hands, nausea, mouth sores, lung damage, low white and red cell and platelet count, hair loss, asthma, allergic reaction, skin pigmentation.

☐ **BUSULFAN (Myleran):** Low red and white cell and platelet count, susceptibility to infection and bleeding, lung damage, hyperpigmentation of skin, nausea and vomiting, hair loss, change in menstrual cycle, gynecomastia, cataracts.

☐ **CARMUSTINE (BCNU; BiCNU):** Nausea and vomiting; low red and white cell and platelet count; susceptibility to infection and bleeding; discomfort in vein during injection; affects liver; mouth sores, lowers blood pressure, affects lungs and kidney.

☐ **CISPLATIN (Platinol, CPDD, CPD, DDP):** Nausea and vomiting, low red and white cell and platelet count; diarrhea; hair loss, neurological damage (hearing loss, numbness, tingling and muscle weakness in extremities); kidney damage.

☐ **CYCLOPHOSPHAMIDE (Cytoxan, CTX, endoxan, neosar):** Nausea and vomiting, metallic taste, low red and white cell and platelet count; susceptibility to infection and bleeding; hair loss; irritation of bladder (blood; cystitis); lung scarring.

☐ **CHLORAMBUCIL (Leukeran, CHl, Clb):** Low red and white cell and platelet counts, susceptibility to infection and bleeding, nausea, sterility, liver damage.

☐ **CYTARABINE (Ara-C; cytosine arabinoside, cytosar):** Nausea and vomiting; fever, bone pain, conjunctivitis, rash, low red and white cell and platelet count; susceptibility to infection and bleeding; mouth sores, diarrhea, liver damage,neurotoxicity.

☐ **DACTINOMYCIN (Actinomycin-D, Cosmegen):** Nausea, vomiting, fatigue, fever, diarrhea, low white and red cell and platelet count, hair loss, skin pigmentation, mouth sores, tissue damage from extravasation or leakage at infection site, photosensitivity, susceptibility to infection and bleeding.

☐ **DAUNORUBICIN (Cerubidine):** Low red and white cell and platelet counts, susceptibility to infection and bleeding; tissue damage from extravasation or leakage from vein; heart damage; fever; loss of hair; red urine; malaise, diarrhea

☐ **DIETHYLSTILBESTROL (DES):** Nausea, fluid retention; in women — uterine bleeding; increase in calcium in blood, in men — breast enlargement, higher voice; loss of libido; headache, anxiety, insomnia, skin rash; lethargy.

☐ **DOXORUBICIN HYDROCHLORIDE (Adriamycin, adria):** Nausea and vomiting, low red and white cell and platelet counts; susceptibility to infection and bleeding, hair loss, tissue damage from extravasation or leakage from vein; mouth sores, heart damage; orange-red urine; diarrhea

☐ **ETOPOSIDE (Vepesid, VP-16):** Nausea, vomiting, low red and white cell and platelet counts; low blood pressure, hair loss, unconsciousness.

☐ **FLOXURIDINE (FUDR):** Nausea, vomiting, diarrhea, mouth sores, low red and white cell and platelet count; skin pigmentation; photosensitivity.

☐ **FLUOROURACIL (5-FU, FU):** Nausea, vomiting, diarrhea, low red and white cell and platelet count; susceptible to infection, hair loss; skin pigmentation; photosensitivity, conjunctivitis.

☐ **HYDROXYUREA (Hydrea):** Nausea, vomiting, low red and white cell and palelet count; skin rash; susceptibility to infection and bleeding, mouth sores; neurological and psychological disturbances (Hallucinations, seizures), kidney damage.

☐ **OTHER** _____

☐ **IMIDAZOLE CARBOXAMIDE (DTIC, decarbazine):** Nausea and vomiting, flushing, discomfort at injection site; low red and white cell and platelet count, susceptibility to infection and bleeding; flu-like syndrome (fever, muscle aching), hair loss; liver damage.

☐ **LOMUSTINE (CCNU, CeeNU):** Low red and white cell and platelet count; nausea, vomiting, susceptibility to infection and bleeding; hair loss; mouth sores, kidney and liver damage.

☐ **MERCAPTOPURINE (6-MP, Purinethol) nausea,** vomiting, low red and white cell and platelet count; liver damage (jaundice); mouth sores; diarrhea, dry scaling rash.

☐ **MITOTANE (o,p'-DDD, Lysodren):** Nausea, vomiting, neurological disturbances (visual, depression); blood pressure changes; lethargy; adrenal insufficiency.

☐ **METHOTREXATE (MTX, Mexate, amethopterin):** Nausea, vomiting, low red and white cell and platelet count; susceptibility to infection and bleeding, diarrhea, mouth sores, skin rash; liver and kidney damage, hair loss.

☐ **MITHRAMYCIN (Mithracin, Mithi):** Nausea, headache, lethargy, low red and white cell and platelet count, clotting problems, kidney damage; low calcium, susceptibility to infection and bleeds; hair loss; tissue damage from extravasation or leaking at vein; skin rash.

☐ **MITOMYCIN (Mitomycin-C, Mutamycin):** Low red and white cell and platelet counts, nausea, vomiting, lung and heart damage; hair loss, tissue damage from extravasation or leaking at vein.

☐ **NITROGEN MUSTARD (Mustargen):** Nausea, vomiting, diarrhea, metallic taste, low red and white cell and platelet counts, susceptibility to infection and bleeding, tissue damage from extravasation or leakage from vein or catheter, sterility; hair loss; change in menstrual cycle.

☐ **PHENYLALANINE MUSTARD (Alkeran, melphalan):** Nausea and vomiting, low red and white cell and platelet counts, susceptibility to infection and bleeding, skin rash, lung damage.

☐ **PREDNISONE:** Mood swings; gastric irritation and ulcers; changes in appearance — increase in body weight (fluid and salt retention), puffy face, fullness across shoulders, increase in blood sugar, increase in appetite, increased susceptibility to infection.

☐ **PROCARBAZINE HYDROCHLORIDE (matulane):** Nausea, vomiting, low red and white cell and platelet count, susceptibility to infection and bleeding; mouth sores, numbness of fingers, sleepiness; skin rashes; vomiting and dizziness after drinking alcohol or eating cheese.

☐ **STREPTOZOCIN (STZ, zanosar):** Nausea, vomiting, discomfort at site of infusion, chills and fever; low red and white cell count; kidney damage; low blood sugar.

☐ **TAMOXIFEN (Novaldex):** Hot flashes; nausea, vomiting; transient low white blood cell and platelet count; susceptible to infection; vaginal spotting or discharge; tumor pain or flare; headache, dizziness, light-headedness; skin rash, ankle and hand swelling; increase in calcium level in blood; blurred vision.

☐ **THIOGUANINE (6-TG):** Nausea, vomiting, low red and white cell and platelet count; liver damage (jaundice); mouth sores, diarrhea; susceptibility to infection and bleeding

☐ **TRIETHYLENE THIO PHOSPHORAMIDE (Thiotepa):** Nausea, vomiting; dizziness; headache; low red and white cell and platelet counts; susceptibility to infection and bleeding; change in menstrual cycle; decreased sperm count.

☐ **VINBLASTINE (Velban):** Nausea, vomiting; jaw pain; low red and white cell and platelet counts; susceptibility to infection and bleeding; tissue damage from extravasation and leaking from vein; neurological changes (weakness, numbness and tingling, foot drop); mouth sores, constipation, hair loss.

☐ **VINCRISTINE (Oncovin, VCR):** Tissue damage from extravasation or leakage from vein; neurological damage (sensory impairment; jaw pain, foot drop, muscle wasting); constipation; hair loss; inappropriate antidiuretic hormone secretion.

☐ **OTHER:** Possible changes in mentrual cycles

       Possible changes in spermatogenesis

       Possible Sterility

Figure 2–7. (Continued)

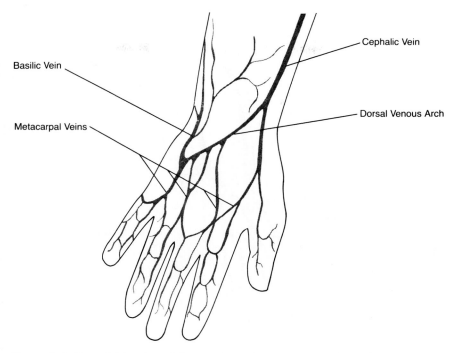

Basilic Vein

Metacarpal Veins

Cephalic Vein

Dorsal Venous Arch

Figure 2–8. Superficial veins of the hand (metacarpal veins) suitable for infusion of nonvesicant chemotherapeutic agents. Use distal veins first, proximal veins later. (From Metheney, N.M.: *Nurses' Handbook of Fluid Balance,* 4th ed. Philadelphia, J.B. Lippincott, 1992, p. 157.)

term intravenous catheter) with clear, occlusive dressing to maintain placement, and allow visualization of site during administration of medications.

e. An I.V. extension tubing primed with normal saline solution may be added to the I.V. access for better manipulation. Connect extension set or I.V. tubing with a blunt cannula or protected needle, to avoid accidental sticks.

f. When administering paclitaxel (Taxol), administer via low sorbing I.V. tubing and extension set with 0.2-μm in-line filter.

g. Assess blood return to assure placement of scalp vein needle or intracath.

h. Instill 5–10 ml of normal saline solution or sterile water for injection to assess patency of vein.

i. Administer chemotherapeutic medication by proper I.V. route (see Figs. 2–4 to 2–7).

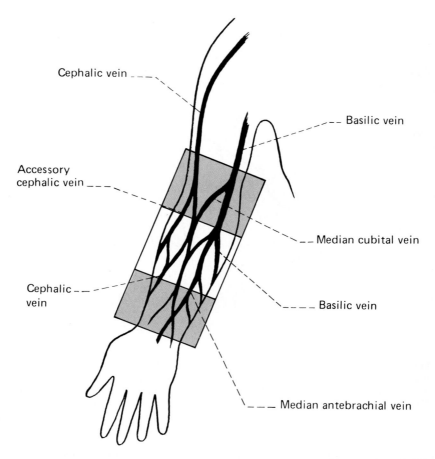

Figure 2–9. Superficial veins of the forearm. □ Preferred site for administration of vesi-cant chemotherapeutic agents. ■ Antecubital veins, which are to be avoided when admin-istering vesicants. (Adapted from Metheney, N.M.: *Nurses' Handbook of Fluid Balance*, 4th ed. Philadelphia, J.B. Lippincott, 1992, p. 157.)

    j. Administer vesicants according to knowledge and hospital or agency policy or variations in Table 2–3.
       (1) Vesicant first.
       (2) Vesicant last.
       (3) Vesicant "sandwiched" between two nonvesicant medica-tions.
    k. Use the two-needle technique when administering a vesicant or irritant medication direct I.V. (draw up medication, change needle, administer medication). This will prevent irri-tation to the vein or surrounding tissue.

Table 2–2   Vesicant and Irritant Chemotherapeutic Medications

GENERIC NAME (BRAND NAME)	DESCRIPTION	LOCAL ANTIDOTE, COMMENTS
Amsacrine (AMSA-PD*)	Vesicant	Hydrocortisone
Carmustine (BiCNU, BCNU)	Irritant	
Cisplatin (Platinol)	Irritant Extravasation of large amount of concentrated solution may produce tissue necrosis.	Treatment is not recommended unless a large amount of highly concentrated solution is extravasated. Sodium bicarbonate (T) Sodium thiosulfate
Dacarbazine (DTIC-Dome)	Irritant	Protect exposed tissue from light following extravasation.
Dactinomycin (Actinomycin-D)	Vesicant	
Daunomycin (Daunorubicin, Cerubidine)	Vesicant	Topical DMSO(T)
Doxorubicin (Adriamycin, Rubex)	Vesicant	Apply cold to site for 24 hr. as tolerated by patient (M). Note: Local infiltration of the site with an injectable corticosteroid and flooding of the site with normal saline has been known to lessen the local reaction.
Epirubicin (Pharmorubicin)	Vesicant	(As for doxorubicin)
Etoposide (VePesid)	Irritant	Local subcutaneous injection of 1–6 ml hyaluronidase (Wydase) 150 U/ml and moderate heat to site (M).
Idarubicin (Idamycin)	Vesicant	(As for doxorubicin)
Mechlorethamine, nitrogen mustard (Mustargen)	Vesicant	Sterile isotonic sodium thiosulfate (⅙ molar): dilute 4 ml sodium thiosulfate injection (10%) with 6 ml sterile water for injection (M). If using sodium thiosulfate 25%, mix water for ⅙ molar solution. Administer 1 ml for each mg extravasated. Apply cold compress.
Mitomycin-C (Mutamycin)	Vesicant	Delayed dermal reactions are possible even if patient is asymptomatic at the time of drug administration. Topical DMSO may be beneficial.

(Continued)

Table 2–2   Vesicant and Irritant Chemotherapeutic Medications
(Continued)

GENERIC NAME (BRAND NAME)	DESCRIPTION	LOCAL ANTIDOTE, COMMENTS
Paclitaxel (Taxol)	Irritant†	Local application of heat
Plicamycin (Mithracin)	Irritant	Application of moderate heat to site (M) Hydrocortisone (T)
Streptozocin (Zanosar)	Irritant	
Teniposide (VM-26, Vumon)	Irritant	(As for etoposide)
Vinblastine (Velban, Velbe, Velsar)	Vesicant	(As for etoposide)
Vincristine (Oncovin, Vincasar)	Vesicant	(As for etoposide)
Vindesine (Eldesine*)	Vesicant	(As for etoposide)

*Available commercially in Canada; investigational in the United States.
(T) = theoretical antidote; (M) = manufacturer-recommended antidote.
†Note: Irritation with paclitaxel is believed to be due to the drug vehicle, Cremophor HL, not a direct response to the drug.

   l. Observe I.V. site after each 1–2 ml to assess for:
     (1) Adequate venous backflow.
     (2) Patency of the vein.
     (3) Signs of infiltration or extravasation.
   m. Flush tubing with 5–10 ml normal saline for injection or sterile water for injection between medications and after final drug has been administered.
   n. Periodically assess client for signs of untoward side effects of medication(s) being administered.
   o. When medication and flush are completed:
     (1) Remove needle or venous catheter.
     (2) Apply adhesive bandage or other sterile dressing to site.
     (3) Instruct the client to raise the extremity for 3–5 minutes after needle or I.V. cannula is withdrawn to reduce chance of local bleeding.
     (4) Gentle pressure may be applied to the site to reduce local bleeding if necessary.
   p. Chart medication and response according to agency policy.
   q. Instruct client to report signs of untoward side effects.
   r. Teach or review with client and significant other self-care measures needed to minimize or prevent untoward side effects of medication(s) administered.

Table 2–3 Controversial Issues in the Administration of Vesicants

ISSUE	SOLUTION	RATIONALE
Administration site	Use antecubital fossa.	Larger veins, easier starts, more rapid infusion.
	Avoid antecubital region.	Mobility of arm restricted. Extensive tissue damage can occur with extravasation.
Cannulation of vein	Larger gauge (#19–21) steel butterfly needle.	Decreases administration time.
	Smaller gauge (#23–25) steel butterfly needle.	Less likely to damage inner wall of vein. Less pain on insertion. Reduced incidence of mechanical or chemical phlebitis.
	Small, thin-walled flexible cannula (20–23 gauge).	Flexibility decreases risk of dislodgement due to movement. Blood flows more easily around cannula, accelerating dilution of medication.
Sequencing of medications	Administer vesicant first.	Vascular integrity decreases over time. Vein more stable and less irritated at the beginning of treatment. Irritating agent may cause venous spasm, pain.
	Administer vesicant last.	Other medications can be administered before irritating effects of vesicant occur. Venous spasm may occur at beginning of I.V. push injection and may be misinterpreted as pain at I.V. site.
Thermal management of site	Apply heat.	Increased blood flow to area promotes reabsorption of remaining vesicant. Facilitates dispersion of antidote in subcutaneous tissue.
	Do not apply heat.	Increases metabolic demands and may increase cell destruction.
	Apply cold.	Constricts peripheral veins, decreases absorption of extravasated medication. Slows metabolism and reduces ability of agent to cause cell destruction. Minimizes local pain.

Safe Disposal of Cytotoxic Agents and Related Materials

1. Outcome (ONS, 1988, module 2, p. 9; modules 3, 4, p. 10): Health care personnel, the patient, and the environment will be protected from unnecessary exposure to potentially hazardous substances.
2. Nursing measures:
    a. Dispose of waste (vials, ampules, syringes, needles, I.V. bags and tubings, connectors, gauze, gown, mask, gloves) properly, according to the agency's hazardous waste procedures.
    b. Place sharp objects in a puncture-resistant, leakproof cardboard or plastic container.
    c. Dispose of needles intact—do not break.
    d. Leave unused portions of antineoplastic agents in vial or ampule and dispose of in plastic bag lined with absorbent material.
    e. Secondary I.V. (piggyback) bags and lines used for chemotherapy administration may be rinsed by "backflowing" one bagful of the main I.V. solution and allowing it to run before disconnecting and discarding secondary bag and line.
    f. Place the leak-proof, puncture-proof container with sharp objects and other contaminated equipment (e.g., gowns, masks, gloves, absorbent pads) in a sealable 4-mil polyethylene or 2-mil polypropylene bag. Bags for hazardous drug disposal should be colored differently from other hospital trash bags.
    g. Mark or label the outside of the container "Caution: Chemotherapy" or "Biohazard."
    h. Discard gloves after each use or after a medication spill.
    i. Avoid skin contact when removing gloves.
    j. Wash hands thoroughly after removing gloves.
    k. Report accidental contact with chemotherapeutic agents according to agency policy.
    l. Hazardous drug-related waste containers should be disposed of separately from other hospital trash and should be disposed of in accordance with applicable Environmental Protection Agency (EPA), state, and local regulations for hazardous waste, at an incinerator or licensed sanitary landfill for toxic wastes.
    m. Place linen contaminated with bodily secretions of patients who have received antineoplastic agents during the preced-

ing 48 hours in specially marked laundry bags, placed inside an impervious bag labeled "Caution: Chemotherapy" or "Biohazard."

Recommendations for Clean-up of Chemotherapy Spills

1. Outcome: Health care personnel, the patient, and the environment will be protected from unnecessary exposure to potentially hazardous substances (ONS, 1988, module 2, p. 9; modules 3, 4, p. 10).
2. Procedure:
    a. Clean-up should be carried out by trained personnel and with proper equipment.
    b. The area should be identified with a warning sign to limit access to the area.
    c. A "spill kit" is recommended by the American Society of Hospital Pharmacists, U.S. Department of Labor Occupational Safety and Health Administration (OSHA), and Oncology Nursing Society (American Society of Hospital Pharmacists, 1990, U.S. Department of Labor Occupational Safety and Health Administration, [in press]). This kit should be clearly labeled and kept in or near preparation and administration areas. The kit should contain:
        (1) A powered air-purifying respirator (PAPR), with high-efficiency particulate air (HEPA) filter or half mask respirator.
        (2) Chemical splash goggles.
        (3) Two pairs of gloves.
        (4) Utility gloves.
        (5) A low-permeability gown.
        (6) Disposable coveralls and shoe covers.
        (7) Two sheets (12" × 12") of incinerable absorbent material.
        (8) Two 250-ml and 1-liter spill control pillows.
        (9) A sharps container.
        (10) A small scoop to collect broken glass fragments.
        (11) Two large hazardous drug waste-disposal bags.
        (12) Cytotoxic warning labels.
    d. Clean-up materials should be disposed of in a sealed, properly labeled bag.
    e. The spill and clean-up should be documented properly by persons exposed and reported to appropriate departments.

Recommended Institutional Policies

1. ONS standards:
   a. Health care personnel will be protected from unnecessary exposure to potentially hazardous substances.
   b. Health care personnel will be kept informed of current information as it becomes available (ONS, 1988, p. 11).

A written Hazard Communication Program is now legally required per OSHA's Code of Federal Regulations 29CFR-1910.1200 (Hazard Communication System, Right To Know Law). Under this newly expanded federal law, each hospital, agency, or physician's office is responsible for the development, implementation, and maintenance of comprehensive written policies and procedures describing containment, collection, and disposal of cytotoxic waste materials, and a staff education program. Personnel at each agency or institution where chemotherapy is prepared and/or administered must develop and regularly review the following:

1. Procedures for preparing and dispensing chemotherapeutic medications.
2. Procedures to be followed in case of accidental contact.
3. Plans for staff education, including:
   a. An initial program for all employees who prepare or administer chemotherapy.
   b. An orientation program for new employees.
   c. A program for periodic review and update of procedures for proper handling and disposal of chemotherapeutic agents.
   d. Periodic evaluation of procedures for handling chemotherapeutic agents as part of the facility's quality assurance program.
   e. A written hazard communication program.

Training records must be maintained and should include the following information:

1. Dates of training sessions.
2. Contents or a summary of information covered in the session.
3. Names and qualifications of the person(s) conducting the training session.
4. Names and job titles of all persons attending the training session.

Training records should be maintained for three years from the date on which the training occurred.

Recommendations for course content and a clinical practicum on this subject can be found in the 1988 ONS Cancer Chemotherapy Guidelines (Module I, pp. 2–12) and OSHA instruction on hazardous drug handling (in press).

Measures to Be Taken When Caring for the Client Who Is Receiving or Has Recently Received Chemotherapy

1. Use appropriate protective apparel to protect against contamination:
   a. Disposable gloves.
   b. Disposable gowns.
   c. Disposable plastic-backed paper absorbent pads.
   d. Waste disposal bags with cytotoxic drug warning labels.
2. Handle urine and other excreta from clients receiving chemotherapy carefully and avoid splattering during disposal.
3. Dispose of linen contaminated with bodily secretions in a properly labeled water-soluble laundry bag for the first 48 hours after chemotherapy administration.
4. Provide staff orientation and training about these procedures.

Guidelines for preparation and administration of parenteral antineoplastic agents are summarized in Table 2–4.

Extravasation

1. Definitions:
   a. Extravasation—Infiltration or leakage of an intravenous chemotherapeutic agent into the local tissue surrounding the administration site. May result in local tissue damage.
   b. Flare reaction—A raised, red streak along the course of a vein, which may be mistaken for extravasation (see Table 2–5 for differentiation).
   c. Irritant—A medication that may produce pain and inflammation at the administration site, or along the path of the vein by which it is administered.
   d. Vesicant—A medication that has the potential to cause cellular damage or tissue destruction if leakage into subcutaneous tissue occurs.

(Text continued on page 62)

Table 2-4 Directions for Reconstitution and Administration of Parenteral Antineoplastic Medications

FOR ALL DRUGS: Use of gown, gloves, mask, and (when indicated) splash goggles should be standard procedure during preparation and administration of ALL chemotherapeutic agents, to avoid exposure by inhalation or direct contact of medication or droplets. Should accidental contact occur, the following measures must be taken: Skin—wash immediately and thoroughly with soap and water. Mucous membranes—wash thoroughly with water. Eyes—immediately irrigate for 15 minutes with normal saline solution or water.

GENERIC NAME (BRAND NAME)	AVAILABILITY	INITIAL DILUTION	FURTHER DILUTION/ ADMINISTRATION	ADDITIONAL INFORMATION
Amsacrine (AMSA-PD) (investigational)	Ampule 75 mg in 1.5 ml with vial of diluent (L-lactic acid).	Aseptically transfer 1.5 ml solution from the ampule to the vial of L-lactic acid diluent. The resulting red–orange solution contains 5 mg amsacrine per ml. A glass syringe is preferred for transfer to avoid reaction between the solution and the syringe (plastic syringe may be used provided solution does not remain in syringe longer than 15 min.).	Transfer the desired dose to 500 ml dextrose in water solution. Do not dilute in saline-containing solutions, as amsacrine is incompatible with solutions containing chloride ions and may result in precipitation. Infuse over 1 hr.	Prepare using a glass syringe. Protect I.V. solution from direct sunlight. Use within 24 hr. when stored at room temperature, or within 72 hr. when stored under refrigeration. VESICANT—Assess I.V. site for pain, burning.

Asparaginase (L-Asparaginase, Elspar, Kidrolase, L-ASP)	Vial—10,000 I.U. with 80 mg mannitol.	Reconstitute with 5 ml sterile water for injection or sodium chloride injection. Solution will contain 2000 I.U. per ml. Solution should be clear. Can be administered via Y-site or direct I.V. For I.V. drip, see next column. For I.M. administration: Add 2 ml sodium chloride for injection to vial.	Dilute further with sodium chloride for injection or 5% dextrose in water. Solution should be clear. Use within 8 hr. after preparation. Administer through sidearm of running I.V. over 30 min.	Assist with intradermal skin test before administration of full dose. If filter is used, recommended size is 5.0 μm. Administration via the 0.2-μm filter can result in loss of potency.
Bleomycin (Blenoxane)	Vial—15 Units.	Intramuscularly (I.M.) or subcutaneously (S.C.). Dissolve contents of vial in 1–5 sterile or bacteriostatic water for injection, sodium chloride injection, or 5% dextrose injection.	For I.V. push: Dissolve contents of the vial in 5 ml or more of normal saline solution or 5% dextrose in water, and administer slowly over a period of 10 min. or as a continuous infusion.	Stable for 24 hr. after preparation. Because of possibility of anaphylaxis, assist with administration of test dose of 1–2 Units prior to first two doses. NOTE: Anaphylactoid reaction more common in the patient being treated for lymphoma.
Carmustine (BiCNU, BCNU)	Vial—100 mg with vial of sterile diluent (3 ml dehydrated alcohol injection, USP).	Add supplied diluent, then add 27 ml sterile water for injection. Solution will contain 3.3 mg/ml. Solution should be clear and colorless.	Administer by I.V. drip only over 1–2 hr. Dilute initial solution with 0.9% sodium chloride injection or 5% dextrose injection.	Skin contact may result in hyperpigmentation.

(Continued)

45

Table 2–4 Directions for Reconstitution and Administration of Parenteral Antineoplastic Medications (Continued)

GENERIC NAME (BRAND NAME)	AVAILABILITY	INITIAL DILUTION	FURTHER DILUTION/ ADMINISTRATION	ADDITIONAL INFORMATION
Carboplatin (Paraplatin)	Vial—50 mg, 150 mg, 450 mg.	Immediately before use, reconstitute contents of vial with diluent (sterile water for injection, dextrose 5% in water [D5/W], or sodium chloride for injection). To 50 mg add 5 ml; to 150 mg add 15 ml; to 450 mg add 45 ml; for a concentration of 10 mg/ml.	Dilute with D5/W or sodium chloride for injection. Common concentration for administration—1–4 mg/ml. Administered over 30 min. May be further diluted to concentrations as low as 0.5 mg/ml.	Do not use aluminum needles in preparation or administration.
Cisplatin (Platinol) (Platinol-AQ)	Vial—10 mg, Vial—50 mg, 100 mg.	For Platinol: Add sterile water for injection: 10 ml to 10 mg vial, 50 ml to 50 mg vial. Each ml will contain 1 mg cisplatin in clear, colorless solution. (NOTE: Platinol-AQ is in solution form.)	Administer by I.V. infusion only over 6–8 hr. in 1–2 L of 5% dextrose in ⅓ to ½ normal saline, with 37.5 g mannitol. DO NOT infuse in just 5% dextrose in water.	Store reconstituted solution at room temperature; a precipitate will form if refrigerated. IRRITANT—Extravasation of a large amount of concentrated solution may result in local tissue necrosis. Hydrate client before and after cisplatin infusion with additional I.V. fluids.

Drug	Available Forms	Reconstitution	Dilution	Notes
Cladribine (Leustatin, 2-chlorodeoxyadenosine, 2-CDA)	Vial—10 ml (1 mg/ml). Clear, colorless solution.	(None required.)	To prepare a single daily dose, add the calculated dose to 500 ml 0.9% sodium chloride injection USP. DO NOT use D5/W as diluent, as this may increase degradation. Administer as a continuous infusion over 24 hr. Repeat daily × 7 days. To prepare a 7-day infusion, see manufacturer's directions.	NOTE: Contains no antimicrobial preservative or bacteriostatic agent. Must be prepared under aseptic technique. Do not mix with other I.V. drugs or additives or infuse simultaneously via a common I.V. line.
Cyclophosphamide (Cytoxan, Endoxan, Neosar, Proctytox, CTX)	Vial—100 mg, 200 mg, 500 mg, 1 gm, 2 gm. Lyophilized—100 mg, 200 mg, 500 mg, 1 gm, 2 gm.	Dilute with sterile water for injection or bacteriostatic water for injection (paraben preserved only) 5 ml to 100 mg; 10 ml to 200 mg; 25 ml to 500 mg; 50 ml to 1 gm; 100 ml to 2 gm. Shake to dissolve. Contains 20 mg/ml. Can be administered I.V. push.	May be further diluted in: 5% dextrose in water; 5% dextrose in 0.9% sodium chloride solution; 5% dextrose in Ringer's injection; lactated Ringer's injection; sodium chloride 0.45%; or ⅙ molar lactate solution.	Note: Lyophilized powder dissolves more rapidly. If bacteriostatic water is used as initial diluent, solution should be used within 24 hr. if stored at room temperature, or within 6 days under refrigeration.

(Continued)

Table 2–4 Directions for Reconstitution and Administration of Parenteral Antineoplastic Medications (Continued)

GENERIC NAME (BRAND NAME)	AVAILABILITY	INITIAL DILUTION	FURTHER DILUTION/ ADMINISTRATION	ADDITIONAL INFORMATION
Cytarabine (Cytosar-U, Cytosine, Ara-C, Tarabine)	Vial—100 mg, 500 mg, 1 gm, 2 gm.	For intravenous use: Add supplied diluent (bacteriostatic water for injection with benzyl alcohol 0.945%) 5 ml to 100 mg (solution contains 20 mg cytarabine/ ml); 10 ml to 500 mg (solution contains 50 mg cytarabine/ml), 10 ml to 1 gm or 20 ml to 2 gm (solution contains 100 cytarabine/ml). For intrathecal use: Reconstitute with preservative-free 0.9% sodium chloride for injection and use immediately.	I.V. injection, or infusion further diluted in 1000 ml 5% dextrose solution or 0.9% sodium chloride solution. Administer over 8–24 hr.	Discard if solution is not clear. Prepare and administer with gown and gloves on.
Dacarbazine (DTIC-Dome, DTIC)	Vial—100 mg, 200 mg.	Add sterile water for injection: 9.9 ml to 100 mg; 19.7 ml to 200 mg. Solution contains 10 mg dacarbazine per ml.	Administer by I.V. push or by I.V. infusion in 5% dextrose solution or 0.9% sodium chloride injection: 1–200 mg in 50 ml over 30 min.; 200–500 ml in 100 mg over 60 min.; over 500 mg in 150 ml over 2 hr.	Solution stable for 8 hr. at room temperature or 72 hr. under refrigeration. Protect from light. Discard if solution turns pink or precipitate noted. IRRITANT—Assess I.V. site for pain, burning. Manufacturer recommends local application of heat should extravasation occur.

Dactinomycin (Cosmegen, Actinomycin-D, ACT-D)	Vial—0.5 mg with 20 mg mannitol (gold-colored powder).	Add 1.1 ml preservative-free sterile water for injection for a solution containing 500 mcg (0.5 mg) per ml. Solution will be clear and golden-yellow.	For I.V. drip: Add to infusion solutions of 5% dextrose injection or sodium chloride injection. For I.V. push: Administer into sideport of freely flowing I.V. of 5% dextrose solution or 0.9% sodium chloride for injection.	VESICANT—Assess I.V. site for pain, burning.
Daunorubicin (Cerubidine, Daunomycin)	Vial—20 mg with 100 mg mannitol (red lyophilized powder).	Add 4 ml sterile water for injection and agitate vial gently until powder has completely dissolved. Contains 5 mg daunorubicin per ml. Solution will be red-colored.	May further dilute in 10–15 ml sterile normal saline solution and administer via sideport of freely flowing I.V. or: Administer I.V. drip in 50–100 ml 5% dextrose injection or sodium chloride injection over 20–30 min.	Prepare with gown and gloves. Flush area for 15 min. if accidental contact occurs. VESICANT—Assess I.V. site for pain, burning.
Doxorubicin (Adriamycin RDF)	Vial—10 mg, 20 mg, 50 mg, 150 mg (red-orange lyophilized powder).	Add sodium chloride for injection: 5 ml to 10 mg, 10 ml to 20 mg, 25 ml to 50 mg vial, 75 ml to 150 mg vial. Solutions contain 2 mg/ml. Bacteriostatic diluents are not recommended.	Administer slowly into a large vein via Y-site of a freely flowing I.V. of dextrose in water or normal saline solution over 3–5 min. or longer. May be further reconstituted in 5% dextrose injection or sodium chloride injection and administered as a continuous infusion via a control pump over 24 to 96 hr.	To prevent pressure buildup in vial, withdraw appropriate volume of air before adding diluent. Incompatible with heparin. VESICANT—Assess I.V. site for pain, burning. NOTE: Symptoms may not always be present with extravasation. If extravasation is suspected: discontinue infusion and start in another vein. Apply cold to site.
(Adriamycin PFS)	Vial—10 mg in 5 ml, 20 mg in 10 ml, 50 mg in 25 ml, 200 mg in 100 ml (multi-dose vial) (2 mg/25 ml).	No further dilution required.		

(Continued)

Table 2–4 Directions for Reconstitution and Administration of Parenteral Antineoplastic Medications (Continued)

GENERIC NAME (BRAND NAME)	AVAILABILITY	INITIAL DILUTION	FURTHER DILUTION/ ADMINISTRATION	ADDITIONAL INFORMATION
Epirubicin hydrochloride (Pharmorubicin)	Vial—10 mg, 20 mg, 50 mg, 100 mg (red–orange lyophilized powder).	Add sodium chloride injection: 5 ml for 10 mg vial, 25 ml for 50 mg vial. Shake vial until contents are dissolved. Final solution contains 2 mg/ml. Bacteriostatic diluents are not recommended by manufacturer.	No further dilution required. Administer into tubing of freely flowing I.V. over no less than 3–5 min.	Incompatible with heparin. VESICANT—Avoid extravasation.
Epoetin alfa (erythropoietin, Epogen, Procrit, EPO)	Vial—2,000, 3,000, 4,000, 10,000 U/ml.	(None necessary.)	(None necessary.)	DO NOT shake vial during preparation, as this may denature the glycoprotein and render drug biologically inactive. Administer subcutaneously. Contains no preservative—do not re-enter vial, discard unused portion. Do not administer in conjunction with other drug solutions.
Etoposide (VP-16-213, VePesid)	Ampule—100 mg in 5 ml; 150 mg in 7.5 ml (20 mg/ml).	None required.	Dilute in 5% dextrose injection or 0.9% sodium chloride injection to a concentration of 0.2 or 0.4 mg per ml. Administer over 30–60 min.	Discard if precipitate seen. IRRITANT—Assess I.V. site for pain, burning.

Filgrastim (Neupogen, G-CSF)	Vial—300 µg in 1 ml; 480 µg in 1.6 ml (300 µg/ml).	(None required.)	Note: No further solution necessary for S.C. administration. For I.V. administration: Reconstitute with 5% dextrose in water.	Do not shake vial during preparation.
Floxuridine (FUDR)	Vial—500 mg.	Reconstitute with 5 ml sterile water for injection. Solution contains 100 mg/ml.	May be further reconstituted in 5% dextrose injection or sodium chloride injection to a volume appropriate to the infusion apparatus used, and administered as a continuous intra-arterial infusion via pump to overcome the pressure in large arteries and insure a uniform rate of infusion (see Chapters 2 and 17). Administer by continuous intra-arterial infusion only, at 0.1–0.6 mg/kg/day.	
Fludarabine phosphate (Fludara)	Vial—50 mg. Lyophilized powder with 50 mg mannitol and sodium hydroxide.	Reconstitute contents of vial with 2 ml sterile water for injection. Each ml contains fludarabine phosphate, 25 mg; mannitol, 25 mg; and sodium hydroxide to adjust to pH of 7.7.	Dilute further with 100–125 ml 5% dextrose in water (D₅W) or 0.9% sodium chloride for injection.	Administer over 30 min. Reconstituted solution may be stored at room temperature and ambient light. Use within 8 hr. after preparation (contains no preservative). If the eyes are accidentally exposed, irrigate immediately.

(Continued)

Table 2–4 Directions for Reconstitution and Administration of Parenteral
Antineoplastic Medications (Continued)

GENERIC NAME (BRAND NAME)	AVAILABILITY	INITIAL DILUTION	FURTHER DILUTION/ ADMINISTRATION	ADDITIONAL INFORMATION
5-Fluorouracil (Adrucil, 5-FU)	Ampule—500 mg in 10 ml (colorless to faint yellow solution).	None required.	May be further diluted in 500 ml or 1000 ml 5% dextrose solution. Administer by slow push into sideport of freely flowing I.V., or diluted in 500–1000 ml 5% dextrose solution over 8–12 hr.	Protect from light. Store at room temperature. Low temperature will cause precipitation.
Goserlin acetate implant (Zoladex)	3.6 mg implant in preloaded syringe.	(None necessary.)	Administer S.C. into the upper abdominal wall.	Local anesthesia may be administered prior to administration. NOTE: The syringe cannot be used for aspiration—do not aspirate prior to injecting. If the injecting needle penetrates a large blood vessel, blood will be seen instantly in the syringe chamber. If this occurs, withdraw the needle and inject at another site, using a new syringe. After insertion of the needle and before injecting, change direction of needle so that it parallels the abdominal wall. After injecting, remove needle and apply bandage to site.

Idarubicin (Idamycin)	Vial—5 mg, 10 mg.	Immediately before use, reconstitute contents of vial with 0.9% sodium chloride for injection. Add 5 ml to 5 mg vial; 10 ml to 10 ml vial, for a final concentration of 1 mg/ml. Bacteriostatic diluents are not recommended.	Administer slowly over 10–15 min. into sideport of freely flowing I.V. infusion of 0.9% sodium chloride injection USP (0.9%) or 5% dextrose injection USP.	Incompatible with heparin. VESICANT—Assess I.V. site for pain, burning. NOTE: Symptoms may not always be present with extravasation. If extravasation is suspected, discontinue infusion, elevate, and apply cold to site.
Ifosfamide (Ifex)	Vial—1 gm, 3 gm (powder).	Dilute with sterile water for injection or bacteriostatic water for injection (benzyl alcohol or parabens preserved)—20 mg to 1 mg vial, 60 mg to 3 mg vial, and shake to dissolve. Reconstituted solutions contain 50 mg ifosfamide/ml.	May be diluted further to achieve concentrations of 0.6 to 20 mg/ml in the following fluids: 5% dextrose injection or sodium chloride injection; lactated Ringer's injection, or sterile water for injection. Administer via I.V. drip over a minimum of 30 min.	Administer with mesna, a uroprotective agent. Do not use if discolored or particulate matter seen in solution.
Interferon alfa (IFN-A, IFN-α, Roferon-A, Intron-A)	Injectable solution—3 million IU/ml; 9 million IU/ml; 18 million IU/ml; 36 million IU/ml. Sterile powder for injection: 18 million IU per vial, with accompanying diluent.	For powdered form ONLY: Reconstitute contents of vial with 3 ml of accompanying diluent. Each ml of reconstituted solution contains 6 million IU interferon alfa.	(None required.)	Do not shake solution. Inspect visually for particulate matter and discoloration. Administer appropriate dose I.M. or S.C. as ordered. Store unopened vials of powder, diluent, or solution at 36°–46°F (2°–8°C). Do not freeze.

(Continued)

Table 2–4 Directions for Reconstitution and Administration of Parenteral Antineoplastic Medications (Continued)

GENERIC NAME (BRAND NAME)	AVAILABILITY	INITIAL DILUTION	FURTHER DILUTION/ ADMINISTRATION	ADDITIONAL INFORMATION
Mechlorethamine hydrochloride (Mustargen, nitrogen mustard, HN2)	Vial—10 mg (white powder).	Inject 10 ml sterile water or sodium chloride into vial. With needle still in the rubber stopper, shake vial several times to dissolve medication. Solution contains 1 mg/ml. Do not use if solution discolored. Mechlorethamine is unstable in solution form. Prepare immediately prior to administration.	Do not dilute further. Inject into sideport of freely flowing I.V. over 3–5 min. or longer. INTRACAVITARY ADMINISTRATION: Techniques vary (see Table 2–1).	Should medication accidentally come in contact with eye(s), irrigate immediately with copious amounts of water for at least 15 min. followed by a 2% sodium thiosulfate solution. Administer immediately after preparation, as drug is unstable once reconstituted. VESICANT—Assess I.V. site for pain and/or burning. If leakage of drug is obvious, prompt infiltration of the area with sterile isotonic sodium thiosulfate (1/6 molar) and application of ice for 6–12 hr. may minimize the local reaction. NEUTRALIZATION OF EQUIPMENT AND UNUSED SOLUTION: Soak equipment, such as gloves, I.V. tubing, and I.V. bags, in aqueous solution containing equal volumes of 5% sodium thiosulfate and 5% sodium bicarbonate for 45 min., then rinse and discard.

Melphalan for injection (Alkeran)	Vial—50 mg with 10 ml vial sterile diluent.	Reconstitute with 10 ml of supplied diluent and shake vigorously until a clear solution is obtained. This provides 5 mg melphalan/ml.	After initial reconstitution, immediately dilute dose to be administered in 0.9% sodium chloride injection to a concentration not greater than 0.45 mg/ml.	Administer over a minimum of 15 min. Complete administration within 60 min. of reconstitution. Do not refrigerate reconstituted product or a precipitate will form.
Mesna (Mesnex)	Vial—200 mg in 2 ml, 400 mg in 4 ml, 1 gm in 10 ml.	(None required.)	Reconstitute with 5% dextrose in water (D_5W), 5% dextrose and sodium chloride for injection. D_5NS or 0.9% sodium chloride injection (NS), for a final concentration of 20 mg mesna/ml fluid.	Administer as an I.V. bolus dose. Administer 20% of the mesnex dose at the time of ifosfamide administration, and 4 and 8 hr. later. Refrigerate after reconstitution and use within 6 hr. Use a new ampule for each administration. Mesnex is not compatible with cisplatin.

(Continued)

55

Table 2-4 Directions for Reconstitution and Administration of Parenteral Antineoplastic Medications (Continued)

GENERIC NAME (BRAND NAME)	AVAILABILITY	INITIAL DILUTION	FURTHER DILUTION/ ADMINISTRATION	ADDITIONAL INFORMATION
Methotrexate (Folex, Mexate, Mexate-AQ, MTX)	Vial—20, 50, 100, 250 mg and 1 gm (golden yellow powder). Also available in solution (25 mg/ml): vials—2, 4, 10 ml (golden yellow solution).	For I.V. or I.M. administration: Reconstitute 20 or 50 ml preservative-free 5% dextrose solution or sodium chloride for injection to a concentration no greater than 25 mg/ml. Reconstitute 1 gm vial with 19.4 ml to a concentration of 50 mg/ml. Solution will be golden yellow. For intrathecal administration: Reconstitute immediately prior to use with appropriate preservative-free solution, such as 0.9% sodium chloride injection to a concentration of 1–2.5 mg/ml (see Chap. 5 for intrathecal administration).	For slow I.V. push: 5–149 mg. For I.V. infusion: dilute further with 5% dextrose solution. Infusion volumes and rates vary widely.	Store powder or reconstituted solution at room temperature.

Drug	How supplied	Preparation	Administration	Special considerations
Mitomycin (Mutamycin, Mitomycin-C)	Vial—5 mg, 20 mg, 40 mg with mannitol.	Add sterile water for injection: 10 ml to 5 ml vial; 40 ml to 20 ml vial. Solution contains 0.5 mg mitomycin per ml, and will be purple-colored. If powder does not dissolve, allow to stand until solution is obtained.	Administer via Y-site of freely flowing I.V. over 10 min.	Protect from light after reconstitution. VESICANT—may cause thrombophlebitis or extravasation. Monitor I.V. site for pain, burning. NOTE: Extravasation may occur without pain or burning sensation.
Mitoxantrone (Novantrone)	Vial (2 mg/ml)— 20 mg in 10 ml, 25 mg in 12.5 ml, 30 mg in 15 ml (dark blue solution).	Add to 0.9% sodium chloride solution or 5% dextrose in water to a concentration of 0.5 mg/ml.	Administer by I.V. infusion over 15–30 min.	Incompatible with heparin. Vein may turn blue owing to color of medication. Flush vein with 50 ml normal saline before and after administration.
Paclitaxel (Taxol)	Ampule—30 mg in 5 ml polyoxyethylated castor oil (Cremophor EL) 50% and dehydrated alcohol USP 50%.	Dilute contents of ampule in 0.9% sodium chloride injection, 5% dextrose injection, 5% dextrose in 0.9% sodium chloride, or 5% dextrose in Ringer's injection to a final concentration of 0.3–1.2 mg/ml.	None required.	Use diluted solution within 8 hr. after preparation. Must be prepared in glass or polyolefin container. Do not use if excessive particulate matter observed in solution. Note: Solution may show haziness; however, no significant loss in potency has been noted. Administer as a continuous infusion over 6–24 hr. via polyethylene tubing, a low sorbing extension set, and a 0.2-μm in-line filter with a microporous membrane. Avoid use of plasticized PVC containers or administration sets. VESICANT—Cremophor vehicle can cause tissue damage.

(Continued)

Table 2–4 Directions for Reconstitution and Administration of Parenteral Antineoplastic Medications (Continued)

GENERIC NAME (BRAND NAME)	AVAILABILITY	INITIAL DILUTION	FURTHER DILUTION/ ADMINISTRATION	ADDITIONAL INFORMATION
Plicamycin (Mithracin)	Vial—2500 mcg plicamycin plus 100 mg mannitol.	Add 4.9 ml sterile water for injection to vial, and shake to dissolve. Solution contains 500 µg mithramycin per ml. (NOTE: 1 mg = 1000 µg.)	Dilute appropriate dose in 1 L 5% dextrose injection or sodium chloride injection, and administer by slow I.V. infusion over 4–6 hr.	Potent irritant. May cause thrombophlebitis or extravasation. Assess I.V. site for pain, burning. Should either occur, discontinue infusion and restart at another site. Application of moderate heat to the site may help to disperse the medication and minimize discomfort and local tissue irritation.
Streptozocin (Zanosar, STZ)	Vial—1 gm.	Add 9.5 ml 5% dextrose injection USP, or 0.9% sodium chloride injection USP. The resulting pale gold solution will contain 100 mg of streptozocin and 22 mg citric acid/ml.	Administer slow I.V. push into Y-site of freely flowing I.V. May be diluted further in up to 500 ml 5% dextrose injection USP, or 0.9% sodium chloride injection USP, and administered as an I.V. infusion.	VESICANT—May cause severe local irritation at I.V. site. Avoid extravasation. Assess site for pain, burning. Protect reconstituted solution from light. Maximum storage time after reconstitution—12 hr. (contains no preservative).
Teniposide (Vumon, VM-26)	Ampule—50 mg in 5 ml.	None required—prepared as a solution.	Add to 100–150 ml 0.9% sodium chloride for injection.	Administer over 30–60 min. into sidearm of freely flowing I.V. Do not administer if precipitate is noted. Avoid extravasation. IRRITANT—Assess site for pain or burning.

Thiotepa	Vial—15 mg.	Add 1.5 ml sterile water for injection for solution containing 10 mg/ml. Solution should be clear to slightly opaque.	For I.V. infusion: Add diluted medication to 50 ml dextrose, sodium chloride, Ringer's solution, or lactated Ringer's solution. For intravesical administration: Add 60 mg thiotepa to 30–60 ml sterile water for injection. For intratumor administration: Dilute dose in sterile water for injection, 10 mg per ml. For intracavitary administration: See package insert.	After intracavitary administration: Turn patient q 15 min. for 1 hr. to assure distribution of medication. Use solution as soon as possible after preparation. Do not use if grossly opaque or if precipitate seen.
Vinblastine (Velban, Velbe, Velsar, VBL)	Vial—10 mg.	Add 10 ml sodium chloride for injection (preserved with phenol or benzyl alcohol). Solution contains 1 mg vinblastine per ml.	Administer direct I.V. or via sideport of freely flowing I.V. over 1 min. Do not dilute in large volumes or administer over prolonged periods of time.	Administer 5–10 ml sodium chloride injection prior to I.V. push to assure patency of vein. VESICANT—Assure proper positioning of needle by drawing back for blood return after each 1–2 ml is administered. Should extravasation accidentally occur, application of moderate heat and hyaluronidase may reduce cellulitis. Should accidental contamination of the eye occur during preparation or administration, rinse immediately and thoroughly with water or saline.

(Continued)

Table 2-4 Directions for Reconstitution and Administration of Parenteral Antineoplastic Medications (Continued)

GENERIC NAME (BRAND NAME)	AVAILABILITY	INITIAL DILUTION	FURTHER DILUTION/ ADMINISTRATION	ADDITIONAL INFORMATION
Vincristine (Oncovin, Vincasar PFS, VCR)	Oncovin: Vial—1 mg, 2 mg, 5 mg (1 mg/ml). Hyporets (prefilled syringes)—1 mg in 1 ml, 2 mg in 2 ml. Vincasar PFS: Vial—1 mg in 1 ml.	Prediluted. NOTE: Do not add additional fluid to vial prior to removal of the desired dose.	Administer directly into vein, via sideport of freely flowing I.V. over 1 min. Do not dilute in large volumes or administer over prolonged periods of time.	VESICANT—Assess site for extravasation. Should leakage into surrounding tissue occur: Administer remaining portion of medication into another vein. Local injection of hyaluronidase and application of moderate heat to site helps disperse the medication and may reduce local discomfort and possibility of cellulitis.

| Vindesine sulfate (Eldisine) | 5 ml vial with 5 mg vindesine sulfate and 25 mg mannitol. Sodium hydroxide and/or sulfuric acid have been added to adjust pH. | Add 5 ml bacteriostatic normal saline solution for 1 mg/ml. Reconstituted solution is stable for 24 hr. at room temperature, or 14 days under refrigeration at 2–8°C. | No further dilution necessary. | The solution may be injected directly into a vein or into the sideport of a freely flowing I.V. Vindesine should not be mixed with other chemotherapeutic agents or medications in the same vessel. VESICANT—Local tissue damage may occur with extravasation. Draw back to assure blood return after each 1–2 ml. Assess site for pain, infiltration. Should either be noted or suspected: Discontinue administration. Inject remaining portion into another vein. Inject hyaluronidase locally, then elevate extremity above the level of the heart for a few minutes in an attempt to reduce intravenous pressure and prevent post-injection leakage of the medication. Apply moderate heat in an attempt to help disperse the medication and reduce discomfort. Assess the site on a continuing basis. |

Note: All chemotherapeutic medications should be prepared using a Luer-Lok syringe.

Table 2–5 Comparison of Flare Reaction and Extravasation for All Vesicants (see Table 2–2)

FEATURE	FLARE REACTION	EXTRAVASATION
Agents responsible	Daunorubicin, Doxorubicin	All Vesicants
Appearance	Raised, red streak usually occurs within minutes, most commonly along vein line of infusion. Resembles hivelike patches.	Redness not always present at time of extravasation; usually occurs 6–12 hr. later.
Blood return	Usually good.	Usually absent or sluggish.
Subjective symptoms	May experience pain.	Usually experiences an itching sensation, not pain.
Duration	Raised, red streak usually disappears in 30–90 min. after drug infusion.	Swelling does not dissipate for several days.

Adapted from Wood, L.S., and Gullo, S.M.: I.V. vesicants: How to avoid extravasation. Am. J. Nurs. 93(4):42–46, 1993.

Medications that may be irritant or vesicant agents are listed in Table 2–2.

2. Outcomes (ONS, 1992, p. 2):
   a. The incidence of extravasation is reduced.
   b. Potential extravasations are detected early and treated according to the most current literature available.
   c. Undue harm to the patient is minimized or prevented due to early and knowledgeable intervention.
3. Nursing management:
   a. Be familiar with vesicant medications and hospital or agency policy for reporting and intervention.
   b. Administer vesicant medications in larger veins of the arm, midway between wrist and elbow joints (see Fig. 2–9).
   c. Assess status of I.V. by:
      (1) Drawing back to assess blood return after each 1 to 2 ml of a vesicant chemotherapeutic agent is administered.
      (2) Instructing the client to report pain or burning at the I.V. site.
   d. If extravasation of a vesicant chemotherapeutic agent occurs or is suspected, the following measures should be taken:
      (1) Discontinue chemotherapy, leaving I.V. cannula in place.
      (2) Aspirate residual medication and blood via I.V. tubing.

Note: If unable to aspirate residual drug from I.V. cannula, remove cannula.

(3) Instill the antidote through the existing cannula (see Table 2–2). If cannula has been removed, inject the antidote subcutaneously into the extravasation area using a 25-g needle.

(4) Avoid applying pressure to the area.

(5) Apply sterile occlusive dressing.

(6) Apply heat or cold as indicated (see Tables 2–2, 2–3).

(7) Elevate the affected arm.

(8) Notify physician of extravasation.

(9) Observe the site regularly for pain, erythema, induration, and/or tissue necrosis.

(10) Document incident. Extravasation record (Fig. 2–10) may be used. If it is not available, document in nursing note and include:

  (a) Date.
  (b) Time.
  (c) Size and type of I.V. needle or cannula.
  (d) Insertion site.
  (e) Medication(s) administered.
  (f) Sequence of chemotherapeutic agents.

Table 2–6   Suggested Contents of an Emergency Extravasation Tray*

Disposable latex gloves (talc-free, 0.007–0.009″ thick)
Needles—18 gauge; 25 gauge; filter needles (2 each)
Syringes—tuberculin; 3 cc; 5 cc; 10 cc; 20 cc
One-inch paper tape; 2 sterile 4 × 4s; 6 alcohol wipes; 4 Telfa pads; hot pack; cold pack.
Local anesthetic—Lidocaine, ethyl chloride.
Diluent—1 each: 30 ml bacteriostatic 0.9% sodium chloride injection; 30 ml bacteriostatic water.
Hydrocortisone or other steroid cream—1% (optional)
Antidotes—10% sodium thiosulfate (10 ml)
  Hydrocortisone solution (100-ml vial)
  Sodium bicarbonate 1 mEq/ml 50 ml
  Dexamethasone 4 mg/ml
  Dimethyl sulfoxide 50–100% topical
  Hyaluronidase 150 U (store in refrigerator)
Extravasation record form
Policy and procedure for extravasation management

*Kit should always be available when a vesicant medication is being administered. Restock supplies and medications after each use.

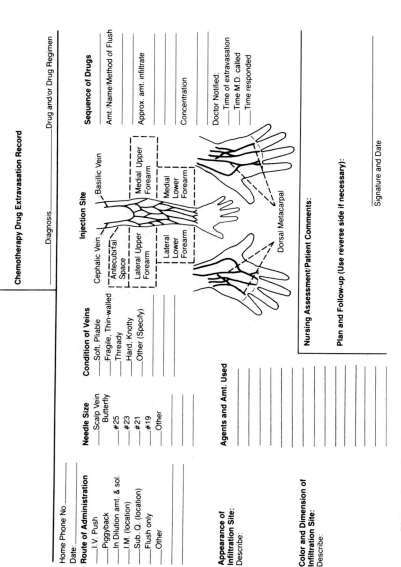

Figure 2–10. Sample extravasation record. (Reproduced with permission of Stanford University Hospital and Clinics. Stanford Medical Center, Stanford, CA.)

(g) Approximate amount of medication.
(h) Subjective symptoms reported by client.
(i) Nursing assessment of site.
(j) Nursing interventions.
(k) Physician notification and intervention.
(l) Instructions given to client.
(m) Follow-up measures.
(n) Nurse's signature.
(Note: A photograph of the site may be required.)

An extravasation tray or kit should be kept in an area accessible to the nurse administering chemotherapy. Suggested contents of the extravasation tray are specified in Table 2–6.

References

American Society of Hospital Pharmacists: ASHP technical assistance bulletin on handling cytotoxic drugs. Am. J. Hosp. Pharm. 47:1033–1049, 1990.

Laidlaw, J.L., et al.: Permeability of latex and polyvinyl chloride gloves to antineoplastic drugs. Am. J. Hosp. Pharm., 41:2618–2623, 1984.

Oncology Nursing Society: *Cancer Chemotherapy Guidelines: Recommendations for the Management of Vesicant Extravasation, Hypersensitivity and Anaphylaxis*. Pittsburgh, Oncology Nursing Society, 1992.

Oncology Nursing Society: *Cancer Chemotherapy Guidelines Module I: Recommendations for Cancer Chemotherapy Course Content*. Pittsburgh, Oncology Nursing Society, 1988.

Oncology Nursing Society: *Cancer Chemotherapy Guidelines Module II: Recommendations for Nursing Practice in the Acute Care Setting*. Pittsburgh, Oncology Nursing Society, 1988.

Oncology Nursing Society: *Cancer Chemotherapy Guidelines Module III: Recommendations for Nursing Practice in the Outpatient Setting*. Pittsburgh, Oncology Nursing Society, 1988.

Oncology Nursing Society: *Cancer Chemotherapy Guidelines Module IV: Recommendations for Nursing Practice in the Home Care Setting*. Pittsburgh, Oncology Nursing Society, 1988.

Speyer, J.L., and Sorich, J.: Intraperitoneal carboplatin: Rationale and experience. Semin. Oncol., Suppl. 2, 19(1):107–113, 1992.

U.S. Department of Health and Human Services, Occupational Safety and Health Administration: *Recommendations for the Safe Handling and Disposal of Hazardous Drugs* (OSHA Instruction CPL–2–2.20B CH–4). Washington, D.C., U.S. Department of Health and Human Services, Occupational Safety and Health Administration, draft.

Recommended Readings

Preparation and Administration

Ashley, B.W., and Cross-Skinner, S.: Oncology nursing care delivery issues in the ambulatory setting. Curr. Issues Cancer Nurs. Pract. 1(1):1–10, 1992.

Berman, A., Chisholm, L., de Carvahlo, M., et al.: Cancer chemotherapy: Intravenous administration (Programmed Instruction). Cancer Nurs. 16(2):145–160, 1993.

Curran, C.F., Luce, J.K., and Page, J.A.: Doxorubicin-associated flare reactions. Oncol. Nurs. Forum 17:387–389, 1990.

Gallelli, J.F.: Issues and risks associated with handling antineoplastic drugs. J. Pharm. Pract. 4:72–76, 1991.

Goodman, M.: Delivery of cancer chemotherapy. In Baird, S.B., et al. (eds.): *Cancer Nursing: A Comprehensive Textbook* (pp. 296–298). Philadelphia, W.B. Saunders, 1991.

Gullo, S.M.: Safe handling of antineoplastic drugs: Translating the recommendations into practice. Oncol. Nurs. Forum 15:595–601, 1988.

Gullo, S.: Safe handling of chemotherapy. Oncol. Nurs. Forum 17(11):113–116, 1990.

Office of Occupational Medicine: *Work Practice Guidelines for Personnel Dealing with Cytotoxic (Antineoplastic) Drugs.* Washington, D.C., Office of Occupational Medicine, U.S. Department of Labor, 1986.

Power, L.A., et al.: Update on safe handling of hazardous drugs and the advice of experts. Am. J. Hosp. Pharm. 5:1051–1060, 1990.

Schulmeister, L.: Developing guidelines for bleomycin test dosing. Oncol. Nurs. Forum 16:205–207, 1989.

Stevens, K.R.: Safe handling of cytotoxic drugs in home chemotherapy. Semin. Oncol. Nurs. 5(2[Supp 1]):15–20, 1989.

U.S. Department of Health and Human Services: *Recommendations for the Safe Handling of Parenteral Antineoplastic Drugs.* Washington, D.C., U.S. Department of Health and Human Services, Public Health Service, 1986.

Valanis, B., et al.: Comparison of antineoplastic drug handling policies of hospitals with OSHA guidelines: A pilot study. Am. J. Public Health 80:480–481, 1990.

Valanis, B., et al.: Staff members compliance with their facility's antineoplastic drug handling policy. Oncol. Nurs. Forum 18:571–576, 1991.

Valanis, B., et al.: Acute symptoms associated with antineoplastic drug handling among nurses. Cancer Nurs. 16(4):288–295, 1993.

Wiseman, K.C., and Wachs, J.E.: Policies and practices used for the safe handling of antineoplastic drugs. Am. Acad. Occup. Health Nurs. J. 38:517–523, 1990.

Wong, R.J.: Glove selection for handling cytotoxic and hazardous drugs. Am. J. Hosp. Pharm. 47:1033–1049, 1990.

Wroblewski, S.: Chemotherapy spills on carpet. Oncol. Nurs. Forum 17:764, 1990.

Extravasation

Alberts, D.S., and Dorr, R.T.: Case report: Topical DMSO for mitomycin induced skin ulceration. Oncol. Nurs. Forum 18:693–695, 1991.

Beason, R.: Antineoplastic vesicant extravasation. J. Intravenous Nurs. 3(2):111–114, 1990.

Dorr, R.T.: Antidotes to vesicant chemotherapy extravasation. Blood Rev. 4:41–60, 1990.

McCaffrey, D., and Engeking, C.: Ten fallacies associated with the nature and management of chemotherapy extravasation. Progressions 2(4):3–10, 1990.

Petus, F.T., et al.: Mitoxantrone extravasation injury. Cancer Treat. Rep. 71:992–993, 1987.

Rudolph, R., and Larson, D.L.: Etiology and treatment of chemotherapy agent extravasation injuries: A review. J. Clin. Oncol. 5:1116–1126, 1987.

Tsavaris, N.B., et al.: Prevention of tissue necrosis due to accidental extravasation of cytotoxic drugs by a conservative approach. Cancer Chemother. Pharmacol. 30:330–333, 1992.

Wood, S., and Gullo, S.: IV vesicants: How to avoid extravasation. Am. J. Nurs. 93:42–46, 1993.

Alternative Modes of Administration

Almadrones, L., et al.: Problems associated with administration of intraperitoneal therapy using the Port-A-Cath system. Oncol. Nurs. Forum 17:75–80, 1990.

Chisholm, L., et al.: Cancer chemotherapy: Alternative administration routes (Programmed Instruction). Cancer Nurs. 16(3):237–246, 1993.

Doane, L.S.: Delivering intraperitoneal chemotherapy in ovarian cancer. Today's OR Nurse 14(9):11–18, 1992.

Doane, L.S., et al.: How to give peritoneal chemotherapy. Am. J. Nurs. 90(4):58–64, 1990.

Ensminger, W.D.: Regional chemotherapy. Semin. Oncol. 20(1):3–11, 1993.

Herr, H.W.: Intravesical therapy. Hematol. Clin. North Am. 6:117–127, 1992.

Hoff, S.T.: Nursing perspectives on intraperitoneal chemotherapy. J. Intravenous Nurs. 14:309–314, 1991.

Howell, S.B., et al.: A phase II trial of intraperitoneal cisplatin and etoposide for primary treatment of ovarian epithelial cancer. J. Clin. Oncol. 8:137–145, 1990.

Kirmani, S., et al.: A phase II trial of intraperitoneal cisplatin and etoposide as salvage treatment for minimal residual ovarian carcinoma. J. Clin. Oncol. 9:649–657, 1991.

Lamm, D.L., et al.: A randomized trial of intravesical doxorubicin and immunotherapy with Bacillus Calmette-Guérin for transitional cell carcinoma of the bladder. N. Engl. J. Med. 325:1205–1209, 1991.

LeBouton, J.: Nursing aspects of Bacillus Calmette-Guérin immunotherapy for superficial bladder cancer. Urol. Nurs. 10(4):9–14, 1990.

Malloy, J.: Administration of intraperitoneal chemotherapy: A new approach. Nursing 21(1):58–62, 1991.

Malstrom, H., Larsson, D., Simonsen, E.: Phase I study of intraperitoneal carboplatin as adjuvant therapy in early ovarian cancer. Gynecol. Oncol. 39:289–294, 1990.

Markman, M., et al.: Phase II trial of intraperitoneal mitoxantrone in the management of refractory ovarian cancer. J. Clin. Oncol. 8:146–150, 1990.

Markman, M., et al.: Phase I trial of intraperitoneal Taxol: A gynecologic oncology group study. J. Clin. Oncol. 10:1485–1491, 1992.

Markman, M., et al.: Phase II trial of weekly or biweekly intraperitoneal mitoxantrone in epithelial ovarian cancer. J. Clin. Oncol. 9:978–982, 1991.

Reich, B., et al.: A trial of Taxol administered by the intraperitoneal route: A gynecologic oncology group study. J. Clin. Oncol. 10:1485–1491, 1992.

Schnellhammer, P.F., et al.: Bacillus Calmette-Guérin for superficial transitional cell carcinoma of the bladder. J. Urol. 135:261–264, 1986.

Zook-Enck, D.: Intraperitoneal therapy via the Tenckhoff catheter: Prevention and management of complications. J. Intravenous Nurs. 13:375–382, 1990.

Continuous Infusion

Atiq, O.T., et al.: Treatment of unresectable primary liver cancer with intrahepatic fluorodeoxyuridine and mitomycin C through an implantable pump. Cancer 69:920–924, 1991.

Schulmeister, L.: An overview of continuous infusion chemotherapy. J. Intravenous Nurs. 15:315–322, 1992.

Chapter *3*

Chemotherapeutic Agents Used in the Treatment of Cancer

Linda Tenenbaum, R.N., M.S.N., O.C.N.

This chapter includes information about medications used in the treatment of cancer. All material is presented in table form for easy reference. Medications are categorized according to their pharmaceutical classifications.

Each table categorizes the category and describes the mechanisms of action of medications in that category.

Column 1 includes:

1. The generic names, listed alphabetically within each category.
2. Brand name(s). Brand names for the United States and Canada are included.
3. The abbreviation, if commonly used.
4. Forms and doses available.

Photographs of medications are not included in this book. The reader is referred to *Facts and Comparisons*, the *Physicians' Desk Reference* (in the United States), or the *Compendium of Pharmaceuticals and Specialties* (in Canada).

Column 2 includes:

1. Routes of administration.
2. Sample dosage regimens.

When the recommended dosage for the child varies from the adult dosage, both are listed.

Column 3 includes:

1. Types of cancer for which the medication is administered. This includes uses that are recommended in the manufacturers' literature as well as those under clinical investigation.

Column 4 includes:

1. Toxicities of the medication. The most common toxicities appear first. Toxicities that occur 20–25 per cent of the time or more appear in **bold print.**

Easy-reference charts summarizing toxicities can be found in Appendix G.

Column 5 includes:

1. Nursing interventions specific to administration of the medication, or care of the client receiving the medication. General nursing interventions for problems related to chemotherapy may be found in the tables in Section II (pages 210 through 219).

Categories of Chemotherapeutic Agents

Chemotherapeutic agents are classified into the categories listed below. The generic name is given first, followed by brand names and abbreviation (if any).

1. **Alkylating agents** (Table 3–1):
   - busulfan (Myleran)
   - carboplatin (Paraplatin)
   - chlorambucil (Leukeran)
   - cisplatin (Platinol, CIS-DDP)
   - cyclophosphamide (Cytoxan, Endoxan, Neosar, Procytox, CTX)
   - dacarbazine (DTIC-Dome, DTIC)
   - ifosfamide (Ifex)
   - mechlorethamine hydrochloride (Mustargen, nitrogen mustard, HN2)
   - melphalan (Alkeran, L-Pam, Phenylalanine mustard)
   - thiotepa, triethylene thiophosphoramide (Thiotepa)
2. **Nitrosoureas** (Table 3–2):
   - carmustine (BiCNU, BCNU)
   - lomustine (CeeNU, CCNU)
   - streptozocin (Zanosar)

3. **Antimetabolites** (Table 3–3):
   - cladribine (Leustatin)
   - cytarabine, cytosine arabinoside (Cytosar-U, Ara-C, Tarabine)
   - floxuridine (FUDR)
   - fludarabine (Fludara)
   - 5-fluorouracil (Adrucil, 5-FU)
   - 5-fluorouracil topical (Efudex, Fluoroplex)
   - mercaptopurine (Purinethol, 6-MP)
   - methotrexate, abitrexate (Folex, Mexate, Mexate-AQ, Uromitexan, MTX)
   - pentostatin (Nipent, 2-deoxycoformycin, 2-DCA)
   - thioguanine (Lanvis, 6-TG)
4. **Mitotic inhibitors** (Table 3–4):
   - docetaxel (Taxotere, investigational)
   - etoposide (VePesid, VP-16-213)
   - paclitaxel (Taxol)
   - teniposide (Vumon, VM-26)
   - vinblastine (Velban, Velbe, Velsar, VLB)
   - vincristine (Oncovin, Vincasar, VCR)
   - vindesine (Eldisine)
5. **Antitumor antibiotics** (Table 3–5):
   - bleomycin (Blenoxane)
   - dactinomycin (Cosmegen, Actinomycin-D, ACT-D)
   - daunorubicin hydrochloride (Cerubidine, Daunomycin, DNR)
   - doxorubicin hydrochloride (Adriamycin, Rubex, ADR)
   - epirubicin hydrochloride (Pharmorubicin)
   - idarubicin (Idamycin)
   - mitomycin (Mutamycin, Mitomycin-C)
   - mitoxantrone hydrochloride (Novantrone)
   - plicamycin (Mithracin)
6. **Miscellaneous cancer chemotherapeutic agents** (Table 3–6):
   - altretamine (Hexalen, Hexastat, hexamethylmelamine, HMM)
   - amsacrine (AMSA-PD, amsidine, amsidyl, M-AMSA)
   - asparaginase (Elspar, Kidrolase, L-ASP)
   - estramustine phosphate sodium (Emcyt)
   - hydroxyurea (Hydrea)
   - levamisole (Ergamisol)
   - mesna (Mesnex)
   - mitotane (Lysodren)
   - procarbazine (Matulane, Natulan)
7. **Steroids and hormonally active agents** (Table 3–7):
   a. Adrenal corticosteroids
      - cortisone acetate (Cortone)
      - prednisone (Deltasone, Orasone, SK-Prednisone)
      - prednisolone (Cortalone, Delta-Cortef)

- dexamethasone (Decadron, Dexone, Hexadrol, SK-Dexamethasone)
- methylprednisolone sodium succinate (Medrol)
  b. Adrenal cortical steroid inhibitor
- aminoglutethamide (Cytadren)
  c. Estrogens
- chlorotrianisene (TACE)
- conjugated estrogens (Premarin, Progens)
- diethylstilbestrol diphosphate (Stilphostrol, DES)
- esterified estrogens (Estratab, Menest)
- estradiol (Estrace)
- estradiol valerate (Delestrogen, Estraval, Femogex, Gynogen, Menoval, Pro-val, Valergen)
- ethinyl estradiol (Estinyl)
  d. Progestational agents
- medroxyprogesterone acetate (Provera)
- megestrol acetate (Megace)
  e. Antiestrogens
- tamoxifen citrate (Nolvadex, Tamofen)
- toremifene (Investigational)
  f. Androgens
- dromostanolone proprionate (Drolban)
- fluoxymesterone (Android-F, Halotestin, Ora-Testryl, Ultandrogen)
- methyltestosterone (Android, Metandren, Oreton methyl, Primotest forte, Testred)
- testolactone (Teslac)
- testosterone (Android-5, Android-10, Android-25, Estratest)
- testosterone cypionate (Andronate, Depotestosterone, Testred cypionate)
- testosterone enanthate (Andro-L.A., Delatestryl, Everone, Malogex, Testoject-EP, Testrin)
- testosterone proprionate (Malogen, Testex)
  g. Antiandrogens
- flutamide (Eulexin, Euflex)
  h. Luteinizing hormone releasing hormone (LHRH) agonists
- goserelin acetate (Zoladex)
- leuprolide acetate (Lupron, Lupron Depot)

Combination Chemotherapy

Combination chemotherapy is the use of two or more chemotherapeutic agents administered together in treating a form of cancer. In this manner one agent may act synergistically with others in the combination. The combination usually includes medications from different categories of chemotherapeutic agents, with varying modes and times of action and toxicities. The first combination chemotherapy, used in the 1960s for treatment of Hodgkin's disease, was MOPP (Table 3–8). This and similar combinations are administered today for treatment of Hodgkin's disease and non-Hodgkin's lymphomas.

Medications in the MOPP combination include:

M—Mechlorethamine (Mustargen, nitrogen mustard), an alkylating agent that is cell cycle–nonspecific. The primary toxicities are myelosuppression (nadir at 7 to 14 days) and nausea and vomiting. Mechlorethamine is administered intravenously on the first and eighth days of the course of therapy.

O—Oncovin (vincristine), a *Vinca* alkaloid, cell cycle–specific to the M phase. Primary toxicities are mild nausea and vomiting and neurotoxicity. Vincristine is administered intravenously on the first and eighth days of the course of therapy.

P—Procarbazine (Matulane), which is in the miscellaneous category. Like mechlorethamine, procarbazine is cell cycle–nonspecific. The primary toxicities are myelosuppression (nadir at 3 to 8 weeks) and neurotoxicity. Procarbazine is administered orally on days 1 through 14 of the course of therapy.

P—Prednisone, a corticosteroid, also cell cycle–nonspecific. Toxicities are rare and include sodium and fluid retention. Prednisone produces an alteration in the cellular environment. It is administered orally on days 1 through 14 of the course of therapy.

Combination chemotherapy regimens have improved treatment response by the use of two alternating, equally effective combinations. Sample combinations are listed in Table 3–9.

Table 3-1 Alkylating Agents

Produce breaks in DNA molecule and crosslinking of strands.
Interfere with DNA replication and transcription.
Cell cycle–nonspecific.

MEDICATION AND FORMS AVAILABLE	DOSAGE RANGE	INDICATIONS	TOXICITY Note: All alkylating agents may be carcinogenic, teratogenic	NURSING INTERVENTIONS
Busulfan (Myleran) AVAILABLE: Tablets—2 mg.	**P.O.:** REMISSION INDUCTION: **Adult:** 4–8 mg daily until leukocyte count falls to approximately 15,000/μL. **Adult or child:** approximately 60 μg/kg of body weight or 1.8 mg/m² daily until leukocyte count falls to approximately 15,000/μL. MAINTENANCE: 1–3 mg daily.	Chronic granulocytic (myelocytic) leukemia—palliative therapy, preoperative treatment for bone marrow transplant.	**Myelosuppression,** mild N & V, A*, hyperuricemia, ovarian and sperm suppression, gynecomastia, alopecia, hyperpigmentation, cataract formation. "Busulfan lung syndrome," hypersensitivity reaction (both rare—see Chapter 13).	Administer antiemetic as ordered. Monitor complete blood count and report severe myelosuppression. Discontinue therapy if there is a precipitous fall in leukocyte count. Assess for dyspnea, cough. Assess lung sounds. Monitor BUN, creatinine, uric acid and report elevations. Encourage increased fluid intake. Administer allopurinol if ordered to relieve symptoms of hyperuricemia.

74

Carboplatin (Paraplatin, CBCDA) AVAILABLE: Vial—50 mg, 150 mg, 450 mg.	**I.V.:** Metastatic carcinoma of ovary: single agent—360 mg/m² on day 1 every 4 weeks; in combination—300 mg/m² on day 1 every 4 weeks × 6 cycles (with cyclophosphamide 600 mg/m²). Testicular carcinoma: investigational; intraperitoneal (investigational). First-line treatment for carcinoma of ovary in combination with cyclophosphamide; carcinoma of lung, head, and neck; testicular carcinomas (seminoma and non-seminoma).	**Myelosuppression, N, V*, electrolyte disturbances (hyponatremia, hypomagnesemia, hypocalcemia, hypokalemia), ↑ alkaline phosphatase,** ↑ hepatic enzymes (ALT, AST), ↑ bilirubin. Pain, asthenia (under 10%). ↑ BUN, serum creatinine. Peripheral neuropathies, cardiovascular, genitourinary, respiratory toxicities, hearing loss, alopecia, hypersensitivity reaction (HSR). NOTE: Myelosuppression of platelets may be prolonged and severe in patients previously treated with other antineoplastic agents.	Premedicate with antiemetic as ordered. Assess complete blood count, creatinine clearance, AST, ALT, total bilirubin, alkaline phosphatase. Dose reduction may be required for the client with neutrophils <2,000/mm³, platelets <100,000/mm³, or creatinine clearance <60 ml/min, or in patients previously treated with other antineoplastic agents. Assess for hearing loss, peripheral neuropathies, HSR. NOTE: Unlike cisplatin, clients receiving carboplatin do not require pretreatment hydration or post-treatment hydration or forced diuresis unless they are dehydrated.

(Continued)

Table 3–1 Alkylating Agents (Continued)

MEDICATION AND FORMS AVAILABLE	DOSAGE RANGE	INDICATIONS	TOXICITY Note: All alkylating agents may be carcinogenic, teratogenic	NURSING INTERVENTIONS
Chlorambucil (Leukeran) AVAILABLE: Tablets—2 mg.	P.O.: Hodgkin's disease (adult): 0.2 mg/kg/day for 3–6 weeks. Non-Hodgkin's lymphomas, chronic lymphocytic leukemia: 0.1 mg/kg/day for 3–6 weeks, as a single daily dose. Child: 0.1–0.2 mg/kg or 4.5 mg/m².	Chronic lymphocytic leukemia, lymphomas, giant follicular lymphomas, Hodgkin's disease. Carcinoma of prostate, breast, testicle, ovary; multiple myeloma, choriocarcinoma.	M, N, V, A (rare).* Urticaria, ovarian, and sperm suppression, amenorrhea. Pulmonary fibrosis, hepatotoxicity (both rare). Seizures (rare).	Administer on an empty stomach 1 hr. before breakfast or bedtime to reduce nausea. Administer antiemetic as ordered. Assess lung sounds, assess for dyspnea. Have client report cough or difficulty breathing. Monitor liver function studies.
Cisplatin (Platinol, Platinol-AQ, CIS, DDP) AVAILABLE: Vial—10 mg, 50 mg, 100 mg†	I.V.: Metastatic testicular tumors: 20 mg/m² days 1–5 every 3 weeks for three courses. Metastatic carcinoma of ovary: 50–100 mg/m² over 6–8 hours q 3 weeks. Advanced carcinoma of bladder: 50–70	Testicular cancer, carcinoma of ovary, bladder. Non–small cell carcinoma of lung, squamous cell carcinoma of head and neck, osteogenic sarcoma, germ cell tumors. Carcinoma of prostate, bladder, esophagus, endometrium, and	N, V (severe), M,* hyperuricemia, nephrotoxicity, A, D, electrolyte disturbances (hypomagnesemia, hypocalcemia, hypokalemia, hyponatremia, hypophosphatemia), ototoxicity. Peripheral neuropathy. Anaphylaxis (rare), tet-	Administer antiemetics as ordered. Provide adequate hydration before and after cisplatin infusion to reduce risk of nephrotoxicity by encouraging client to drink 2,000–3,000 ml fluid/day, or administering I.V. fluids beginning 4 hours

mg/m² q 3–4 weeks. Note: Dose reduction may be required with total leukocyte count <2,000/mm³ or with marked granulocytopenia.

cervix, renal cell carcinoma.

any, hyperuricemia, SIADH (syndrome of inappropriate antidiuretic hormone).

prior to therapy, and for 24 hours after administration to maintain urinary output of at least 100 ml/hr; administering cisplatin in 1,000–2,000 ml chloride-containing solution over 6–8 hours; and administering mannitol or lasix if ordered. Do not infuse via aluminum needle or connections. Notify physician if creatinine clearance <60 ml/min. Administer parenteral antiemetic regimen prior to and following administration. Monitor BUN, creatinine and creatinine clearance, uric acid, electrolytes, AST, ALT. Assess serum electrolytes, uric acid. Assess for HSR, have emergency medications on hand (see Chapter 13). Perform periodic audiometric testing. Maintain I.V. flow and administer diuretic following administration to maintain adequate renal output of at least 125 ml/hr.

(Continued)

Table 3–1 Alkylating Agents (Continued)

MEDICATION AND FORMS AVAILABLE	DOSAGE RANGE	INDICATIONS	TOXICITY Note: All alkylating agents may be carcinogenic, teratogenic	NURSING INTERVENTIONS
Cyclophosphamide (Cytoxan, Endoxan, Neosar, Procytox, CTX) AVAILABLE: Tablets—25 mg, 50 mg. Vial—100 mg, 200 mg, 500 mg, 1 gm, 2 gm. Lyophilized—100 mg, 200 mg, 500 mg, 1 gm, 2 gm.	**P.O., I.V., I.M.** INDUCTION: 40–50 mg/kg (1500–1800 mg/m²) I.V. in divided doses over 2–5 days. MAINTENANCE: 1–5 mg/kg P.O. daily. I.V. 10–15 mg/kg q 7–10 days or 3–5 mg/kg twice weekly. (Dose may require reduction during course of radiation therapy.) PULSE THERAPY: 20–40 mg/kg I.V. twice weekly q 3 weeks as tolerated. Intraperitoneal, intrapleural.	Malignant lymphomas (stages III, IV), Hodgkin's disease, lymphocytic lymphoma (nodular or diffuse), mixed-cell type lymphoma, histiocytic lymphoma, Burkitt's lymphoma, leukemias (lymphocytic, granulocytic, acute myelogenous and myelocytic, acute lymphoblastic [stem-cell] leukemia in children and adults). Wilms' tumor, osteogenic sarcoma, neuroblastoma (disseminated disease), rhabdomyosarcoma, mycosis fungoides (advanced disease), choriocarcinoma. Adenocarcinoma of ovary, carcinoma of breast, lung, prostate, retinoblastoma, carcinoma of head and neck, multiple myeloma.	**M, N, V, A,** D.* **Alopecia,** dermatitis. Ovarian and sperm suppression, amenorrhea. Hyperpigmentation of skin and nails. Sterile hemorrhagic cystitis, SIADH, hyponatremia. Cardiotoxicity; may potentiate cardiotoxic effects of doxorubicin, daunorubicin, epirubicin. Pulmonary fibrosis with high doses over a prolonged period. Hepatotoxicity (rare). Metallic taste, nasal stuffiness, runny eyes. If infused too fast: headache, dizziness, diaphoresis, and flushing.	To minimize nausea: Administer antiemetic as ordered prior to administration. To minimize damage to bladder wall: Encourage P.O. fluid intake of 2–3 L for 1 day prior to and 2 days following administration. Assess urinary output, BUN, creatinine. Assess quality and regularity of pulse. Assess lung sounds. Have client report cough or dyspnea. Monitor complete blood count. (Note: Dose may be reduced with total leukocyte count below 2,000/mm³ or with marked neutropenia.) For intrapleural or intraperitoneal or intrapleural administration, see Table 2–1.

Dacarbazine (DTIC-Dome, DTIC)

AVAILABLE:
Vial—100 mg, 200 mg.

I.V.:
For metastatic malignant melanoma: 2–4.5 mg/kg daily × 10 days q 4 weeks or 250 mg/m² I.V. × 5 days q 3 weeks. Hodgkin's disease: 150 mg/m² × 5 days q 4 weeks (in combination with other effective agents) or 375 mg/m² on day 1 q 15 days (in combination with other effective agents).

Metastatic malignant melanoma, Hodgkin's disease (as a second-line therapy in combination with other effective agents), sarcomas.

N, V (severe), M, A.*
Pain or burning at infusion site, alopecia. Elevation of hepatic and renal function test values. Facial flushing and facial paresthesias, erythema, urticaria, photosensitivity. Flu-like syndrome (fever, malaise, and myalgia), D* (rare). IRRITANT.

To reduce nausea: Restrict food intake for 4–6 hr prior to administration. Administer antiemetics as ordered. Administer via Y-site of freely flowing I.V. Instruct client to report pain or burning at I.V. site. Local pain or burning may be alleviated by application of heat to site. Monitor temperature and report elevation. Monitor lab. values for hepatic and renal function. Instruct client to avoid exposure to sunlight while receiving therapy.

Ifosfamide (Ifex)

AVAILABLE:
Vial—1 gm, 3 gm.

I.V.:
1.2–2.5 gm/m² daily × 5 days q 3–4 weeks; 1.2, 1.8, 2.0 gm/m² daily; or 5 gm q 3–4 weeks.

Germ cell testicular cancer (third-line therapy), sarcomas, carcinoma of lung, non-Hodgkin's lymphomas.

Hematuria, sterile hemorrhagic cystitis, M, N, V, A, D, S,* **alopecia.**
Central nervous system toxicity, including somnolence, confusion, hallucinations, depressive psychosis, fatigue, weakness, lethargy, coma. S. (Note: Microscopic hematuria is common, gross hematuria is less common.)

Administer antiemetic as ordered prior to administration.
To minimize damage to bladder wall:
Encourage P.O. fluid intake of 2–3 L for 1 day prior to and 2 days following administration. Obtain urinalysis prior to each dose. If erythrocytes in urine >10/high-power field, medication may be withheld.

(Continued)

Table 3–1 Alkylating Agents (Continued)

MEDICATION AND FORMS AVAILABLE	DOSAGE RANGE	INDICATIONS	TOXICITY Note: All alkylating agents may be carcinogenic, teratogenic	NURSING INTERVENTIONS
				Administer in A.M. to prevent accumulation of the medication in the bladder at night. Administer Mesna I.V. bolus in dosage equal to 20% of ifosfamide dose at time of ifosfamide administration, and repeat 4 and 8 hr later. Instruct client to empty bladder before going to bed at night, and during the night should he awaken. Assess urinary output, BUN, mental status, and neurological function.
Mechlorethamine hydrochloride (Mustargen, nitrogen mustard, HN2) AVAILABLE: Vial—10 mg.	**I.V.:** Total dose for each course 0.4 mg/kg of body weight. Administer as a single dose or in divided doses of 0.1–0.2 mg/kg/day. **Intracavitary:** 0.2–0.4 mg/kg. (Note: Dosage should be based on ideal day body weight.)	Hodgkin's disease (Stage III, IV—palliative treatment), chronic lymphocytic leukemia, chronic granulocytic (myelocytic) leukemia, bronchogenic carcinoma and resultant intrapleural effusions, mycosis fungoides, lymphosarcoma, polycythemia vera.	**N, V (severe), M,** A, D.* Pain or thrombophlebitis at infusion site. Alopecia, weakness, jaundice, ovarian and sperm suppression, amenorrhea, vertigo, tinnitus, ototoxicity, metallic taste, anaphylaxis. VESICANT— local tissue damage may occur with extravasation.	Avoid contact of medication with skin or eyes during preparation or administration. To reduce nausea: Premedicate with antiemetic as ordered. Assess infusion site and instruct client to report pain or discomfort at I.V. site.

Melphalan (Alkeran, L-PAM, Phenylalanine mustard)

AVAILABLE:
Tablets—2 mg (white).
Vial—50 mg with 10 ml vial sterile diluent.

P.O.:
Multiple myeloma: 6 mg daily or 2 mg t.i.d.
INDUCTION: 10 mg daily × 7–10 days.
MAINTENANCE: 2 mg/day when >4,000 and platelet count >100,000 OR:
INDUCTION: 0.15 mg/kg daily × 7 days followed by a rest period of at least 2 weeks.
MAINTENANCE: ≤0.05 mg/day when leukocyte count >4,000 and platelet count >100,000 OR:
INDUCTION: 0.25 mg/kg daily × 4 days OR 0.20 mg/kg × 5 days. Repeat q 4–6 weeks if granulocyte and platelet levels are within normal ranges.
PULSE THERAPY: 6 mg q d 2 mg t.i.d. × 2–3 weeks, then discontinue for up to 4 weeks until leukocytes and platelets rise, and repeat cycle.
BONE MARROW TRANS-PLANTATION: 4 mg/kg × 4 days.
I.V.: multiple myeloma—palliative treatments when oral therapy not appropriate. 16 mg/m² q 2 weeks × 4 doses, then q 4 weeks.
Epithelial carcinoma of ovary:
0.2 mg/kg daily × 5 days q 4–5 weeks.

Multiple myeloma, epithelial carcinoma of ovary, carcinoma of breast, osteosarcoma, chronic lymphocytic leukemia, chronic myelocytic (granulocytic) leukemia. Malignant melanoma.

M, N, V (moderate).* Alopecia, maculopapular rash, urticaria, ovarian and sperm suppression, pulmonary fibrosis (rare).

Administer on an empty stomach to reduce nausea. Monitor leukocytes and platelets q 2 weeks. Assess lung sounds. Have patient report cough or dyspnea.

Table 3–1 Alkylating Agents *(Continued)*

MEDICATION AND FORMS AVAILABLE	DOSAGE RANGE	INDICATIONS	TOXICITY Note: All alkylating agents may be carcinogenic, teratogenic	NURSING INTERVENTIONS
Thiotepa (Thiotepa) AVAILABLE: Vial—15 mg.	**I.V.:** INITIAL DOSE: 0.4 mg/kg. MAINTENANCE DOSE: 0.3 mg/kg q 1–4 weeks. **Intratumor:** INITIAL DOSE: 0.6–0.8 mg/kg. MAINTENANCE: 0.07–0.8 mg/kg q 1–4 weeks. **Intravesical:** 30–60 mg or 10–30 mg/m² in 30–60 ml distilled water once a week for 3–4 weeks, or 6–8 weeks. **Intracavitary:** 0.6–0.8 mg/kg.	Adenocarcinoma of breast, ovary; malignant effusions, superficial papillary adenocarcinoma of the bladder, Hodgkin's disease, lymphomas, lymphosarcomas.	**M, N, V, A.**[*] Localized pain at infusion site, ovarian and sperm suppression, amenorrhea, hyperpigmentation, headache, dizziness, hives, skin rash, fever, HSR (rare).	Monitor for rash, hives, temperature elevation, HSR. FOR CARCINOMA OF BLADDER: May be introduced by indwelling (Foley) catheter. Encourage client to change position every 15 min while chemotherapy solution is being retained (usually 2 hr). See Table 2–1. FOR INTRACAVITARY ADMINISTRATION, see Table 2–1.

[*]A = anorexia, D = diarrhea, M = myelosuppression, N = nausea, S = stomatitis, V = vomiting.
†Note: 100 mg dose available only in cisplatin-AQ.

Table 3-2 Nitrosoureas

May be classified as a subcategory of alkylating agents.
Act in same manner as alkylating agents.
Cross blood-brain barrier.

MEDICATION AND FORMS AVAILABLE	DOSAGE RANGE	INDICATIONS	TOXICITY	NURSING INTERVENTIONS
Carmustine (BiCNU, BCNU) AVAILABLE: Vial—100 mg with 3 ml sterile diluent.	I.V.: 150–200 mg/m² q 6 weeks as a single dose, or 75–100 mg/m²/day on 2 successive days. TOPICAL (investigational): solution or ointment applied daily or b.i.d. × 6–8 weeks.	Primary and metastatic tumors of the central nervous system, Hodgkin's disease, non-Hodgkin's lymphomas, multiple myeloma, induction phase of acute myelocytic (granulocytic) leukemia, malignant melanoma, hepatocellular carcinoma. Mycosis fungoides.	**N, V** (severe), **M.*** Burning or pain at I.V. site. Flushing of skin and/or burning of eyes (with rapid infusion). Renal, hepatic failure (usually reversible), pulmonary fibrosis, ovarian, sperm suppression. With accidental contact of reconstituted solution with skin: hyperpigmentation.	Premedicate with antiemetic. Avoid contact with skin during preparation and administration. Administer in 150 ml D₅W over 1–2 hr. Decrease I.V. rate for severe pain, and observe site. Assess I.V. site for signs of irritation. Decrease rate of infusion and inform physician if client reports severe pain. Monitor creatinine, BUN, SGOT, SGPT, LDH, alkaline phosphatase, and bilirubin, and report elevations. Monitor creatinine clearance and report reduction. Monitor I & O. Stomatitis measures (see Table 10–4).

(Continued)

83

Table 3–2 Nitrosoureas (Continued)

May be classified as a subcategory of alkylating agents.
Act in same manner as alkylating agents.
Cross blood-brain barrier.

MEDICATION AND FORMS AVAILABLE	DOSAGE RANGE	INDICATIONS	TOXICITY	NURSING INTERVENTIONS
Lomustine (CeeNU, CCNU) AVAILABLE: Capsules—10, 40, 100 mg.	**P.O.** (adult or child): 130 mg/m² as a single dose q 6 weeks. (Lower dose [100 mg/m²] is indicated with compromised bone marrow function).	Primary and metastatic tumors of the central nervous system, Hodgkin's disease, multiple myeloma, malignant melanoma, gastric adenocarcinoma, colorectal adenocarcinoma, hepatocellular carcinoma, carcinoma of pancreas.	**M, N, V, A,** S.* Ovarian, sperm suppression, renal failure, alopecia, hepatotoxicity, nephrotoxicity, pulmonary toxicity. Neurological reactions (disorientation, lethargy, ataxia, dysarthria).	Premedicate with antiemetic. Regimen may include sedative and/or hypnotic to help client sleep through major side effects. Avoid food or beverage intake for 2 hr after medication is administered to avoid nausea. Stomatitis measures (see Table 10–4.) Monitor BUN, creatinine, SGOT, SGPT, LDH, alkaline phosphatase, and bilirubin, and report elevations. Monitor creatinine clearance and report reduction.

| Streptozocin (Zanosar)

AVAILABLE:
Vial—1 gm. | 1 gm/m^2 weekly for 4 weeks, or 500 mg/m^2 daily × 5 days q 6 weeks, or until maximum response or treatment-limiting toxicity is reached.
Maximum single dose—1500 mg/m^2. | Metastatic islet cell carcinoma of the pancreas. | **Renal toxicity, M, N, V,** D,* hepatotoxicity, abnormalities of glucose tolerance. | Assess urine output, BUN, creatinine. Assess for and report hyperglycemia, hypophosphatemia, increase in BUN, creatinine, decreased creatinine clearance, and proteinuria, as dose may require reduction. (Note: Proteinuria is one of the first signs of renal toxicity.) Monitor and report altered hepatic function (hypoalbuminemia, increased SGOT, LDH). |

*A = anorexia, D = diarrhea, M = myelosuppression, N = nausea, S = stomatitis, V = vomiting.

Table 3–3 Antimetabolites

Structurally similar to metabolites necessary for cell function and replication.
Cell cycle–specific to S phase.

MEDICATION AND FORMS AVAILABLE	DOSAGE RANGE	INDICATIONS	TOXICITY	NURSING INTERVENTIONS
Cladribine (Leustatin, 2-CDA) AVAILABLE: Vial—1 mg/ml.	**I.V.:** Hairy cell leukemia: 0.09 mg/kg/day for 7 days by continuous I.V. infusion.	Hairy cell leukemia.	Fever ≥100° F, myelosuppression, (particularly neutropenia, anemia), fatigue, nausea. Bacterial, viral, fungal infections. (NOTE: Infections severe in first month, mild–moderate in subsequent months of therapy.) Rash, malaise, V, A, D,* abnormal breath sounds, cough, myalgia, arthralgia, edema, tachycardia. (NOTE: From day 15 to the last follow-up visit, the only events reported by >5% of patients were fatigue, headache, rash, cough, and malaise.) **With high doses:** Irreversible paraparesis/quadraparesis, acute nephrotoxicity, severe myelosuppression.	Monitor temperature and complete blood counts and report alterations. Assess I.V. site for swelling, redness, or pain. Assess complete blood count, lung sounds, respirations, renal and neuro. status, and report abnormalities.

Drug	Use	Dose	Side Effects	Nursing Considerations
Cytarabine (Cytosar-U, Tarabine, Ara-C) AVAILABLE: Vial—100 mg, 500 mg, 1 gm, 2 gm (light yellow powder).	Acute myelocytic leukemia, acute lymphocytic leukemia, including prophylaxis or treatment of central nervous system metastases. Chronic myelocytic leukemia (blast phase), erythroleukemia. Hodgkin's disease, non-Hodgkin's lymphomas.	I.V.: REMISSION–INDUCTION: acute non-lymphocytic leukemias: 100 mg/m² daily by continuous infusion for 7 days, or 100 mg/m² q 12 hr for 7 days. High-dose: 3 gm/m² over 60 minutes q 12 hr × 12 doses. INTRATHECAL: 5–75 mg/m², frequency varies (see Tables 2–2 and 3–1).	**Myelosuppression, N, V, A, S, D.*** Hepatic dysfunction, anal inflammation, fever, rash. Thrombophlebitis or pain at I.V. site. Renal dysfunction (urinary retention), neuritis, pruritus, conjunctivitis, anaphylaxis, pulmonary toxicity. Peeling of skin may occur if administered with radiation therapy. Ara-C syndrome (fever, myalgia, bone pain, maculopapular rash, conjunctivitis, and malaise) occurring 6–12 hr after administration.	Administer antiemetics as ordered. Assess infusion site for burning, pain, and slow rate should this occur. Encourage P.O. fluid intake unless contraindicated. Stomatitis measures (see Table 10–4). Monitor hepatic, renal function, complete blood count. Monitor urinary output. See Chapter 5 for intrathecal and intracavitary administration. Note: Nausea and vomiting may be severe if cytarabine is administered in combination with methotrexate. Corticosteroids may be administered for prevention or treatment of Ara-C syndrome.
Floxuridine (FUDR) AVAILABLE: Vial—500 mg.	Gastrointestinal adenocarcinoma with metastases to liver, gallbladder, and/or bile ducts.	INTRAARTERIAL ONLY: 0.1–0.6 mg/kg daily. (0.4 mg/kg daily by continuous hepatic artery infusion (see Table 2–1).	Same as fluorouracil, plus abdominal cramps and pain, regional enteritis, duodenitis, gastritis, glossitis, fever, lethargy.	Administer via volumetric pump. Monitor complete blood count, hepatic function and report alterations. Report severe responses; dose may be reduced or temporarily discontinued. See information on pumps, ports, regional perfusion.

(Continued)

Table 3–3 Antimetabolites (Continued)

MEDICATION AND FORMS AVAILABLE	DOSAGE RANGE	INDICATIONS	TOXICITY	NURSING INTERVENTIONS
Fludarabine phosphate (Fludara) AVAILABLE: Vial—50 mg lyophilized powder.	**Adult:** Chronic lymphocytic leukemia (CLL): **I.V.:** 25 mg/m² daily for 5 days. Repeat every 28 days. Lymphoma: 15–40 mg/m² daily for 5 days every 28 days. (NOTE: The safety and effectiveness of fludarabine in children has not been established.)	B-cell chronic lymphocytic leukemia that is unresponsive to standard therapy or has progressed despite treatment. Non-Hodgkin's lymphoma (investigational).	**M, N,* fever,** chills, weakness, paresthesias, malaise, fatigue, myalgia, V, A, D, S,* edema, rash, pruritus, cough, dyspnea, gastrointestinal bleed, hyperglycemia, gonadal suppression, tumor lysis syndrome, agitation, confusion, visual disturbances, anaphylaxis, coma.	Assess complete blood count, assess for temperature elevation or other signs of infection. Avoid sources of infection. Assess for dyspnea or cough. (NOTE: Pulmonary toxicity may be treated with corticosteroid therapy; dose may be modified or withheld with severe hematological or neurotoxicity.)
5-Fluorouracil (Adrucil, 5-FU) AVAILABLE: Ampule—500 mg in 10 ml (faint yellow solution).	**I.V.:** INDUCTION: 12 mg/kg or 480 mg/m² daily for 4 days (maximum daily dose—800 mg): If no toxicity, administer 6 mg/kg (or 240 mg/m²) on days 6, 8, 10, and 12. MAINTENANCE: Repeat first course every 30 days or: administer 10–15 mg/kg/week as a single dose.	Carcinoma of colon, rectum, stomach, pancreas, breast, and ovary, hepatocellular carcinoma.	**M, N, V, D, S, A.* Alopecia, esophagopharyngitis,** dermatitis. Photosensitivity manifested by hyperpigmentation and/or erythema. Nail changes. Phlebitis, darkening of veins used for administration.	Stomatitis measures (see Table 10–4). Instruct client to avoid exposure to direct sunlight. Assess for maculopapular rash. Note: Rash more common on extremities, less frequently seen on trunk.

Topical forms (Efudex, Fluoroplex) AVAILABLE: Topical solution—Fluoroplex 1%, Efudex 2%, 5%. Cream—Fluoroplex 1%, Efudex 5%.	Apply sufficient medication to cover involved skin areas twice daily. Treatment period usually lasts 2–6 weeks.	Carcinoma of skin, actinic (solar) keratosis, superficial basal cell carcinoma.	Pain, pruritus, burning, inflammation, hyperpigmentation.	Instruct client/family to apply medication with a nonmetallic applicator or fingertips and wash hands carefully. Gloves must be worn during application. Instruct client to avoid prolonged exposure to sunlight or other forms of ultraviolet radiation during treatment.
Mercaptopurine (Purinethol, 6-MP) AVAILABLE: Tablets—50 mg.	**P.O.:** INDUCTION and CONSOLIDATION (adult or child): 2.5 mg/kg/day. MAINTENANCE (adult or child): 1.5–2.5 mg/kg once daily.	Acute leukemias (blast phase), chronic myelogenous leukemia.	M, hyperuricemia, S, N (occasional), V, A. Cholestatic jaundice, other hepatotoxicity (rare), immunosuppression.	Monitor urine, hepatic function. Administer allopurinol if ordered. Note: Dose of mercaptopurine must be reduced if administered with allopurinol. Stomatitis measures (see Table 10–4).

(Continued)

Table 3-3 Antimetabolites (Continued)

MEDICATION AND FORMS AVAILABLE	DOSAGE RANGE	INDICATIONS	TOXICITY	NURSING INTERVENTIONS
Methotrexate (Folex, Mexate, Mexate-AQ, MTX) AVAILABLE: Tablets—2.5 mg. Low sodium, preservative-free powder—20, 50, 100, 250 mg, 1 gm. Preservative-free liquid (25 mg/ml)—50, 100, 200, 250 mg, 1 gm. Preserved isotonic liquid (25 mg/ml)—2 ml. Tablets, yellow; powder and liquid amber.	**P.O., I.M., I.V.** intraarterial: Doses vary greatly with condition treated. (See prescribing information.) (NOTE: For high dose methotrexate see Box 19-4.) **INTRATHECAL:** 12 mg/m² or empirical dose of 15 mg q 2 to 5 days until CSF count returns to normal, followed by 1 additional dose.	Hodgkin's disease, lymphomas, acute lymphoblastic and myelocytic leukemias, choriocarcinoma, central nervous system metastases (prophylaxis or treatment). Carcinoma of ovary, lung, cervix, testicle, and breast. Lymphosarcoma, osteosarcoma, epidermoid carcinoma of head and neck. Advanced stages of mycosis fungoides. (NOTE: FDA approved for treatment of arthritis.)	Myelosuppression, **S, M, N, G.I. ulceration,** V, A, D.* alopecia. Taste alterations, blurred vision, transient paresis, dizziness, malaise. Fatigue, fever, infertility, azotemia, renal failure, pruritus, erythema, photosensitivity, hepatotoxicity, pneumonitis. (NOTE: Headaches and/or seizures may occur with intrathecal administration.)	Avoid skin contact or inhalation during preparation. Provide adequate hydration before and after administration. Monitor complete blood count. Stomatitis measures (see Table 10-4). Instruct patient to avoid exposure to sunlight. For high-dose methotrexate (greater than 250 mg/m² I.V.): Maintain alkaline urine (pH 6.8 or higher). Monitor renal function, I & O. Administer calcium leucovorin "rescue" as ordered by physician within 12-24 hr after methotrexate. For intrathecal administration, see Table 2-1.

Pentostatin (Deoxycoformycin, Nipent) AVAILABLE: Vial—10 mg.	I.V.: Hairy cell leukemia: 4 mg/m² every week or every other week or 4 mg/m² weekly for 3 consecutive weeks, alternating with α interferon 3,000,000 U S.C. daily × 4 weeks. Repeat entire cycle 7 times over 14 months.	Hairy cell leukemia refractory to α interferon therapy. Chronic lymphocytic leukemia, mycosis fungoides, adult T-cell lymphoma.	**M, N, V,* rash, fatigue, fever,** chills, D,* cough, upper respiratory infection, conjunctivitis, tachycardia, headache, hypersensitivity reaction, hepatotoxicity, renal toxicity, headache, paresthesias, lethargy, somnolence, anxiety, confusion, depression.	Hydrate patient before administration with 500–1,000 ml 5% dextrose in 0.45% normal saline as ordered. Monitor neurological status, vital signs. Administer 500 ml 5% dextrose in 0.45% normal saline after administration as ordered. Monitor complete blood count, renal and hepatic function, and report alterations. Administer allopurinol if ordered to prevent hyperuricemia secondary to tumor lysis.
Thioguanine (Lanvis, 6-TG) AVAILABLE: Tablets—40 mg.	P.O.: 2 mg/kg daily. May increase cautiously to 3 mg/kg daily after 4 weeks.	Acute myelocytic (granulocytic) leukemia, chronic granulocytic leukemia.	**M,** hyperuricemia, N (occasional), V, A, D, S,* hepatotoxicity.	Provide adequate hydration. Stomatitis measures (see Table 10–4). Monitor hepatic function (SGOT, SGPT, alkaline phosphatase) and report elevations.

*A = anorexia, D = diarrhea, M = myelosuppression, N = nausea, S = stomatitis, V = vomiting.

Table 3–4 Mitotic Inhibitors

Bind to substances necessary for formation of mitotic spindle, preventing cell division.
Vincristine, vinblastine, and vindesine are cell cycle–specific to M phase (some action in late G_2 phase).
Teniposide and etoposide are cell cycle–specific to G_2 phase and block DNA production.

MEDICATION AND FORMS AVAILABLE	DOSAGE RANGE	INDICATIONS	TOXICITY	NURSING INTERVENTIONS
Etoposide (VePesid, VP-16-213) AVAILABLE: Vial—100 mg in 5 ml; 150 mg in 7.5 ml (clear yellow solution). Capsule—50 mg.	**I.V.:** Carcinoma of lung: 35 mg/m² × 4 days to 50 mg/m² × 5 days q 3–4 weeks. Testicular carcinoma: 50–100 mg/m² days 1 through 5 or 100 mg/m² on days 1, 3, and 5 q 3–4 weeks. **P.O.:** Carcinoma of lung: Administer 2× the I.V. dose, rounded to the nearest 50 mg.	Refractory testicular tumors, small cell (oat cell) carcinoma of lung, carcinoma of breast, Hodgkin's disease, non-Hodgkin's lymphomas.	**M, N, V**, A, S, D*†. **Alopecia, hyperuricemia.** Orthostatic hypotension (with rapid I.V. administration). Paresthesias. Anaphylaxis (rare), aftertaste, fever, rash, pruritus, constipation, abdominal pain, dysphagia. Hepatotoxicity, metabolic acidosis (with higher doses).	Administer antiemetic as ordered prior to therapy. Administer I.V. dose by drip over 30–60 min. Instruct client to move slowly and gradually when arising to sitting or standing position. Stomatitis measures (see Table 10–4). Assess for signs of anaphylaxis (wheezing, bronchospasm, hypotension, tachycardia). Have emergency medications (adrenaline, epinephrine 1:1000, Benadryl) and oxygen on hand. Note: Capsules are to be stored under refrigeration at 2–8°C. (36–46°F.).

| Paclitaxel (Taxol)

AVAILABLE:
Ampule—6 mg/ml in 5 ml ampule | I.V.:
135 mg/m^2 administered over 24 hr q 3 weeks. | Metastatic carcinoma of ovary, after failure of first-line chemotherapy. | **Myelosuppression, N, V, D, S, M,* alopecia. Hypersensitivity reactions (HSR). Mild HSR: flushing, skin rash, urticaria, pruritus, diaphoresis, tachycardia.** Severe HSR: hypotension requiring treatment, tachycardia, dyspnea or bronchospasm requiring bronchodilators, angioedema, or generalized urticaria.
NOTE: Allergic response more common during first or second course of treatment, and may occur as early as 1–3 min after beginning taxol, or as late as 12 hr after completing taxol treatment. (NOTE: Alopecia may include loss of eyebrows, eyelashes, pubic and axillary hair). Taste alterations. Local erythema, swelling, and discomfort, along the course of injected vein. | Administer as a continuous infusion over 6–24 hr. Preceded by prophylactic antiallergic regimen: dexamethasone 20 mg P.O. or I.V. 12 and 6 hr before administration; diphenhydramine 50 mg I.V. 30–60 min prior to administration; and cimetidine 300 mg or ranitidine (50 mg) 30–60 min before taxol. Obtain baseline V/S and EKG before initiating infusion. Assess respiratory and neurologic status. EKG. Monitor V/S q 15 min during first hour, hourly for three additional hours, then q 4 hr. Monitor for and report neutropenia, as this may require dose alteration. |

(Continued)

Table 3–4 Mitotic Inhibitors (Continued)

MEDICATION AND FORMS AVAILABLE	DOSAGE RANGE	INDICATIONS	TOXICITY	NURSING INTERVENTIONS
			Fatigue, headache, elevation of hepatic and renal function tests, serum triglyceride level. Pain or burning, especially in the feet, sensory loss, paresthesias, loss of deep tendon reflexes (DTRs). NOTE: neuropathic symptoms more common in patients with history of prior alcohol use. Transient myalgias and arthralgias. Bradycardia. Ventricular tachycardia (rare).	
Teniposide (VM-26, Vumon) AVAILABLE: Ampule—50 mg in 5 ml.	**I.V.:** Acute lymphocytic leukemia: Combination: 165 mg/m^2 in solution twice weekly. Neuroblastoma (single agent): 130–180 mg/m^2 in solution once weekly. Combination: 100 mg/m^2 in solution every 21	Acute lymphocytic leukemia. Neuroblastoma, non-Hodgkin's lymphoma (second-line therapy in combination).	**M, Alopecia,** N, V, D, A, S.* Phlebitis may occur if medication is not adequately diluted. Fever, hepatotoxicity (mild), hypotension may occur with rapid administration. VESICANT—Local tissue damage may occur with extravasation.	Administer antiemetic as ordered prior to therapy. Administer at a concentration of 0.2 mg/ml in 0.9% sodium chloride for injection or 5% dextrose in water over 30–60 min. Assess I.V. for patency prior to administration. Assess site fre-

days. Non-Hodgkin's lymphoma: single agent: 30 mg/m^2 in solution daily × 5–10 days, or 50–100 mg/m^2 in solution once weekly. Combination: 60–70 mg/m^2 in solution once weekly.

Cardiotoxicity, renal toxicity, anaphylaxis (rare).

quently during administration. Monitor I.V. rate (if too fast client may develop postural hypotension). Assess for hypersensitivity (fever, rash, wheezing, hypotension, tachycardia). Have emergency medications (Benadryl, adrenaline, epinephrine 1:1000) and oxygen on hand.

Vinblastine (Velban, Velbe, Velsar, VLB)

AVAILABLE:
Vial—10 mg.

I.V., P.O.:
Adult:
3.7–11.1 mg/m^2 (start at low dose, increase with each successive dose, at least 7 days apart). Maximum single dose 18.5 mg/m^2.
Child:
2.5–7.5 mg/m^2 (scheduling as above). Maximum single dose 12.5 mg/m^2. May be administered as a continuous infusion over 24 hr.

Hodgkin's disease (Stages III, IV), lymphocytic and histiocytic lymphomas. Mycosis fungoides (advanced stages), advanced carcinoma of testis. Carcinoma of breast and choriocarcinoma that are unresponsive to other therapies. Squamous cell carcinoma of the head and neck, Kaposi's sarcoma.

M,* alopecia, jaw pain, bone pain, pain at tumor site, malaise, hypertension, constipation. N, V, S, A, D, rectal bleeding. Constipation may cause abdominal cramps or lead to paralytic ileus. Ovarian and sperm suppression, numbness, paresthesias, peripheral neuritis, loss of DTRs, headache, mental depression, seizures. Anaphylaxis and bronchospasm (rare).
(NOTE: Toxicity may be enhanced in the presence of hepatic insufficiency.)
VESICANT—Local tissue damage may occur with extravasation.

Administer antiemetic as ordered. Flush with normal saline before and after administration. Assess for neurotoxicity: loss of DTRs or hand grasps, paresthesias, peripheral neuropathy, headache, malaise, and jaw pain. Assess stool and auscultate abdomen for bowel sounds. Monitor mental status. Assess respiration, lung sounds, vital signs for signs of bronchospasm. (NOTE: This is a rare occurrence and may be more likely to occur when vinblastine is administered with mitomycin.)

(Continued)

95

Table 3-4 Mitotic Inhibitors (Continued)

MEDICATION AND FORMS AVAILABLE	DOSAGE RANGE	INDICATIONS	TOXICITY	NURSING INTERVENTIONS
Vincristine (Oncovin, Vincasar PFS, VCR) AVAILABLE: Vial—1 mg, 2 mg, 5 mg (1 mg/ml). Oncovin also available in Prefilled Syringes, 1 mg in 1 ml, 2 mg in 2 ml.	I.V.: Adult: 1.4 mg/m² weekly. Child: 2.0 mg/m² weekly.	Acute lymphocytic leukemia, Hodgkin's disease, non-Hodgkin's lymphomas, neuroblastoma, Wilms' tumor, small-cell (oat cell) carcinoma of lung, carcinoma of breast, uterine cervix, colorectal carcinoma, acute granulocytic leukemia, chronic granulocytic leukemia (blast phase). Ewing's sarcoma, osteogenic sarcoma, medulloblastoma, systemic mycosis fungoides, multiple myeloma, malignant melanoma, lymphosarcoma, rhabdomyosarcoma, Kaposi's sarcoma.	**Alopecia, peripheral neuropathy (paresthesias, neuritic pain, loss of deep tendon reflexes),** muscle wasting. N, V, A, S, D.*† **Constipation**—may lead to paralytic ileus, especially in young child. Mild myelosuppression, ovarian and sperm suppression, SIADH. May have rise in serum uric acid level with treatment for acute leukemia. Bone pain (may be severe), abdominal pain. Anaphylaxis (rare). VESICANT—Local tissue damage can occur with extravasation. (NOTE: Toxicity may be enhanced in the presence of hepatic insufficiency.)	For direct I.V. or via Y-site of freely flowing I.V.: Administer over 1 min. Avoid extravasation. Observe for and report paresthesias, muscle weakness, alterations in deep tendon reflexes, foot drop, and difficulty walking. Assess stool. Administer cathartic, stool softener and/or bulk laxative as ordered. Assess fluid and electrolyte balance: intake, output, blood, and urine sodium.

| Vindesine (Eldisine) (Investigational in U.S.—commercially available in Canada) AVAILABLE: Vial—5 mg lyophilized powder (with mannitol, 25 mg). | I.V.: Adult: 3 mg/m² q 7–10 days for 8 cycles. Child: 4 mg/m² q 7–10 days for 8 cycles or 2 mg/m²/day on 2 consecutive days followed by 5–7 days without the medication for 8 cycles. | Acute lymphocytic leukemia (child), blast crisis of acute myelocytic leukemia, non–small cell carcinoma of lung, carcinoma of breast, esophagus, non-Hodgkin's lymphomas. | **M*, alopecia, peripheral neuropathy, numbness, tingling, loss of deep tendon reflexes,** N, V, A, D†, S. Jaw pain, mental depression, constipation (may lead to paralytic ileus) abdominal pain, SIADH (see Table 12–6). Generalized musculoskeletal pain, chills, fever, malaise, macular rash, pain at tumor site. VESICANT—Local tissue damage may occur with extravasation. | Administer antiemetic as ordered. Check vein patency before and during administration. Should extravasation occur: Discontinue medication. Apply heat and hyaluronidase to site. Elevate site above level of heart. Assess site for pain, swelling. (See extravasation measures, Chapter 2.) Administer stool softeners and/or cathartics as ordered. Assess peripheral neurological status and report alterations. Stomatitis measures (see Table 10–4). Assess fluid and electrolyte status and report alterations. |

*A = anorexia, D = diarrhea, M = myelosuppression, N = nausea, S = stomatitis, V = vomiting.
†Note: Diarrhea may be a sign of intestinal obstruction.

Table 3–5 Antitumor Antibiotics

Bind with DNA to inhibit synthesis of DNA and RNA. Cell cycle–nonspecific.

MEDICATION AND FORMS AVAILABLE	DOSAGE RANGE	INDICATIONS	TOXICITY	NURSING INTERVENTIONS
Bleomycin (Blenoxane) AVAILABLE: Vial—15 U.	**S.C., I.M., I.V.:** Hodgkin's disease (INDUCTION), lymphosarcoma, reticulum-cell sarcoma, squamous cell carcinoma or carcinoma of the testes: 0.25–0.5 U/kg weekly or biweekly. Hodgkin's disease (MAINTENANCE): 1 U daily or 5 U weekly. (NOTE: Cumulative lifetime dose not to exceed 400 U.)	Hodgkin's disease, lymphomas, lymphosarcoma, carcinoma of the testes (embryonal cell, choriocarcinoma, teratocarcinoma). Squamous cell carcinoma of the head and neck (mouth, tongue, buccal mucosa, gingiva, larynx), cervix, vulva, and penis. Carcinoma of the lung with pleural infiltration, malignant melanoma, reticulum cell sarcoma.	**Hyperpigmentation, erythema, rash, striae, vesiculation, photosensitivity, alopecia, M, N, V, A, S,** * myelosuppression (rare). Fever, chills. Pulmonary toxicities (pneumonitis, pulmonary fibrosis). Nailbed changes, desquamation of hands and soles of feet. Renal, hepatic toxicities, pain at tumor site. Hypersensitivity reaction (HSR) (rare).	Administer test dose (usually 1–2 U) I.M. as ordered. Assess client for HSR (fever >101F°, chills, wheezing, hypotension, mental confusion). Have emergency medications available (see Table 13–9). (Note: Acetaminophen may be administered to avert fever). Provide adequate hydration with hyperpyrexia. Assess pulmonary function and report alterations (see Chapter 13). Stomatitis Measures (Table 10–4). Monitor renal, hepatic function. Monitor creatinine clearance and report decrease. Dose may need to be decreased with inadequate creatinine clearance. (NOTE: Anaphylaxis is more common in clients being treated for lymphoma.)

Dactinomycin (Cosmegen, Actinomycin-D, ACT-D)

AVAILABLE:
Vial—500 mcg (0.5 mg) with 20 mg mannitol (yellow lyophilized powder).

I.V.
Adult:
500 μg (0.5 mg) daily for a maximum of 5 days.
Child:
15 μg (0.015 mg) per kg daily for 5 days, or 2500 μg (2.5 mg) over a 1 week period.
Adult and Child: A second course may be given after at least 3 weeks provided all signs of toxicity have disappeared.
Reduce dosage if radiation therapy has been administered.
REGIONAL PERFUSION:
Upper extremity: 35 μg (0.035 mg) per kg. Lower extremity or pelvis: 50 μg (0.05 mg) per kg.

Wilms' tumor, testicular carcinoma, metastatic choriocarcinoma, Ewing's sarcoma, rhabdomyosarcoma, sarcoma botryoides, metastatic nonseminomatous testicular carcinoma.

M, N, V, D, A, S,* Alopecia, erythema, pharyngitis, esophagitis, hyperpigmentation of previously irradiated skin areas (radiation recall) may occur. Hypocalcemia, rash, acne, malaise, fatigue, myalgia, ovarian and sperm suppression.
VESICANT—Local tissue damage may occur with extravasation.
With regional perfusion, may have edema, venous thrombosis of involved extremity.

Administer antiemetic prior to medication. May be administered by slow I.V. push or into Y-site of a freely flowing I.V. Administer with no filter or below in-line filter. Assess I.V. site for burning or other sign of extravasation. Assess renal function, blood count. Stomatitis measures (see Table 10–4). With regional perfusion, assess extremity for circulatory alterations or edema.

(Continued)

99

Table 3–5 Antitumor Antibiotics (Continued)

MEDICATION AND FORMS AVAILABLE	DOSAGE RANGE	INDICATIONS	TOXICITY	NURSING INTERVENTIONS
Daunorubicin hydrochloride (Cerubidine, Daunomycin, DNR) AVAILABLE: Vial—20 mg with 100 mg mannitol (red powder).	IV: Adult: In combination with cytarabine for nonlymphocytic leukemias: 45 mg/m²/day on days 1, 2, and 3 of the first course, and days 1 and 2 of subsequent courses.† Acute lymphocytic leukemia. Child, age 2 years and above: 25 mg/m² on day 1 of each week in combination with vincristine and prednisone. May repeat dose ×2 if necessary to obtain complete remission. Under age 2 years, or <0.5 m² BSA: administer 1.0 mg/kg. Maximum lifetime dose: Adult: 550 mg/m². Child over age 2 years: 300 mg/m². Child under age 2 years: 10 mg/kg.	Remission induction in acute nonlymphocytic leukemia in adults, acute lymphocytic leukemia in child or adult.	**M, N, V,** (mild) D, S.* Mucositis, **alopecia,** cardiotoxicity, radiation recall, hyperuricemia, fever, chills, rash. Ovarian and sperm suppression. Hypersensitivity reaction (HSR) (rare).	Obtain baseline EKG. Administer antiemetic as ordered. Administer via I.V. sidearm into rapidly flowing I.V. Assess I.V. site for burning or other signs of extravasation. Monitor hepatic, renal laboratory values. Inform client that urine will be red-orange in color. Stomatitis measures (see Table 10–4).

Doxorubicin (Adriamycin PFS, Adriamycin RDF, Rubex, ADR)

AVAILABLE:
Vial—10 mg, 20 mg, 50 mg, 150 mg (red powder if RDF or red solution if PFS). Adriamycin PFS also available in 200 mg multidose vial.

I.V.:
Adult:
60–75 mg/m² q 3 weeks or 20 mg/m² once weekly or 30 mg/m² daily × 3 days q 4 weeks.
Maximum lifetime dose 550 mg/m². Reduce to 400 mg/m² for persons who have received cyclophosphamide or radiation therapy to the mediastinum.
Child:
30 m²/m² × 3 days every 4 weeks.
INTRAVESICAL (bladder): 30–60 mg/m² in sterile distilled water (1 mg/ml).

Hodgkin's disease, non-Hodgkin's lymphomas, acute lymphoblastic leukemia, acute myeloblastic leukemia, carcinoma of ovary, thyroid, breast, stomach, prostate, endometrium. Small-cell (oat cell) carcinoma of the lung. Wilms' tumor, hepatocellular carcinoma, multiple myeloma, neuroblastoma, squamous cell carcinoma of head and neck, transitional cell carcinoma of bladder, germ cell tumors, mesothelioma, renal cell carcinoma, rhabdomyosarcoma, osteosarcoma, mycosis fungoides. Papillary cell carcinoma of the bladder.

Alopecia, S, N, V, M,* mucositis, A, D,* esophagitis, phlebosclerosis, especially when small veins are used, erythematous streaking along vein of administration. VESICANT—Local tissue damage may occur with extravasation. Facial flushing if administered too rapidly. Radiation recall, cardiac arrhythmias. CHF may occur with prolonged administration. Photosensitivity. Hyperpigmentation of nailbeds and dermal creases (especially in children), hyperuricemia. Hypersensitivity reaction (HSR) including fever, chills, urticaria, flu-like syndrome, HSR, hepatotoxicity. Ulceration and necrosis of the colon, especially the cecum. Conjunctivitis and lacrimation (rare), anaphylaxis (rare).
Dysuria, urgency, abdominal discomfort. N, V.*

Administer via Y-site of freely flowing I.V. over 3–5 min. A large vein is the preferred administration site. Check for blood return frequently. Assess I.V. site. Inform client that urine will be red-orange for 2–3 days after therapy. Monitor cardiac rhythm, EKG, and report irregularities. Monitor serum bilirubin and report elevation above 1.2 mg/dl as dose may require reduction. Instruct client to avoid exposure to sunlight during course of therapy. Stomatitis measures (see Table 10–4).

(Continued)

Table 3–5 Antitumor Antibiotics *(Continued)*

MEDICATION AND FORMS AVAILABLE	DOSAGE RANGE	INDICATIONS	TOXICITY	NURSING INTERVENTIONS
Epirubicin hydrochloride (Pharmorubicin RDF) AVAILABLE: Vial—10 mg, 20 mg, 50 mg (red-orange lyophilized powder).	I.V.: 75–90 mg/m^2 q 3 weeks (may be divided over 2 days) or 12.5–25 mg/m^2 weekly.	Metastatic carcinoma of lung, breast, ovary, stomach, acute leukemias, Hodgkin's disease, lymphomas.	**M, N, V**, S, D,* **alopecia** (partial or complete), radiation recall, urticaria and streaking along vein, phlebitis, fever, headache, cardiotoxicity. VESICANT—Local tissue damage may occur with extravasation. (NOTE: Toxicity may be enhanced by hepatic impairment.)	Administer antiemetic as ordered. Assess liver function studies. Dose may be altered with increase in values. Stomatitis measures (see Table 10–4). See guidelines for safe preparation and handling (Chapter 2). Assess I.V. site for pain. If it occurs or if blood return is poor, stop I.V. and restart at another site.

Idarubicin (Idamycin)	I.V.: Acute myeloid leukemia (adults): INDUCTION: 12 mg/m² daily for 3 days, in combination with Ara-C.	Acute myeloid leukemia (adults).	**M, N, V, D, S,* alopecia, mucositis, abdominal cramps,** urticaria, rash, local reaction at injection site, fever, headache, peripheral neuropathy, congestive heart failure, arrhythmias, chest pain, myocardial infarction. (NOTE: Cardiac symptoms more common in persons over age 60 or those with pre-existing cardiac disease). VESICANT—local tissue damage may occur with extravasation.	Administer antiemetics as ordered. Administer over 10–15 minutes into tubing of freely flowing I.V., preferably into a large vein. Check for blood return and assess I.V. site frequently. Inform client that urine may be red-orange for up to 3 days after therapy. Assess vital signs, cardiac, rhythm, EKG, and report abnormalities. Assess complete blood count, AST, ALT, serum bilirubin, BUN, creatinine, uric acid, and report abnormalities. Stomatitis measures (Table 10–4).
AVAILABLE: Vial—5 mg, 10 mg (orange-red lyophilized powder).				
Mitomycin (Mutamycin, Mitomycin-C)	I.V.: 15–20 mg/m² q 6–8 weeks. INTRAVESICAL (bladder): 20–60 mg in sterile distilled water (1 mg/ml) t.i.w.	Adenocarcinoma of pancreas, colon, stomach. Carcinoma of breast, bladder, lung, malignant melanoma, esophageal carcinoma and other carcinomas of the head and neck.	**M, alopecia, S, A,** N, V, D.* Malaise, fever, chills, headache, drowsiness, blurred vision. Pulmonary, renal toxicity. HUS (hemolytic uremic syndrome). VESICANT—Local tissue damage may occur with extravasation.	Administer antiemetic as ordered. Administer into Y-site of freely flowing I.V. Avoid extravasation. Monitor BUN, urine output, and creatinine clearance. Inform physician if serum creatinine is elevated as dose may be withheld. Assess for signs of pulmonary dysfunction (dyspnea, nonproductive cough). Stomatitis measures (see Table 10–4).
AVAILABLE: Vial—5 mg, 20 mg, 40 mg with mannitol (10 mg in 5 mg vial, 40 mg in 20 mg vial, 80 mg in 40 mg vial).				

(Continued)

103

Table 3–5 Antitumor Antibiotics (Continued)

MEDICATION AND FORMS AVAILABLE	DOSAGE RANGE	INDICATIONS	TOXICITY	NURSING INTERVENTIONS
Mitoxantrone hydrochloride (Novantrone) AVAILABLE: Vial (2 mg/ml)—20 mg, 25 mg, 30 mg (dark blue concentrate for injection).	I.V.: 10–14 mg/m^2 q 3 weeks. Decrease dose to 10–12 mg/m^2 when used in combination with other antineoplastic agents. INDUCTION: 12 mg/m^2 days 1–3. May repeat course in event of incomplete antileukemic response. CONSOLIDATION: 12 mg/m^2 days 1 and 2 beginning approximately 6 weeks after final induction. Administer second course approximately 4 weeks after first course.	Carcinoma of breast, acute nonlymphocytic leukemia in adults (initial treatment), lymphomas.	M, N, V, D, S, fever, alopecia, hyperuricemia, blue-green urine. Bluish discoloration may occur along vein. Phlebitis near infusion site, abdominal pain, hepatic, renal, pulmonary toxicities, headache, conjunctivitis. Cardiac arrhythmias may occur in client who has received anthracyclines. Allergic reaction (hypotension, urticaria, dyspnea, rash) may occur.	Alert client and family of possible discoloration or phlebitis along vein. Assess cardiac status and report alterations if client has received daunorubicin, doxorubicin, epirubicin, or idarubicin prior to mitoxantrone administration. Monitor vital signs, AST, ALT, BUN, creatinine, uric acid and report alterations.

| Plicamycin (Mithracin)

AVAILABLE:
Vial—2.5 mg (2500 mcg) with 100 mg mannitol (yellow powder). | I.V.:
Testicular tumors: 25–35 mcg/kg for 8–10 days. May repeat course of therapy at monthly intervals. For hypercalcemia/hypercalciuria: 25 mcg/kg × 3–4 days. | Testicular tumors, hypercalcemia, hypercalciuria. | N, V, D, A, S, M,* hypocalcemia, hypokalemia, hypophosphatemia. (NOTE: Severe thrombocytopenia and hypocalcemia may result in prolonged clotting time and hemorrhage.) Rash, facial flush, phlebitis, hepatic, renal toxicity, headache, lethargy, depression. VESICANT—Local tissue damage may occur with extravasation. | Contraindicated for client with: Impaired bone marrow function. Thrombocytopenia. Susceptibility to bleeding from other causes. Administer antiemetic as ordered. Administer in 500 ml D$_5$W or normal saline over 1 to 2 hr or 4 to 6 hr. Monitor prothrombin time, clotting time, platelets, PTT, and blood electrolytes AST, ALT, LDH, alkaline phosphatase, serum bilirubin, BUN, creatinine, proteinuria, or increased retention of BSP dye and report alterations. (NOTE: Bleeding problems may begin with an episode of epistaxis and/or hematemesis.) Assess for signs of hypocalcemia (muscle cramping or weakness, tingling of extremities). Stomatitis measures (see Table 10–4). |

*A = anorexia, D = diarrhea, M = myelosuppression, N = nausea, S = stomatitis, V = vomiting, BSA = body surface area.
†For persons over age 60, dose may be reduced to 30 mg/m².

Table 3–6 Miscellaneous Antineoplastic Agents

MEDICATION AND FORMS AVAILABLE	DOSAGE RANGE	INDICATIONS	TOXICITY	NURSING INTERVENTIONS
Altretamine (Hexalen), formerly known as hexamethylmelamine AVAILABLE: Capsules—50 mg.	Palliative treatment of ovarian cancer following first-line therapy with cisplatin and/or alkylating agent-based combination: 260 mg/m² /day in 4 divided doses administered P.C. and H.S. for 14 or 21 days of each 28-day cycle, in four divided doses.	Persistent or recurrent ovarian cancer that is nonresponsive to first-line agents.	**Myelosuppression, N, V, A,** * **peripheral neuropathy,** fatigue, skin rash, central nervous system symptoms (mood disorders, agitation, confusion, ataxia, dizziness, vertigo, seizures, Parkinsonian-like symptoms). May cause severe orthostatic hypotension when administered with antidepressants of the monamine oxidase (MAO) inhibitor class. Carcinogenic at high doses.	Administer antiemetics as ordered. Monitor complete blood count, granulocytes. Drug may be temporarily discontinued and restarted at 200 mg/m² if leukocyte count <2,000 mg/mm³, granulocytes <1,000 mg/mm³, or platelets <75,000/mm³. Assess for evidence of infection or bleeding. Instruct patient to report tingling or numbness in extremities promptly. Administer pyridoxine as ordered to ameliorate symptoms of peripheral neuropathy.

Drug	Use	Dose	Indications	Side Effects	Nursing Implications
Aminoglutethimide (Cytadren) AVAILABLE: Tablets—250 mg.	**P.O.:** Adults: 250 mg four times a day (preferably at 6-hr intervals). May increase in increments of 250 mg daily at intervals of 1–2 weeks to a total daily dose of 2 gm.	Adrenal carcinoma, metastatic carcinoma breast.	**Lethargy, somnolence,** maculopapular rash, N, V,* dizziness, ataxia, fever, hyponatremia, hyperkalemia. May cause orthostatic hypotension, adrenal insufficiency, hypothyroidism. Headache and hepatotoxicity (both rare).	Most clients require glucocorticoid replacement therapy. Teach client importance of taking replacement therapy regularly. Note: Dexamethasone cannot be used as replacement since aminoglutethimide accelerates metabolism of dexamethasone. Replacement of choice is hydrocortisone. Monitor blood pressure, serum electrolytes, assess for and report edema or other side effects.
Amsacrine (AMSA-PD, M-AMSA) AVAILABLE: Ampule—75 mg with vial of L-lactic acid diluent.	**I.V.:** **Acute Leukemias:** 75–125 mg/m² daily × 5 days.	Remission-induction in acute adult leukemia refractory to conventional therapy.	M, N, V, S, D,* mucositis, dysphagia, abdominal pain, pain and local phlebitis at infusion site if not adequately diluted, hepatotoxicity, alopecia, cardiac irregularities when administered with low serum K⁺. Local tissue damage may occur with extravasation (rare). Discoloration of urine (orange) and/or skin (yellow) may occur. Pruritus, rash, urticaria, fever, headache, dizziness, confusion, seizures.	Administer in 500 ml D,W over 60–90 min or longer. Administer antiemetic as ordered. Assess serum K⁺ prior to administration. Dose may be reduced or delayed if hypokalemia is present. Assess liver function studies, report alterations to physician. Monitor temperature for elevation during infusion. Stomatitis measures (see Table 10–4).

(Continued)

Table 3–6 Miscellaneous Antineoplastic Agents (Continued)

MEDICATION AND FORMS AVAILABLE	DOSAGE RANGE	INDICATIONS	TOXICITY	NURSING INTERVENTIONS
L-Asparaginase (*E. coli* strain) (Elspar, Kidrolase, L-ASP) AVAILABLE: Vial—10,000 I.U. with 80 mg mannitol.	**I.V., I.M.:** INDUCTION: 200 IU/kg daily × 28 days, or 1000 IU/kg daily for 10 days, beginning on day 22 of the treatment period, or 6000 IU/m² I.M. on days 4, 7, 10, 13, 16, 19, and 22 of the treatment period.	Acute lymphocytic leukemia. Remission-induction, chronic lymphocytic leukemia. Lymphosarcoma, reticulosarcoma, Hodgkin's disease.	N, V (severe),* hepatotoxicity, hyperglycemia, pancreatitis, depressed fibrinogen and clotting factors, azotemia, renal failure. Somnolence, personality alterations, hallucinations, depression, lethargy, confusion, fever, anaphylaxis. Toxicity may be increased when administered with or immediately prior to vincristine and prednisone.	Prior to administration: Administer acetaminophen 1/2 to 1 hr before infusion if ordered, obtain baseline temperature, assist with intradermal skin test if indicated. Administer via sideport of freely flowing I.V. over 30–45 min. May be administered via 5 µ filter. *Do not administer* through 0.2 µ filter. During infusion, assess for temperature elevation, signs of anaphylaxis (wheezing, arthralgia, restlessness, tachycardia, hypotension, dyspnea, facial flushing, hives). Have emergency medications (Benadryl, adrenalin, epinephrine 1:1000, hydrocortisone) on hand. If administered I.M., have KVO I.V. running should administration of emergency I.V. medications be required. Monitor hepatic function tests.

Estramustine phosphate (Emcyt)	**P.O.:** 14 mg/kg daily (one 140 mg capsule for each 10 lb or 22 kg of body weight), administered in 3 or 4 divided doses.	Metastatic and/or progressive carcinoma of prostate.	Breast tenderness, sodium and fluid retention, gynecomastia, hepatotoxicity, A, N, D, V, M.* Thrombophlebitis, dyspnea, leg cramps, lethargy, insomnia, headache, hypertension.	Prepare client for alterations and tenderness of breast. Administer at least 1 hr before or 2 hr after meals. Instruct patient to swallow capsules with a glass of water and avoid milk products, calcium-rich foods, or medications containing calcium (e.g.: some antacids), as this may impair absorption of estramustine. Instruct client not to cross legs. Assess circulation, assess for dyspnea, edema, thrombophlebitis. Monitor blood sodium level and blood pressure.
AVAILABLE: Capsules—140 mg.				
Hydroxyurea (Hydrea)	**P.O. (for CML):** 20–30 mg/kg/day as continuous therapy. For solid tumors: 80 mg/kg as a single dose every third day, or 20–30 mg/kg/day.	Resistant chronic myelocytic leukemia, malignant melanoma, inoperable carcinoma of ovary, squamous cell carcinoma of head and neck (excluding the lip).	M, N, V, A, S,* constipation or diarrhea, renal impairment, dysuria, maculopapular rash, facial erythema, fever, chills, malaise. Alopecia (rare).	Administer as 1 dose to maintain adequate blood levels of medication. Stomatitis measures (see Table 10–4). *If client is unable to swallow capsule:* Open and empty capsule into a glass of water, stir, and have client swallow immediately. Monitor I & O, BUN, creatinine, uric acid. Encourage P.O. fluid intake. Administer allopurinol if ordered.
AVAILABLE: Capsule—500 mg.				

(Continued)

109

Table 3–6 Miscellaneous Antineoplastic Agents (Continued)

MEDICATION AND FORMS AVAILABLE	DOSAGE RANGE	INDICATIONS	TOXICITY	NURSING INTERVENTIONS
Mitotane (Lysodren) AVAILABLE: Tablets—500 mg.	**P.O.:** Start at 2–6 gm daily, increase to 10 gm/day administered in 3 or 4 divided doses. If not tolerated, reduce dose and gradually increase until maximal tolerated dose is achieved.	Inoperable carcinoma of the adrenal cortex.	**N, V, A, D,* lethargy, somnolence, dizziness, vertigo,** rash, visual blurring, diplopia, retinopathy, hematuria, hemorragic cystitis, albuminuria, hypertension, orthostatic hypotension, flushing.	Assess client and report side effects. Physician may wish to reduce dose or temporarily discontinue therapy if side effects become severe. May require corticosteroid replacement therapy with severe adrenocortical insufficiency.

| Procarbazine (Matulane, Natulan)

AVAILABLE:
Capsules—50 mg. | P.O. (adult):
First week:
2–4 mg/kg/day to the nearest 50 mg. Then:
4–6 mg/kg/day to the nearest 50 mg until leukocyte count is below 4000/mm³ or platelets below 100,000/mm³, or until maximum response is obtained.
Maintenance:
1–2 mg/kg/day. In combination (e.g.: MOPP regimen): 100 mg/m²/day × 14 days. Child—Dose highly individualized and rarely used. 50 mg/m²/day × 1 week then 100 mg/m²/day until maximum clinical response obtained or leukopenia or thrombocytopenia occur. | Hodgkin's disease, non–small cell carcinoma of lung, primary neoplasms of the brain, malignant melanoma, multiple myeloma. | **N, V, M, D,** A, S.* Myalgia, arthralgia, chills, fever, dry mouth, constipation, fatigue, lethargy, drowsiness, alopecia, dermatitis, pruritus, hyperpigmentation, neuropathies, paresthesias, headache, dizziness, apprehension, depression, confusion, facial flushing. May potentiate action of narcotics, sedatives, tranquilizers. | Administer antiemetic as ordered. To avoid headache and flushing related to hypertension, teach client to avoid alcoholic beverages or foods high in tyramine. Use central nervous system depressants with caution. Teach client to check with oncologist before taking any new medication. Assess for toxicity and report to physician. Stomatitis measures (see Table 10–4). Administer pyridoxine 50 mg P.O. daily if ordered to prevent neurotoxic effects. |

*A = anorexia, D = diarrhea, M = myelosuppression, N = nausea, S = stomatitis, V = vomiting.

Table 3-7 Hormonal Agents

MEDICATION AND FORMS AVAILABLE	DOSAGE RANGE	INDICATIONS	TOXICITY	NURSING INTERVENTIONS
Glucocorticoids				
Prednisone (Apo-Prednisone, Deltasone [Liquid Pred Syrup], Ora-sone, SK-Prednisone) AVAILABLE: Tablets—1, 2, 2.5, 5, 10, 20, 25, 50 mg. Oral solution—5 mg/ml.	**P.O.:** 40–100 mg/m²/day.	For palliative management of leukemias and lymphomas in adults and acute leukemias in children. Mycosis fungoides. Hypercalcemia associated with cancer of the breast, multiple myeloma, and lymphomas. Hodgkin's disease.	***For All Glucocorticoids:*** **Sodium, fluid retention,** nausea, vomiting. May have gastrointestinal bleeding or peptic ulcer. Hyperglycemia, glycosuria, pancreatitis, hypokalemia, hypercalcemia, alkalosis, muscle weakness, or cramping. With rapid infusion of I.V. steroids: vein irritation, anorectal twitch. With long-term use: glaucoma, cataract formation, osteoporosis, cushingoid appearance, mental alterations (euphoria, psychosis). (NOTE: Steroids may mask signs of infection.)	***For All Glucocorticoids:*** Monitor for hyperglycemia. Monitor Na⁺, K⁺, Ca⁺, I & O. Assess for fluid retention (edema, weight gain). To reduce gastric irritation administer with meals or with milk; administer antacids if ordered. Assess mental status. Avoid falls and potential fractures. Encourage routine eye examinations. Prevent infection. Assess for signs of local infection. Monitor temperature and blood pressure for elevation. Gradually taper dose when discontinuing therapy.
Prednisolone Prelone syrup (Cortalone, Delta-Cortef) AVAILABLE: Tablets—5 mg.	**P.O.:** 40–60 mg/m²/day.			
Prednisolone sodium phosphate (Hydeltrasol, Pediapred oral liquid, Key-Pred, Solu-Prednisolone) AVAILABLE: Vial—20 mg/ml.	**I.M., I.V.:** Dose same as P.O. prednisolone.	Acute and chronic leukemias in adults, acute leukemia in children.		

Hydrocortisone, cortisol (Cortef, Hydrocortone)

Dose varies with type and severity of disease.

AVAILABLE:
Tablets—5, 10, 20 mg.
Vial—25 mg/ml, 50 mg/ml.

Hydrocortisone sodium succinate (A-Hydrocort, Solu-Cortef)

I.M., I.V.:
(injection or infusion):
Dose varies with type and severity of disease.

AVAILABLE:
Vial—100 mg, 250 mg, 500 mg, 1 gm.

Leukemias and lymphomas (adults), acute leukemias (children), mycosis fungoides.

As for prednisone, prednisolone.

Methylprednisolone (Medrol)

P.O.:
Dose varies with type and severity of disease.

AVAILABLE:
Tablets—2, 4, 8, 16, 24, 32 mg.

(Continued)

Table 3–7 Hormonal Agents (Continued)

MEDICATION AND FORMS AVAILABLE	DOSAGE RANGE	INDICATIONS	TOXICITY	NURSING INTERVENTIONS
Methylprednisolone sodium succinate (A-methaPred, Solu-Medrol) AVAILABLE: Vial—40 mg, 125 mg, 500 mg, 1 gm, 2 gm.	**I.M., I.V.:** Dose varies with type and severity of disease.	Leukemias and lymphomas (adults), acute leukemias (children), mycosis fungoides.		
Dexamethasone (Decadron, Dexone, Hexadrol, SK-Dexamethasone) AVAILABLE: Tablets—0.25, 0.5, 0.75, 1.5, 2, 4, 6 mg. Oral solution—0.5 mg/ml. Vial—4, 10, 20, 24 mg/ml. Prefilled syringe—4, 10, 20 mg.	**P.O., I.V., I.M.** (for relief of symptoms related to cerebral edema): 4–10 mg initially, 4–8 mg q 6 hr until symptoms subside. Premedication for radiation therapy: 5–12 mg. Antiemetic: 8–10 mg.	To relieve cerebral edema related to primary or metastatic tumors. May also be administered as premedication before cerebral irradiation, or as an antiemetic agent prior to or following radiation or chemotherapy administration.		

Estrogens

		For All Estrogens:	For All Estrogens:
Chlorotrianisene (TACE) AVAILABLE: Capsules—12, 25, 72 mg.	Carcinoma of prostate: 12–25 mg daily.	Gynecomastia, breast tenderness, areolar pigmentation. Sodium, fluid retention. N, V,* M (mild)* to postmenopausal females. Thrombophlebitis—may result in embolus. Partial alopecia, hirsutism, deepening of voice, alterations in libido. Cholestatic jaundice. Hypertension, hyperglycemia, erythema, headache. Client may report increased bone pain and pain at tumor site. (Note: Bone pain and tumor pain usually indicate good tumor response to therapy.) If administered during pregnancy, vaginal carcinoma may occur in female offspring.	Advise client about possible breast and libido changes and assess emotional responses to sexual alterations (see Chapter 9). Instruct client about possibility of fluid retention and advise about maintaining decreased sodium intake. Assess vital signs and weight and report increasing blood pressure and/or weight gain (may indicate edema). Instruct client to report warmth and tenderness in calf region (may indicate thrombophlebitis).
Conjugated estrogens (Premarin, Progens) AVAILABLE: Tablets—0.3, 0.625, 0.9, 1.25, 2.5 mg. Ampules—40 mg with 2 ml sterile diluent.	P.O.: Carcinoma of breast: 10 mg t.i.d. Carcinoma of prostate: 1.25–2.5 mg t.i.d.	Palliative therapy for progressive, inoperable carcinoma of the breast in selected males and postmenopausal females. Inoperable, progressive carcinoma of the prostate.	
Esterified estrogens (Estratab, Menest) AVAILABLE: Tablets—0.3, 0.625, 1.25, 2.5 mg.	Carcinoma of breast: 10 mg t.i.d. Carcinoma of prostate: 1.25–2.5 mg t.i.d.		
Diethylstilbestrol diphosphate (Stilphostrol, DES) AVAILABLE: Tablets—50 mg. Ampules—0.25 gm in 5 ml.	P.O.: Carcinoma of prostate: 50 mg t.i.d. initially, increase in advanced cases to 200 mg or more t.i.d. as tolerated. Alternate dose: I.V.: 0.5–1 gm for 5 days or more, then reduce dose to 0.25–0.5 gm weekly or b.i.w.	Palliative therapy in advanced cancer of the breast in postmenopausal female. Palliative therapy of carcinoma of the prostate.	

(Continued)

115

Table 3–7 Hormonal Agents (Continued)

MEDICATION AND FORMS AVAILABLE	DOSAGE RANGE	INDICATIONS	TOXICITY	NURSING INTERVENTIONS
Estradiol (Estrace) AVAILABLE: Tablets—1 mg.	Carcinoma of prostate: 1–2 mg. t.i.d. Carcinoma of breast: 10 mg. t.i.d.	Palliative therapy of carcinoma of prostate. Carcinoma of breast in males and postmenopausal females.		
Estradiol valerate (Delestrogen, Estraval, Femogex, Gynogen, Menoval, Proval, Valergen) AVAILABLE: Vials—10 mg, 20 mg, or 40 mg in 10 ml.	**I.M.:** 30 mg or more q 1–2 weeks.	Palliative therapy of carcinoma of prostate and carcinoma of breast in males, and estrogen receptor–positive tumors in females.		
Ethinyl estradiol (Estinyl) AVAILABLE: Tablets—0.02 mg, 0.05 mg, 0.5 mg.	Carcinoma of prostate: 0.5–1 mg t.i.d. Carcinoma of breast (postmenopausal): 1 mg t.i.d.	As above.		

Progestational Agents (Progestins, Progestogens)

Medroxyprogesterone acetate (Depo-Provera) AVAILABLE: Vial, 100 mg/ml–5 ml. 400 mg/ml–2.5 ml and 10 ml., U-Ject 1 ml.	**I.M.:** Initial dose: 400–1000 mg weekly. Later doses may be reduced to 400 mg/month.	Adjuvant therapy and palliative treatment of late-stage and/or inoperable renal cell carcinoma, cancer of endometrium, cancer of breast.	N, V.* Headache, **edema, breast tenderness,** pruritus, urticaria, nervousness, insomnia, somnolence. Amenorrhea or other alteration in menstrual flow, vaginal bleeding or spotting, thrombophlebitis, cholestatic jaundice, pain at injection site.	Administer antiemetics as ordered. Shake vial vigorously before administration to ensure complete suspension of medication. Administer injection deep I.M. Assess for edema, weight gain. Monitor sodium and calcium levels and report elevation. Assess liver function tests, report elevation in liver enzymes, cholesterol. Instruct client not to cross legs.
Megestrol acetate (Megace) AVAILABLE: Tablets—20 mg, 40 mg	**P.O.:** Carcinoma of breast: 40 mg q.i.d. Carcinoma of endometrium: 40–320 mg/day in divided doses.	As above.	As above plus carpal tunnel syndrome, alopecia.	As above.

(Continued)

117

Table 3-7 Hormonal Agents (Continued)

MEDICATION AND FORMS AVAILABLE	DOSAGE RANGE	INDICATIONS	TOXICITY	NURSING INTERVENTIONS
Antiestrogens				
Tamoxifen citrate (Nolvadex, TAM) AVAILABLE: Tablets—10 mg.	**P.O.:** 10–20 mg b.i.d. (morning and evening).	Palliative treatment of advanced estrogen-dependent breast cancer in postmenopausal females. Adjuvant therapy for early carcinoma of the breast in combination with cytotoxic agents.	**Hot flashes, N, V, A.*** Edema, myelosuppression, vaginal bleeding or discharge, menstrual irregularities, pruritus vulvae, hypercalcemia, skin rash. Client may experience flare of disease symptoms (local pain, bone pain) in first few weeks of therapy. Dizziness, light-headedness, headache, depression. Corneal changes, cataracts, retinopathy.	Monitor complete blood count for and report side effects. Administer antiemetic if ordered. Monitor sodium and calcium levels. Assess for pain, edema, vaginal bleeding. Instruct client to avoid bruising. Medicate as ordered for pain, if flare reaction occurs.

Androgens

Drug	Dose	Use	Side Effects	Nursing Implications
Dromostanolone propionate (Drolban) AVAILABLE: Vial—500 mg in 10 ml.	I.M.: 100 mg three times weekly.	Palliative therapy of metastatic cancer of breast in postmenopausal female with hormone-dependent tumor containing estrogen and/or progesterone receptors.	**For All Androgens:** N.* Retention of sodium, chloride, water, calcium, and inorganic phosphates. Masculinism (hirsutism, decreased breast size, deepening of voice, clitoral hypertrophy, patchy alopecia), increased or decreased libido, amenorrhea or menstrual irregularity, cholestatic jaundice. Headache, anxiety, depression. Occasional allergic response. **For Injectable Androgens:** Injection may be painful.	**For All Androgens:** Monitor weight, sodium, and potassium levels. Assess blood pressure for elevation. Assess for weight gain, edema. Assess emotional responses to sexual alterations (see Chapter 9). **For Injectable Androgens:** Inject deep I.M. to minimize local pain at injection site.
Fluoxymesterone (Android-F, Halotestin, Ora-Testryl, Ultandrogen) AVAILABLE: Tablets—2, 5, 10 mg.	P.O.: 10–40 mg daily in divided doses.			
Methyltestosterone (Android, Metandren, Oreton methyl, Primotest forte, Testred) AVAILABLE: Tablet—10 mg, 25 mg. Capsule—10 mg. Buccal tablets—5 mg, 10 mg, 25 mg.	P.O.: 50–200 mg daily. **BUCCAL:** 25–100 mg daily for 4 weeks. May reduce dose if response is evident.			
Testolactone (Teslac) AVAILABLE: Tablets—50 mg.	P.O.: 250 mg q.i.d.	Palliative treatment of androgen-responsive carcinoma of breast in postmenopausal females.		

(Continued)

119

Table 3-7 Hormonal Agents (Continued)

MEDICATION AND FORMS AVAILABLE	DOSAGE RANGE	INDICATIONS	TOXICITY	NURSING INTERVENTIONS
Testosterone cypionate (Andronate, DepoTestosterone, Testred cypionate) AVAILABLE: Vial—100, 200 mg per ml.	**I.M.:** 200–400 mg q 2–4 weeks.	As above.		
Testosterone enanthate injection (Andro L.A. 200, Andryl 200, Delatestryl, Everone, Malogex, Testoject-EP, Testrin). AVAILABLE: Vial—100 mg/ml, 200 mg/ml.	**I.M.:** 200–400 mg q 2–4 weeks.	As above.	As above.	As above.
Testosterone propionate (Malogen, Testex) AVAILABLE: Vial—25, 50, 100 mg/ml.	**I.M.:** 50–100 mg three times a week.	As above.	As above.	As above.

Antiandrogens

Flutamide (Eulexin) AVAILABLE: Capsules—125 mg.	**P.O.:** Carcinoma prostate: 250 mg t.i.d. (every 8 hr) in conjunction with LHRH agonist (e.g., leuprolide).	Carcinoma prostate.	**Hot flashes, loss of libido,** N, V, D,* gynecomastia, galactorrhea, impotence, rash, photosensitivity, confusion, anxiety, nervousness, drowsiness, depression. Elevation of ALT, AST, bilirubin, creatinine.	Assess for side effects, laboratory value elevations. Discuss side effects with patients. Replace fluid lost if diarrhea is present. Assess psychological status, liver function tests.
Goserlin (Zoladex) AVAILABLE: 3.6 mg. implant in pre-loaded syringe.	**S.C.:** Advanced carcinoma prostate: 3–6 mg q 28 days.	Palliative treatment advanced carcinoma prostate.	**Hot flashes,** sexual dysfunction, decreased erections, lethargy, pain at injection site, lower UTI symptoms, edema, sweating, rash, anorexia, dizziness, insomnia, nausea.	(NOTE: Local anesthetic may be given prior to injection: (1) stretch the skin of the upper abdominal wall; (2) inject needle into S.C. tissue. *Do not aspirate prior to injecting.* If the injecting needle penetrates a blood vessel, blood will be seen instantly in the chamber; (3) change direction of the needle so that it parallels the abdominal wall; (4) push in until needle hub touches patient's skin; (5) withdraw needle 1 cm to create space to discharge implant containing medication; (6) depress plunger to discharge implant; (7) withdraw needle; (8) bandage injection site.

(Continued)

Table 3–7 Hormonal Agents (Continued)

MEDICATION AND FORMS AVAILABLE	DOSAGE RANGE	INDICATIONS	TOXICITY	NURSING INTERVENTIONS
Luteinizing hormone releasing hormone (LHRH) Agonists				
Leuprolide acetate (Lupron) AVAILABLE: Kit containing: Vial—2.8 ml with 5 mg Lupron per ml and 14 syringes.	**S.C.:** 1 mg daily as a single dose.	Carcinoma of the prostate.	Hot flashes, N, V,* gynecomastia, breast tenderness, constipation, headache, dizziness, peripheral edema, bone pain, dysuria.	Teach client to self-administer subcutaneous injection daily using a tuberculin syringe. Teach client to rotate injection site.

*A = anorexia, D = diarrhea, M = myelosuppression, N = nausea, S = stomatitis, V = vomiting.

122

Table 3–8 Sample Schedule—MOPP

DAY	1	2	3	4	5	6	7	8	9	10	11	12	13	14	15 THROUGH 28
Mechlorethamine (Mustargen) I.V. 6 mg/m^2	×							×							NO MEDICATIONS ADMINISTERED. Days 15 through 28 constitute a "rest period." This allows time for the hematopoietic system to replenish red and white blood cells and hemoglobin that have been reduced by the myelosuppressive actions of the chemotherapeutic agents.
Vincristine (Oncovin) I.V. 2 mg/m^2	×							×							
Procarbazine P.O. 100 mg/m^2	×	×	×	×	×	×	×	×	×	×	×	×	×	×	
Prednisone P.O. 40 mg/m^2	×	×	×	×	×	×	×	×	×	×	×	×	×	×	

Table 3–9 Combination Chemotherapy Regimens

MEDICATION	ROUTE	DOSE	ADMINISTER ON DAY(S)
Hodgkin's Disease			
ABDIC:			
Doxorubicin (**Adriamycin**)	I.V.	45 mg/m^2	1
Bleomycin	I.V.	5 U/m^2	1–5
Dacarbazine (**DTIC**)	I.V.	200 mg/m^2	1–5
Lomustine (**CCNU**)	I.V.	50 mg/m^2	1
Prednisone	P.O.	40 mg/m^2	1–5
Repeat cycle every 28 days. Refs.: Longo, 1990; Tannir et al., 1983.			
ABVD:			
Doxorubicin (**Adriamycin**)	I.V.	25 mg/m^2	1 and 15
Bleomycin	P.O.	10 U/m^2	1 and 15
Vinblastine	I.V.	6 mg/m^2	1 and 15
Dacarbazine	I.V.	375 mg/m^2	1 and 15
Rest period			16–27
Repeat cycle every 28 days. NOTE: May be administered alternating with MOPP. Ref.: Santoro et al., 1982.			

(Continued)

Table 3–9   Combination Chemotherapy Regimens   (Continued)

MEDICATION	ROUTE	DOSE	ADMINISTER ON DAY(S)
CVPP-CCNU:			
Cyclophosphamide	P.O.	600 mg/m^2	1
Vinblastine	I.V.	6 mg/m^2	1
Procarbazine	P.O.	100 mg/m^2	1–14
Prednisone	P.O.	40 mg/m^2	1–14
Lomustine	I.V.	75 mg/m^2	1 (alternate cycles)
(**CCNU**)			

Repeat cycle every 28 days.
Ref.: Morgenfeld et al., 1979.

MEDICATION	ROUTE	DOSE	ADMINISTER ON DAY(S)
MOPP:			
Mechlorethamine	I.V.	6 mg/m^2	1 and 8
Vincristine	I.V.	1.4 mg/m^2	1 and 8
(**O**ncovin)		(maximum dose 2.0 mg)	
Procarbazine	P.O.	100 mg/m^2	1–14
Prednisone	P.O.	40 mg/m^2	1–14
Rest period			15–28

Repeat cycle every 28 days.
NOTE: May be administered alternating with ABVD.
Ref.: DeVita et al., 1970.

MEDICATION	ROUTE	DOSE	ADMINISTER ON DAY(S)
MVPP:			
Mechlorethamine	I.V.	6 mg/m^2	1 and 8
Vinblastine	I.V.	10 mg/m^2	1, 8, and 15
Procarbazine	P.O.	100 mg/m^2	1–15
Prednisone	P.O.	40 mg/m^2	1–15
Rest period			16–27

Repeat cycle every 28 days.
Ref.: Nicholson et al., 1970.

Non-Hodgkin's Lymphomas

MEDICATION	ROUTE	DOSE	ADMINISTER ON DAY(S)
BACOP:			
Bleomycin	I.V.	5 U/m^2	15 and 22
Doxorubicin	I.V.	25 mg/m^2	1 and 8
(**A**driamycin)			
Cyclophosphamide	I.V.	650 mg/m^2	1 and 8
Vincristine	I.V.	1.4 mg/m^2	1 and 8
(**O**ncovin)		(maximum dose 2.0 mg)	
Prednisone	P.O.	60 mg/day in divided doses	15–28

Ref.: Schein et al., 1976.

Table 3–9 Combination Chemotherapy Regimens (Continued)

MEDICATION	ROUTE	DOSE	ADMINISTER ON DAY(S)
CHOP:			
Cyclophosphamide	P.O.	750 mg/m^2	1
Doxorubicin (**H**ydroxydaunorubicin)	I.V.	50 mg/m^2	1
Vincristine (**O**ncovin)	I.V.	1.4 mg/m^2 (maximum dose 2.0 mg)	1 and 8
Prednisone	P.O.	100 mg/day in divided doses	1–5
Rest period			15–21 or 15–28
Repeat cycle every 21 or 28 days. Ref.: McKelvey et al., 1976.			
CHOP-BLEO:			
Cyclophosphamide	I.V.	1500 mg/m^2	1
Doxorubicin (**H**ydroxydaunorubicin)	I.V.	50 mg/m^2	1
Vincristine (**O**ncovin)	I.V.	1.4 mg/m^2 (maximum dose 2.0 mg)	1 and 8
Prednisone	P.O.	100 mg/day in divided doses	1–5
Bleomycin	I.V.	8 U/m^2	1 and 8
Repeat cycle every 28 days, × 12 cycles. Ref.: Case, 1983.			
COMLA:			
Cyclophosphamide	I.V.	1500 mg/m^2	1
Vincristine (**O**ncovin)	I.V.	1.4 mg/m^2 (maximum dose 2.0 mg)	1, 8, and 15
Methotrexate	I.V.	120 mg/m^2	22, then weekly for 8 weeks
Leucovorin	P.O. or I.V.	25 mg/m^2	q 6 hr × 4 doses beginning 24 hr after methotrexate
Cytarabine (**A**ra-C)	I.V.	300 mg/m^2	22, then weekly for 8 weeks
Repeat cycle every 28 days. Ref.: Sweet et al., 1980.			

(Continued)

Table 3–9   Combination Chemotherapy Regimens   (Continued)

MEDICATION	ROUTE	DOSE	ADMINISTER ON DAY(S)
COP-BLAM:			
Cyclophosphamide	I.V.	400 mg/m^2	1
Vincristine	I.V.	1.4 mg/m^2	1 and 8
(**O**ncovin)		(maximum dose 2.0 mg)	
Prednisone	P.O.	40 mg/day in divided doses	1–10
Bleomycin	I.V.	15 U	14
Doxorubicin	I.V.	1.0 mg/m^2	1
(**A**driamycin)			
Procarbazine	P.O.	100 mg/m^2	1–10

Repeat cycle every 21 days, × 8 cycles.
Ref.: Laurence et al., 1982.

COP-BLAM III:

Cycle A (administer weeks 1, 7, 13, 19, 25, 31):

Cyclophosphamide	I.V. bolus	350 mg/m^{2†}	1
Vincristine	I.V. infusion over 24 hr	1 mg/m^2	1 and 2
(**O**ncovin)		(maximum dose 2.0 mg)	
Procarbazine	P.O.	100 mg/m^2	1–5
Prednisone	P.O.	40 mg/m^2	1–5
Bleomycin	I.V. infusion over 24 hr	4 U/m^2	1–5
Doxorubicin	I.V. bolus	35 mg/mg/m^{2†}	1
(**A**driamycin)			

Cycle B (administer weeks 3, 10, 16, 22, 28, 34):

Vincristine	I.V. bolus	1 mg/m^2	1
Bleomycin	OMIT		

(Administer all other medications as in Cycle A)
†Increase dosage by 5 mg each cycle to a maximum of 50 mg/m^2, based on blood counts.
Ref.: Coleman et al., 1987.

IMVP-16:

Ifosfamide	I.V. infusion	1000 mg/m^2	1–5
Mesna uroprotection	I.V. bolus prior to ifosfamide	800 mg/m^2	1–5
	I.V. infusion concurrent with ifosfamide	4 mg/m^2	
	I.V. infusion over 12 hr after ifosfamide	2.4 mg/m^2	
	Concurrent with ifosfamide		
Methotrexate	I.M.	30 mg/m^2	3 and 10
Etoposide	I.V.	100 mg/m^2	1, 2, 3
(**VP-16**)			

Repeat cycle every 21–28 days.
Ref.: Cabanillas et al., 1983, 1988.

Table 3–9 Combination Chemotherapy Regimens (Continued)

MEDICATION	ROUTE	DOSE	ADMINISTER ON DAY(S)
MOPP, MVPP (See under Hodgkin's disease on preceding pages.)			
MACOP-B:			
Methotrexate	I.V. bolus followed by	100 mg/m^2	Weeks 2, 6, 10
Methotrexate	I.V. drip	300 mg/m^2	Weeks 2, 6, 10
Leucovorin	P.O.	15 mg	q 6 hr × 6 doses beginning 24 hr after methotrexate dose
Doxorubicin (**A**driamycin)	I.V.	50 mg/m^2	Weeks 1, 3, 5, 7, 9, 11
Cyclophosphamide	I.V.	350 mg/m^2	Weeks 1, 3, 5, 7, 9, 11
Vincristine (**O**ncovin)	I.V.	1.4 mg/m^2 (maximum dose 2.0 mg)	Weeks 2, 4, 8, 10, 12
Prednisone	P.O.	75 mg	Daily weeks 1–10 (in divided doses)
Prednisone	P.O.	Taper dose	Over last 15 days
Bleomycin	I.V.	10 U/m^2	Weeks 4, 8, 12
Clotrimoxazole-DS	P.O.	1 Tab. twice daily	Weeks 1–11
CNS Prophylaxis:			
Methotrexate through 8	I.Th.	12 mg	Twice daily week 6
Cytarabine through 8	I.Th.	30 mg/m^2	Twice daily week 6
Ref.: Klimo and Connors, 1987.			
m-BACOD:			
Methotrexate	I.V.	200 mg/m^2	8 and 15
Leucovorin	P.O.*	10 mg/m^2	q 6 hr × 8 beginning 24 hr after methotrexate
Bleomycin	I.V.	4 U/m^2	1
Doxorubicin (**A**driamycin)	I.V.	45 mg/m^2	1
Cyclophosphamide	I.V.	600 mg/m^2	1
Vincristine (**O**ncovin)	I.V.	1 mg/m^2 (maximum dose 2.0 mg)	1
Dexamethasone	P.O.	6 mg/m^2	1–5
*Administer I.V., if necessary.			
Ref.: Shipp et al., 1990.			

(Continued)

Table 3–9 Combination Chemotherapy Regimens (Continued)

MEDICATION	ROUTE	DOSE	ADMINISTER ON DAY(S)
ProMACE:			
Prednisone	P.O.	60 mg/m²	1–14
Methotrexate	I.V. over 12 hr	1500 mg/m²	14
Leucovorin	P.O.	25 mg/m²	Every 6 hr × 4 doses beginning 24 hr after methotrexate
Doxorubicin (Adriamycin)	I.V.	25 mg/m²	1
Cyclophosphamide	I.V.	650 mg/m²	1
Etoposide	I.V.	120 mg/m²	1
Repeat cycle every 28 days.			
Ref.: Fisher et al., 1983.			
ProMACE-CYTABOM:			
Prednisone	P.O.	60 mg/m²	1–14
Vincristine (Oncovin)	I.V.	1.4 mg/m²	8
Methotrexate	I.V.	120 mg/m²	8
Leucovorin	P.O.	25 mg/m²	Every 6 hr × 4 doses beginning 24 hr after methotrexate
Doxorubicin (Adriamycin)	I.V.	25 mg/m²	1
Cyclophosphamide	I.V.	650 mg/m²	1
Etoposide	I.V.	120 mg/m²	1
Cytarabine	I.V.	300 mg/m²	8
Bleomycin	I.V.	5 U/m²	8
Repeat cycle every 21 days.			
Ref.: Fisher et al., 1984.			
Large Cell Lymphoma			
LNH-80:			
INDUCTION (weeks 0, 1, 4):			
Cyclophosphamide	I.V.	1200 mg/m²	1
Doxorubicin	I.V.	75 mg/m²	1
Vindesine	I.V.	2 mg/m²	1 and 5
Bleomycin	I.V.	5 U/m²	1 and 5
Methylprednisolone	I.V.	60 mg/m²	1–5
Methotrexate	Intrathecal	15 mg/m²	With each course

Table 3–9 Combination Chemotherapy Regimens (Continued)

MEDICATION	ROUTE	DOSE	ADMINISTER ON DAY(S)
CONSOLIDATION:			
(weeks 8–10):			
Cytarabine	S.C.	50 mg/m²	q 12 hr × 8 doses
(weeks 12, 14):			
Methotrexate	I.V.	3 mg/m²	with folinic acid rescue
(weeks 16 to 18):			
L-Asparaginase	I.V.	6,000 U/m²	1
(weeks 26 and 30):			
Cyclophosphamide	I.V.	1200 mg/m²	1
Teniposide	I.V.	60 mg/m²	1
Cytarabine	S.C.	100 mg/m²	2–5
Bleomycin	I.V.	5 mg/m²	1
Methylprednisolone	I.V.	60 mg/m²	1–5
Ref.: Coleman et al., 1987.			

Leukemias

Acute Lymphoblastic Leukemia—Remission Induction Therapy

VP plus daunorubicin and L-asparaginase:

Vincristine	I.V.	1.5 mg/m² (maximum dose 2.0 mg)	1, 8, 15, and 22
Prednisone	P.O.	60 mg/m² (to nearest 2.5 mg)	1–28 in 3 divided doses
Daunorubicin	I.V.	50 mg/m²	1, 2, and 3
L-Asparaginase	I.V.	6,000 IU/m²	3, 6, 9, 15, 18, 21, 24, 27
Ref.: Linker, 1987.			

VP plus L-asparaginase:

Vincristine	I.V.	1.5 mg	weekly × 6
Prednisone	P.O.	40 mg/m²	1–42
L-Asparaginase	I.M.	9,000 U/m²	17–28
Ref.: GIMENA, 1989.			

VP plus L-asparaginase and intrathecal methotrexate:

Vincristine	I.V.	1.5 mg/m² (maximum dose 2.0 mg)	1, 8, 15, 22
Prednisone	P.O.	40 mg/m²	Daily × 28 in 3 divided doses
L-Asparaginase	I.M.	6000 IU/m²	Three times weekly × 9 doses
Methotrexate	I.Th.	0–1 yr—6 mg 1–2 yr—8 mg 2–3 yr—10 mg 3 yr and >—12 mg	1 and 14
Ref.: Arndt and Gilchrist, 1992.			

(Continued)

Table 3–9   Combination Chemotherapy Regimens   (Continued)

MEDICATION	ROUTE	DOSE	ADMINISTER ON DAY(S)
Acute Lymphoblastic Leukemia—Consolidation Therapy			
Treatment A (cycles 1, 3, 5, 7):			
Daunorubicin	I.V.	50 mg/m^2	1 and 2
Vincristine	I.V.	2.0 mg	1 and 8
Prednisone	P.O.	60 mg/m^2	1–14
L-Asparaginase	I.M.	12,000 IU/m^2	2, 4, 7, 9, 11, 14
Treatment B (cycles 2, 4, 6, 8):			
Teniposide	I.V.	165 mg/m^2	1, 4, 8, 11
Cytarabine	I.V.	300 mg/m^2	1, 4, 8, 11
Treatment C (cycle 9):			
Methotrexate	I.V.	690 mg/m^2	Over 42 hr
Leucovorin	P.O.	15 mg/m^2	q 6 hr × 12 doses beginning 24 hr after methotrexate

Ref.: Linker et al., 1987.

MEDICATION	ROUTE	DOSE	ADMINISTER ON DAY(S)
Acute Lymphoblastic Leukemia in Adult—Maintenance Therapy			
Start 1 week after cranial irradiation is begun, and continue to relapse, or for at least 3 years of continuous complete remission.			
6-mercaptopurine (6-MP)	P.O.	200 mg/m^2	1–5 every other week
Methotrexate (MTX)	P.O.	7.5 mg/m^2	As 6-MP—omit on days when I.Th. MTX administered
Prednisone	P.O.	40 mg/m^2	Daily × 14 days after last dose of MTX and 6-MP, in 3 divided doses (to nearest 2.5 mg)
Prednisone	P.O.	Taper dose	29–42
L-Asparaginase	I.V.	6000 IU/m^2	4, 7, 10, 13, 16, 19, 22, 25, 28
Methotrexate	I.Th.	0–1 yr—6 mg 1–2 yr—8 mg 2–3 yr—10 mg >3 yr—12 mg	1 and 14

MEDICATION	ROUTE	DOSE	ADMINISTER ON DAY(S)
Acute Lymphoblastic Leukemia in Child			
VP plus daunorubicin and L-asparaginase:			
Induction:			
Vincristine	I.V.	1.5 mg/m^2 (maximum dose 2.0 mg)	1 of each week
Prednisone	P.O.	40 mg/m^2 (in divided doses, to nearest 2.5 mg)	Daily
Daunorubicin	I.V.	25 mg/m^2	1 of each week
L-Asparaginase	I.M.	5000 U/m^2	16–25

Ref.: Tan and Chan, 1987.

Table 3–9 Combination Chemotherapy Regimens (Continued)

MEDICATION	ROUTE	DOSE	ADMINISTER ON DAY(S)
Maintenance			
Vincristine	I.V.	1.5 mg/m^2 (maximum dose 2.0 mg)	1 every 4 weeks
Prednisone	P.O.	40 mg/m^2	1–5 in 3 divided doses (to nearest 2.5 mg)
6-mercaptopurine	P.O.	75 mg/m^2	Once daily
Vincristine	I.V.	1.5 mg/m^2 (maximum dose 2.0 mg)	1 every 4 weeks
Methotrexate	P.O.	20 mg/m^2	1 of each week
Methotrexate	I.Th.	(see above)	1 of every 12th week

Continue treatment for 2–3 years from time of diagnosis.
Ref.: Arndt and Gilchrist, 1992.

Acute Myelogenous Leukemia—Adults

Remission–Induction:
DAT:

Daunorubicin	I.V.	60 mg/m^2	1, 2, and 3
Cytarabine (Ara-C)	I.V. bolus	25 mg/m^2	1
Cytarabine	I.V. infusion	100 mg/m^2	1–7
6-Thioguanine	P.O.	100 mg/m^2 q 12 hr	1–5

Ref.: Wiernik et al., 1979.

Daunorubicin/cytarabine:
Remission–Induction:

Daunorubicin	I.V.	45 mg/m^2	1, 2, and 3
Cytarabine	I.V. infusion over 24 hr	100 mg/m^2	1–7

Note: A second course of therapy may be administered. The client may be a candidate for bone marrow transplantation if remission is achieved.

Consolidation:

Cytarabine	I.V. infusion over 60 min	3 g/m^2	1 and 2
Daunorubicin	I.V.	30 mg/m^2	1 and 2 (following daunorubicin)

Ref.: Beutler, 1987.

(Continued)

Table 3–9 Combination Chemotherapy Regimens (Continued)

MEDICATION	ROUTE	DOSE	ADMINISTER ON DAY(S)
Idarubicin/Cytarabine:			
Induction:			
Idarubicin	I.V.	12 mg/m²	Daily × 3 days
Cytarabine	I.V. bolus	25 mg/m²	1
Cytarabine	I.V. infusion	200 mg/m²	Daily × 5 days
Repeat course × 1 if remission not achieved.			
Consolidation:			
Idarubicin	I.V.	12 mg/m²	Daily × 2 days
Cytarabine	I.V. bolus	25 mg/m²	Day 1
Cytarabine infusion	I.V.	200 mg/m²	Daily × 4 days
Repeat course × 1.			
Perform allogenic or autologous bone marrow transplant when complete remission (CR) occurs.			
Ref.: Berman et al., 1991.			
MTZ-ARA-C			
Induction:			
Mitoxantrone **(MTZ)**	I.V.	12 mg/m²	1–3
Cytarabine **(Ara-C)**	I.V.	100 mg/m²	1–7 as a continuous infusion
If complete remission is not achieved, administer:			
Mitoxantrone **(MTZ)**	I.V.	12 mg/m²	1 and 2
Cytarabine **(Ara-C)**	I.V. continuous infusion	100 mg/m²	1–5
Consolidation:			
Mitoxantrone **(MTZ)**	I.V.	12 mg/m²	1 and 2
Cytarabine **(Ara-C)**	I.V. continuous infusion	100 mg/m²	1–5
Administer for 2 cycles.			
Ref.: Arlin et al., 1990.			
Hairy cell leukemia refractory to β interferon therapy			
Pentostatin	I.V.	4 mg/m²	Every week or every other week OR: weekly for 3 consecutive weeks, alternating with:
Interferon α	S.C.	3,000,000 U	Daily × 4 weeks.
Repeat entire cycle 7 times over 14 months.			
Ref.: Cummings et al., 1991.			

Table 3–9 Combination Chemotherapy Regimens (Continued)

MEDICATION	ROUTE	DOSE	ADMINISTER ON DAY(S)
Multiple Myeloma			
ABCM			
Doxorubicin (**A**driamycin)	I.V.	30 mg/m^2	1
Carmustine (**BCNU**)	I.V.	30 mg/m^2	1
Cyclophosphamide	P.O.	100 mg/m^2	1–4 of 4th week
Melphalan	P.O.	6 mg/m^2	1–4 of 4th week

Repeat cycle every 6 weeks if neutrophils > 1.8 × 10^9/L and platelets > 80 × 10^9/L for a maximum of 12 cycles.
Ref.: Selby, 1992.

VBAP:			
Vincristine	I.V.	1.0 mg/m^2	1
Carmustine (**BCNU**)	I.V.	30 mg/m^2	1
Doxorubicin (**A**driamycin)	I.V.	30 mg/m^2	1
Prednisone	P.O.	100 mg/m^2	1–4

Repeat cycle every 4 weeks.
Ref.: Salmon et al., 1983.

VCAP			
Vincristine	I.V.	1.0 mg/m^2 (maximum dose 1.5 mg)	1
Cyclophosphamide	P.O.	100 mg/m^2	1–4
Doxorubicin (**A**driamycin)	I.V.	25 mg/m^2	1
Prednisone	P.O.	60 mg/m^2	1–4

Alternate every 3 weeks with VMCP.

VMCP			
Vincristine	I.V.	1.0 mg/m^2 (maximum dose 1.5 mg)	1
Melphalan	P.O.	6 mg/m^2	1–4
Cyclophosphamide	P.O.	125 mg/m^2	1–4
Prednisone	P.O.	60 mg/m^2	1–4

Alternate every 3 weeks with VCAP.
Ref.: Salmon et al., 1983.

(Continued)

Table 3–9 Combination Chemotherapy Regimens (Continued)

MEDICATION	ROUTE	DOSE	ADMINISTER ON DAY(S)
Carcinoma of the Bladder (Disseminated)			
CISCA:			
Cisplatin	I.V.	100 mg/m^2	2
Cyclophosphamide	I.V.	650 mg/m^2	1
Doxorubicin	I.V.	50 mg/m^2	1
(**A**driamycin)			
Repeat cycle every 21 days.			
Ref.: Sternberg et al., 1977.			
CMV:			
Cisplatin	I.V.	100 mg/m^2	2
Methotrexate	I.V.	40 mg/m^2	1 and 8
Vinblastine	I.V.	4 mg/m^2	1 and 8
Ref.: Harker et al., 1985.			
MVAC:			
Methotrexate	I.V.	30 mg/m^2	1, 15, 22
Vinblastine	I.V.	3 mg/m^2	2, 15, 22
Doxorubicin	I.V.	30 mg/m^2	2
(**A**driamycin)			
Cisplatin	I.V.	70 mg/m^2	2
Repeat cycle every 28 days.			
Ref.: Sternberg et al., 1985.			
Carcinoma of the Breast			
CAF:			
Cyclophosphamide	P.O.	100 mg/m^2	1–14
Doxorubicin	I.V.	30 mg/m^2	1 and 8
(**A**driamycin)			
5-**F**luorouracil	I.V.	500 mg/m^2	1 and 8
Repeat cycle every 28 days.			
Ref.: Bull et al., 1978.			
CMF(P):			
Cyclophosphamide	P.O.	100 mg/m^2	1–14 OR
	I.V.	600 mg/m^2	1 only
Methotrexate	I.V.	60 mg/m^2	1 and 8
5-**F**luorouracil	I.V.	700 mg/m^2	1 and 8
Prednisone	P.O.	40 mg/m^2	1–14
Rest period			15–28
Repeat cycle every 28 days for 10 cycles.			
Ref.: Canellos et al., 1976.			

Table 3–9 Combination Chemotherapy Regimens (Continued)

MEDICATION	ROUTE	DOSE	ADMINISTER ON DAY(S)
CMF plus Tamoxifen:			
Cyclophosphamide	P.O.	100 mg/m^2	1–14
Methotrexate	I.V.	40 mg/m^2	1 and 8
5-Fluorouracil	I.V.	600 mg/m^2	1 and 8
Tamoxifen	P.O.	10 mg twice daily	1–28
Rest period			15–28
Repeat cycle every 28 days.			
Ref.: Glick et al., 1980.			
CMFVP (CALGB):			
Induction phase (5 weeks)			
AMEND drug doses and schedules as follows:			
Cyclophosphamide	P.O.	80 mg/m^2	Daily
Methotrexate	I.V.	$30–40 \text{ mg/m}^2$	Weekly
5-Fluorouracil	I.V.	500 mg/m^2	Weekly
Vincristine	I.V.	1 mg/m^2 (maximum dose 1.5 mg)	Weekly
Prednisone	P.O.	40 mg/m^2	Daily × 21
Prednisone	P.O.	Taper dose	22–35
Maintenance phase			
Cyclophosphamide	P.O.	100 mg/m^2	1–14
Methotrexate	I.V.	$30–40 \text{ mg/m}^2$	Weekly
5-Fluorouracil	I.V.	500 mg/m^2	Weekly
Vincristine	I.V.	1 mg/m^2 (maximum dose 1.5 mg)	1 and 8
Prednisone	P.O.	40 mg/m^2	Daily × 14
Prednisone	P.O.	Taper dose	15–35
Repeat maintenance cycle every 28 days.			
Ref.: Tormey, 1984.			
Mitoxantrone–cyclophosphamide–fluorouracil			
Mitoxantrone	I.V.	10 mg/m^2	1
Cyclophosphamide	I.V.	500 mg/m^2	1
5-Fluorouracil	I.V.	1000 mg/m^2	1
Repeat cycle every 21 days.			
Ref.: Holmes et al., 1987.			

(Continued)

Table 3–9 Combination Chemotherapy Regimens (Continued)

MEDICATION	ROUTE	DOSE	ADMINISTER ON DAY(S)
Ovarian Cancer (Advanced)			
H-CAP:			
Hexamethylmelamine	P.O.	150 mg/m^2	1–14
Cyclophosphamide	I.V.	350 mg/m^2	1 and 8
Doxorubicin (**A**driamycin)	I.V.	20 mg/m^2	1 and 8
Cisplatin (**P**latinol)	I.V.	60 mg/m^2	1 and 8
Repeat cycle every 28 days for 6 courses. Ref.: Greco et al., 1991.			
PAC-V:			
Cisplatin (**P**latinol)	I.V.	20 mg/m^2	1–5
Doxorubicin (**A**driamycin)	I.V.	50 mg/m^2	1
Cyclophosphamide	I.V.	750 mg/m^2	1
Rest period			6–28
Repeat cycle every 28 days for 6 courses. Ref.: Ehrlich et al., 1983.			
Carcinoma of the Colon			
Ergamisol/5FU:			
Induction—week 1 (3rd–4th week postsurgery):			
Levamisole (Ergamisol)	P.O.	50 mg q 8 hr	1–3
5-Fluorouracil	I.V.	450 mg/m^2	1–5
Week 3 (5th–6th week postsurgery):			
Levamisole (Ergamisol)	P.O.	50 mg q 8 hr	1–3
Maintenance therapy:			
Weeks 5–52 (7th–56th weeks postsurgery):			
5-Fluorouracil	I.V. push	450 mg/m^2	1 each week
Levamisole	P.O.	50 mg q 8 hr	1–3 every 2 weeks
Ref.: Moertel et al., 1990.			
5-Fluorouracil	I.V.	2600 mg/m^2	2 each week
Leucovorin	I.V.	500 mg/m^2	2 each week
5-Phosphonacetyl-L-Aspartic acid	I.V.	250 mg/m^2	1 each week
Repeat cycle weekly.			
Ref.: Ardalan et al., 1991.			
NOTE: This regimen also used in treating carcinoma of the pancreas.			

Table 3–9 Combination Chemotherapy Regimens (Continued)

MEDICATION	ROUTE	DOSE	ADMINISTER ON DAY(S)
Gastric Adenocarcinoma			
ELF:			
Etoposide	I.V. over 50 min	120 mg/m^2	1–3
Folinic acid	I.V. over 10 min	300 mg/m^2	1–3
(**Leucovorin**)			
5-Fluorouracil	I.V.	500 mg/m^2	1–3

(NOTE: This regimen is recommended for patients over 65 years of age, or when doxorubicin is contraindicated.)
Repeat cycle every 21–28 days.
Ref.: Wilke et al., 1991.

FAM:			
5-Fluorouracil	I.V.	600 mg/m^2	1, 8, 29, and 36
Doxorubicin	I.V.	30 mg/m^2	1 and 29
(**Adriamycin**)			
Mitomycin-C	I.V.	10 mg/m^2	30–56

Repeat cycle every 8 weeks.
Ref.: MacDonald et al., 1980.

FAM-BCNU:			
5-Fluorouracil	I.V.	600 mg/m^2	1, 8, 29, and 36
Doxorubicin	I.V.	30 mg/m^2	1 and 29
(**Adriamycin**)			
Mitomycin-C	I.V.	10 mg/m^2	30–56
Carmustine (**BCNU**)			

Repeat cycle every 8 weeks.
Ref.: Beretta et al., 1983.

Carcinoma of the Lung

Non–Small Cell Carcinoma

CAMP:			
Cyclophosphamide	I.V.	300 mg/m^2	1 and 8
Doxorubicin	I.V.	20 mg/m^2	1 and 8
(**Adriamycin**)			
Methotrexate	I.V.	15 mg/m^2	1 and 8
Procarbazine	P.O.	100 mg/m^2	1–10
Rest period			6–28

Repeat cycle every 4 weeks.
Ref.: Bitran et al., 1978.

CAP:			
Cyclophosphamide	I.V.	400 mg/m^2	1
Doxorubicin	I.V.	40 mg/m^2	1
(**Adriamycin**)			
Cisplatin	I.V.	40 mg/m^2	1
(**Platinol**)			
Rest period			2–27

Repeat cycle every 4 weeks.
Ref.: Krook et al., 1984.

(Continued)

Table 3–9   Combination Chemotherapy Regimens   (Continued)

MEDICATION	ROUTE	DOSE	ADMINISTER ON DAY(S)
CEV:			
Cyclophosphamide	I.V.	1000 mg/m²	1
Etoposide	I.V.	50 mg/m²	1
	P.O.	100 mg/m²	2–5
Vincristine	I.V.	1.4 mg/m² (maximum dose 2 mg)	1
Repeat cycle every 3 weeks. Ref.: Comis, 1986.			
Cisplatin/5-FU/-XRT:			
Cisplatin continuous	I.V.	60 mg/m²	1–4 as an infusion
5-Fluorouracil	I.V.	60 mg/m²	1–4
Irradiation	To thorax	200 cGy	Daily
Repeat every 21 days for 4 courses if patient is candidate for surgery, or for 6 courses if inoperable. Ref.: Bonomi, 1991.			
PVP:			
Cisplatin (**P**latinol)	I.V.	60–120 mg/m²	1
Etoposide (**VP**-16-213)	I.V.	80–120 mg/m²	1, 3, 5
Repeat cycle every 21–28 days. Ref.: Klastersky, 1982.			
PE/CAV:			
Cyclophosphamide	I.V.	800 mg/m²	1
Doxorubicin (**A**driamycin)	I.V.	50 mg/m²	1
Vincristine	I.V.	1.4 mg/m² (maximum dose 2.0 mg)	1
ALTERNATE WITH:			
Etoposide	I.V.	100 mg/m²	1, 3, 5
Carboplatin (**P**araplatin)	I.V.	80 mg/m²	1
Administer one cycle every 3–4 weeks. Ref.: Roth, 1992			

Table 3–9   Combination Chemotherapy Regimens   (Continued)

MEDICATION	ROUTE	DOSE	ADMINISTER ON DAY(S)
Squamous Cell Carcinoma of the Cervix			
BIP:			
Bleomycin	I.V.	30 U	1
Ifosfamide	I.V.	5 g/m²	1
Cisplatin	I.V.	50 mg/m²	1
(**P**latinol)			
Mesna	I.V.	3 g/m²	1*
Mesna	I.V.	3 g/m²	1**

*Administer as additive to ifosfamide infusion.
**Administer over 12 hours following ifosfamide infusion.
Repeat cycle every 21 days.
Ref.: Buxton et al., 1989.

Ewing's Sarcoma			
CTX-DOX:			
Induction therapy:			
Cyclophosphamide	I.V. bolus	150 mg/m²	1–7 for cycle 1, then:
(**C**ytoxan)	P.O.	150 mg/m²	1–7 cycles 2, 3, 4, 5
Doxorubicin	I.V. bolus	35 mg/m²	8

Repeat cycle on days 15, 29, 50, 71.
Maintenance therapy (Phase I):

Vincristine	I.V. bolus	1.5 mg/m² (maximum dose 2.0 mg)	Weekly × 11 (**On**covin)
Datinomycin	I.V. bolus	1.5 mg/m² (maximum dose 2.0 mg)	Every 2 weeks × 6 doses

Maintenance therapy (Phase II):
Repeat induction every 21 days for 6 cycles. Phase I repeated after Phase II in patients with metastatic disease.
Ref.: Hayes et al., 1987.

VADRIAC-XRT (for nonmetastatic disease at time of diagnosis):

Vincristine	I.V. bolus	1.5 mg/m² (maximum dose 2.0 mg)	Weeks 0, 3, 6, 9, 16, 20, 24, 28
Doxorubicin	I.V. bolus	30 mg/m²	Weeks 0 and 3
(**Adria**mycin)			
Cyclophosphamide	I.V. bolus	600 mg/m²	Weeks 0 and 3, then:
		1200 mg/m²	Weeks 6, 9, 12, 16, 20, 24, 28
Radiation therapy		1.8 Gy/day (maximum dose 55–60 Gy to primary tumor)	Administer after 3 cycles of chemotherapy

Ref.: Miser et al., 1988.

(Continued)

Table 3–9 Combination Chemotherapy Regimens (Continued)

MEDICATION	ROUTE	DOSE	ADMINISTER ON DAY(S)
VADRIAC-XRT-ABMT (for metastatic disease at time of diagnosis):			
Vincristine	I.V. bolus	2.0 mg/m² (maximum dose 2.0 mg)	Weeks 0, 1, 2, 3, 6, 9, 12, 18
Doxorubicin (**Adria**mycin)	I.V. bolus	45 mg/m² then 30 mg/m² 35 mg/m²	Weeks 0 and 3, then weeks 6, 9, 12, then: week 18
Cyclophosphamide	I.V. bolus	900 mg/m² 1200 mg/m²	Weeks 0, 3, 6, 9, 12 then: week 18
Radiation therapy		1.8 Gy/day (maximum dose 55–60 Gy to primary tumor, 45–50 Gy to metastases)	Administer after 3 cycles of chemotherapy
Total body irradiation (TBI) (Autologous bone marrow transplant (**ABMT**)		4 Gy	Daily × 2 doses in week 18 Week 18

Ref.: Miser et al., 1988.

Soft Tissue Sarcomas (Adult)

A-DIC:			
Doxorubicin (**Adria**mycin)	I.V. bolus	45–60 mg/m²	1
Dacarbazine (**DTIC**)	I.V. over 1 hr	200–250 mg/m²	1–5

Repeat cycle every 21 days.
Ref.: Borden et al., 1987.

Soft Tissue Sarcomas, Rhabdomyosarcomas (Child)

VAC:			
Vincristine	I.V.	2.0 mg/m² (maximum dose 2.0 mg)	Weekly × 12 weeks
Dactinomycin (**A**ctinomycin-D)	I.V.	0.015 mg/kg (15 μg/kg)	1–5
Cyclophosphamide	P.O.	300 mg/m²	Daily for 5–10 days every 6 weeks

Administer for 18–24 months.
Note: Omit cyclophosphamide initially if radiation therapy is directed to areas around the bladder.
Ref.: Wilbur et al., 1975.

Table 3–9 Combination Chemotherapy Regimens (Continued)

MEDICATION	ROUTE	DOSE	ADMINISTER ON DAY(S)
VAC pulse therapy:			
Vincristine	I.V.	2.0 mg/m^2 (maximum dose 2.0 mg)	Weekly × 12 weeks
Dactinomycin (Actinomycin-D)	I.V.	0.015 mg/kg (15 μg/kg)	Days 1–5 in weeks 1 and 13, then every 3 months for 5–6 courses
Cyclophosphamide	P.O.	10 mg/m^2	Daily for 7 days every 6 weeks for 2 years
Ref.: Wilbur et al., 1975.			
Osteogenic Sarcoma			
Bleomycin	I.V.	15 mg/m^2	1 and 2 of postoperative weeks 2, 13, 26, 39, and 42
Cyclophosphamide	I.V.	600 mg/m^2	
Dactinomycin	I.V.	0.6 mg/m^2 (600 μg/m^2	
Methotrexate	I.V.	Starting dose 12 mg/m^2	Over 24 hr Weeks 4, 5, 6, 7, 11, 12, 15, 29, 30, 40, and 45
Leucovorin	I.V.	15 mg	q 6 hr × 12 doses beginning 24 hr after methotrexate
Doxorubicin	I.V.	30 mg/m^2	Weeks 1, 2, 3, 8, and 17
Ref.: Linker et al., 1987.			

References

Ardalan, B., et al.: A Phase I, II study of high-dose 5-fluorouracil and high-dose leucovorin with low-dose phosphonacetyl-L-aspartic acid in patients with advanced malignancies. Cancer 68:1242–1246, 1991.

Arlin, Z., et al.: Randomized multicenter trial of cytosine arabinoside with mitoxantrone or daunorubicin in previously untreated adult patients with acute nonlymphocytic leukemia (ANLL). Leukemia 4:177–183, 1990.

Arndt, C.A.S., and Gilchrist, G.S.: Acute leukemia in childhood. In Rakel, R.E. (ed.): Conn's Current Therapy, 1992 (pp. 361–376). Philadelphia, W.B. Saunders, 1992.

Beretta, C., et al.: FAM/FAM/B polychemotherapy for advanced carcinoma of the stomach (ACS): A randomized study. Proc. Am. Soc. Clin. Oncol. 2:131, 1983.

Berman, E., et al.: Results of a randomized trial comparing idarubicin and cytarabine arabinoside with daunorubicin and cytarabine arabinoside in adult patients with newly diagnosed acute myelogenous leukemia. Blood 77:1666–1674, 1991.

Berman, E., et al.: Intensive therapy for acute lymphoblastic leukemia. Semin. Hematol. 28(Suppl. 4):72–75, 1991.

Beutler, E.: Acute leukemia in adults. In Rakel, R.E. (ed.): Conn's Current Therapy, 1987 (pp. 321–325). Philadelphia, W.B. Saunders, 1987.

Bitran, J.D., et al.: Metastatic non-oat cell bronchogenic carcinoma: Therapy with cyclophosphamide, doxorubicin, methotrexate, and procarbazine (CAMP). JAMA 240:473–476, 1978.

Bonadonna, C., et al.: Combination chemotherapy of Hodgkin's disease with Adriamycin, Bleomycin, Vinblastine and imidazole in combination with MOPP. Cancer 36:252–259, 1975.

Bonomi, P.: Recent advances in etoposide therapy for non-small cell lung cancer. Cancer 67:254–259, 1991.

Borden, E.C., et al.: Randomized comparison of Adriamycin regimens for treatment of metastatic soft tissue sarcomas. J. Clin. Oncol. 5:840–850, 1987.

Bull, J.M., et al.: A randomized comparative trial of Adriamycin vs. methotrexate in combination drug therapy. Cancer 41:1649–1657, 1978.

Buxton, E.J., et al.: The role of ifosfamide in cervical cancer. Semin. Oncol. 16(Suppl. 3):60–67, 1989.

Cabanillas, F., et al.: Sequential chemotherapy and late intensification for malignant lymphomas of aggressive histologic type. Am. J. Med. 74:382–388, 1983.

Cabanillas, F., et al.: Results of recent salvage chemotherapy regimens for lymphoma and Hodgkin's disease. Semin. Hematol. 25:47–50, 1988.

Canellos, G.P., et al.: Combination chemotherapy for advanced breast cancer: Response and effect on survival. Ann. Int. Med. 84:389–392, 1976.

Case, D.C., Jr.: Long-term results of patients with advanced, diffuse non-Hodgkin's lymphoma treated with cyclophosphamide, doxorubicin, vincristine, prednisone, and bleomycin (CHOP-Bleo). Oncology 40:186–191, 1983.

Champlin, R.E., and Gale, R.P.: Acute lymphoblastic leukemia: Recent advances in biology and therapy. Blood 73:2051–2066, 1989.

Coleman, M., et al.: Advances in chemotherapy for large cell lymphoma. Semin. Hematol. 24:8, 1987.

Coleman, M., et al.: COP-BLAM programs: Evolving chemotherapy concepts in large cell lymphoma. Semin. Hematol. 25(2, Suppl. 2):23–33, 1988.

Comis, R.L.: Clinical trials of cyclophosphamide, etoposide, and vincristine in the treatment of small-cell lung cancer. Semin. Oncol. 13:40–44, 1986.

Cummings, F.J., et al.: Phase II trial of pentostatin in refractory lymphomas and cutaneous T-cell disease. J. Clin. Oncol. 9:565–571, 1991.

DeVita, V.T., Jr., Serpick, A.A., and Carbone, E.: Combination chemotherapy in the treatment of advanced Hodgkin's disease. Ann. Int. Med. 73:881–895, 1970.

Duffy, B.A., and Civin, C.I.: Pediatric leukemias and lymphomas. In Niederhuber, J.E.: Current Therapy in Oncology (pp. 527–537). St. Louis, Mosby–Year Book, 1993.

Ehrlich, C.E., et al.: Treatment of advanced epithelial ovarian cancer using cisplatin, Adriamycin and cytoxan—The Indiana University experience. Clin. Obstet. and Gynecol. 10:325–335, 1983.

Einhorn, L.H., and Donohue, J.: Cis-diamminechloro-platinum, vinblastine, and bleomycin combination chemotherapy in disseminated testicular cancer. Ann. Int. Med. 87:93–98, 1977.

Evans, W.K., et al.: Superiority of alternating non-cross-resistant chemotherapy in extensive non-small cell lung cancer. Ann. Int. Med. 107:451–458, 1987.

Fisher, R.I., et al: Randomized trial of ProMACE-MOPP vs. ProMACE-CytaBOM in previously untreated, advanced stage, diffuse aggressive lymphomas. Proc. Am. Soc. Clin. Oncol. 3:242, 1984.

GIMENA Cooperative Group: GIMENA ALL 1083: A multicentric study on adult acute lymphoblastic leukaemia in Italy. Br. J. Hematol. 71:377–386, 1989.

Glick, J.H., et al.: Tamoxifen plus sequential CMF chemotherapy versus Tamoxifen alone in post-menopausal patients with advanced breast cancer: A randomized trial. Cancer 45:735–741, 1980.

Gralla, R., et al.: Enhancing the safety and efficacy of the MVP regimen (mitomycin + vinblastine + cisplatin) in 100 patients with inoperable non-small cell lung cancer (NSCLC). Proc. Am. Soc. Clin. Oncol. 8:227, 1989.

Greco, F., et al.: Advanced ovarian cancer: Brief intensive combined chemotherapy and second-look operation. Obstet. and Gynecol. 58:199–205, 1981.

Greco, F.A., Johnson, D.H., and Hainsworth, J.D.: A comparison of hexamethylmelamine (altretamine), cyclophosphamide, doxorubicin, and cisplatin (H-CAP) vs. cyclophosphamide, doxorubicin, and cisplatin (CAP) in advanced ovarian cancer. Cancer Treat. Rev. 18(Suppl. A):1547–1555, 1991.

Harker, W.G., et al.: Cisplatin, methotrexate and vinblastine (CMV): Chemotherapy regimen for metastatic transitional cell carcinoma of the urinary tract. J. Clin. Oncol. 3:1463–1470, 1985.

Hayes, F.A., et al.: Metastatic Ewing's sarcoma: Remission induction and survival. J. Clin. Oncol. 5:1199–1204, 1987.

Holmes, F.A., et al.: Mitoxantrone, cyclophosphamide-fluorouracil in metastatic breast cancer unresponsive to hormonal therapy. Cancer 59:1992–1999, 1987.

Kantarjian, H.M., et al.: Results of the vincristine, doxorubicin, and dexamethasone regimen in adults with standard- and high-risk acute lymphocytic leukemia. J. Clin. Oncol. 8:994–1004, 1990.

Klastersky, J., et al.: Etoposide and cisplatinum in non-small cell bronchogenic carcinoma. Cancer Treat. Rev. 9(Suppl. A):133–138, 1982.

Klimo, P., and Connors, J.M.: MACOP-B chemotherapy for the treatment of advanced diffuse large cell lymphoma. Ann. Int. Med. 102:596–602, 1985.

Klimo, P., and Connors, J.M.: Updated clinical experience with MACOP-B. Semin. Hematol. 27(Suppl. 1):26–34, 1987.

Kris, M., Gralla, R., and Wertheim, M.: Trial of the combination of mitomycin, vinblastine, and cisplatin) in patients with advanced non-small cell lung cancer. Cancer Treat. Rep. 70:1091–1096, 1985.

Krook, J.E., Fleming, T.R., Eagan, R.T., et al.: Comparison of combination chemotherapy programs in advanced adenocarcinoma-large-cell carcinoma of the lung: A North Central Cancer Treatment Group Study. Can. Treat. Rep. 68:493–498, 1984.

La Rocca, R.V., et al.: Use of Suramin in treatment of prostatic carcinoma refractory to conventional hormonal manipulation. Urol. Clin. N. Am. 18:123–130, 1991.

Laurence, J., et al.: Combination chemotherapy of advanced diffuse histiocytic lymphoma with the six-drug COP-BLAM regimen. Ann. Int. Med. 97:190–195, 1982.

Laurie, J.A.,: Surgical adjuvant therapy of large-bowel carcinoma: An evaluation of levamisole and the combination of levamisole and 5-fluorouracil. J. Clin. Oncol. 7:1447–1456, 1989.

Link, M.P., et al.: The effect of adjuvant chemotherapy on relapse-free survival in patients with osteosarcoma of the extremity. N. Engl. J. Med. 314:1600–1606, 1986.

Linker, C.A.: Improved results of treatment of adult acute lymphoblastic leukemia. Blood 69:1242–1248, 1987.

Longo, D.L.: The use of chemotherapy in the treatment of Hodgkin's disease. Semin. Oncol. 17:716–735, 1990.

Longo, D.L., et al.: Superiority of ProMACE-CytoBOM over PROMACE-MOPP in the treatment of advanced diffuse aggressive lymphoma: Results of a prospective randomized trial. J. Clin. Oncol. *9*:25–38, 1991.

Lund, B., et al.: High-dose platinum consisting of combined carboplatin and cisplatin in previously treated ovarian cancer patients with residual disease. J. Clin. Oncol. *7*:1469–1473, 1989.

Lynch, D.F.: Preoperative and postoperative adjuvant chemotherapy using CISCA (cyclophosphamide, doxorubicin, and cisplatin) in treatment of invasive transitional-cell carcinoma of the bladder. Urol. Clin. N. Am. *18*:543–546, 1991.

MacDonald, J.S., et al.: 5-fluorouracil, doxorubicin, mitomycin (FAM) combination chemotherapy for advanced gastric cancer. Ann. Int. Med. *93*:533–536, 1980.

MacDonald, J.S., and Schnall, S.F.: The role of 5-fluorouracil plus levamisole in the therapy of colon cancer. Prin. Pract. Oncol. Updates *5*(1):1–9, 1991.

McKelvey, E.M., Gottleib, J.A. and Wilson, H.E.: Hydroxodaunomycin (Adriamycin combination in malignant lymphoma. Cancer *38*:1481–1493, 1976.

Miser, J.S., et al.: Preliminary results of treatment of Ewing's sarcoma of bone in children and young adults. J. Clin. Oncol. *6*:484–490, 1988.

Moertel, C.G., et al.: Levamisole and fluorouracil for adjuvant therapy of resected colon carcinoma. N. Engl. J. Med. *322*:352–358, 1990.

Morgenfeld, M., et al.: Combined chemotherapy with CVPP versus CVPP plus CCNU in Hodgkin's Disease. Cancer *43*:1579–1586, 1979.

Nachman, J., et al.: Young adults 16–21 years of age at diagnosis entered on Childrens Cancer Group acute lymphoblastic leukemic protocols. Cancer *71*:3377–3385, 1993.

Natale, R.B., and Wittes, R.E.: Combination cis-platinum and etoposide in small cell lung cancer. Cancer Treat. Rev. *9*(Suppl. A):91, 94, 1982.

Nicholson, W.M., et al.: Combination chemotherapy in generalized Hodgkin's disease. Br. Med. J. *3*:7–10, 1970.

O'Brien, S., et al.: Mitoxantrone and high-dose etoposide for patients with relapsed or refractory acute leukemia. Cancer *68*:691–694, 1991.

Peckham, M.J., et al.: The treatment of metastatic germ cell testicular tumors with bleomycin, etoposide, and cis-platin (BEP). Br. J. Cancer *47*:613–619, 1983.

Preusser, P., et al.: A Phase II study of combination etoposide, doxorubicin, and cisplatin in advanced measurable gastric cancer. J. Clin. Oncol. *7*:1310–1317, 1989.

Rai, K.R., et al.: Treatment of acute myelocytic leukemia: A study by Cancer and Leukemia Group B. Blood *58*:1203–1212, 1981.

Roth, B.J., Johnson, D.H., Einhorn, L.H.: Randomized studies of cyclophosphamide, doxorubicin, and vincristine versus etoposide and cisplatin versus alternation of these two regimens in small cell lung cancer: A phase III trial of the Southeastern Cancer Study Group. J. Clin. Oncol. *10*:282–291, 1992.

Salmon, S.E., et al.: Combination chemotherapy for multiple myeloma: A Southwest Oncology Group study. J. Clin. Oncol. *1*:453–461, 1983.

Santoro, A., et al.: Alternating drug combinations in the treatment of advanced Hodgkin's disease. N. Engl. J. Med. *306*:770–775, 1982.

Schein, P.S., et al.: Bleomycin, adriamycin, cyclophosphamide, vincristine, and prednisone (BACOP): Combination chemotherapy in the treatment of advanced diffuse histiocytic lymphoma with the six-drug COP-BLAM regimen. Ann. Int. Med. *85*:417–425, 1976.

Selby, P.: Multiple myeloma. In Rakel, R.E. (ed.): *Conn's Current Therapy* (pp. 284–287). Philadelphia, W.B. Saunders, 1992.

Shipp, M.A., et al. The m-BACOD combination chemotherapy regimen in large-cell lymphoma: Analysis of the completed trial and comparison with the M-BACOD Regimen. J. Clin. Oncol. *8*:84–93, 1990.

Sternberg, C., Bracken, R., Handel, P., and Johnson, D.: Combination chemotherapy (CISCA) for advanced urinary tract carcinoma. JAMA *38*:2282–2287, 1977.

Sternberg, C., et al.: Preliminary results of M-VAC (methotrexate, vinblastine, adriamycin, and cisplatin) for transitional cell carcinoma of the urothelium. J. Urol. 133:403–407, 1985.

Sweet, D., et al.: Cyclophosphamide, vincristine and methotrexate with leucovorin rescue and cytosine arabinoside (COMLA) combination sequential chemotherapy in the treatment of advanced diffuse histiocytic lymphoma. Ann. Int. Med. 92:785–790, 1980.

Tan, C., and Chan, K.W.: Acute leukemia in childhood. In Rakel, R.E. (ed.): Conn's Current Therapy (pp. 325–330). Philadelphia, W.B. Saunders, 1987.

Tannir, N., et al.: Long-term follow-up with ABDIC salvage chemotherapy of MOPP-resistant Hodgkin's disease. J. Clin. Oncol. 1:432–439, 1983.

Tormey, D.C., Falkson, G., Simon, R.M., et al.: A randomized comparison of two sequentially administered combination regimens to a single regimen in metastatic breast cancer. Cancer Clin. Trials 2:247–256, 1979.

Tormey, D.C., Weinberg, V.E., Leone, E., et al.: A comparison of intermittent vs. continuous administration of adriamycin vs. methotrexate 5-drug chemotherapy for advanced breast cancer: A cancer and leukemia group study. J. Clin. Oncol. 7:231–239, 1984.

Vogl, S.E., et al.: Chemotherapy for advanced cervical cancer with bleomycin, vincristine, mitomycin-C, and cis-diamminidochloroplatinum (II) (BOMP). Cancer Treat. Rep. 64:1005–1007, 1984.

Vose, J.M., et al.: CHLVPP chemotherapy with involved-field irradiation for Hodgkin's disease: Favorable results with acceptable toxicity. J. Clin. Oncol. 9:1421–1425, 1991.

Wiernick, P.H., Glidewell, O.J., Hoaglund, H.C., et al.: A comparative trial of daunorubicin, cytosine arabinoside and thioguanine and a combination of three agents for the treatment of acute myelocytic leukemia. Pediatr. Oncol. 6:261, 1979.

Wilbur, J.R., et al.: Chemotherapy of sarcomas. Cancer 36:765–769, 1975.

Wilke, H., et al.: New developments in the treatment of gastric cancer. Semin. Oncol. 18:61–70, 1991.

Recommended Readings

Advanced Ovarian Cancer Trials Group. Chemotherapy in advanced ovarian cancer: An overview of randomised clinical trials: Advanced Ovarian Cancer Trials Group. Br. Med. J. 303:884–891, 1991.

Alberts, D.S.: IV Alkeran, (melphalan HCl) for injection. In Pinkel, D., et al.: Burroughs Wellcome Co. Oncology Products Current Clinical Guide, 2nd ed. (pp. 47–58). Research Triangle Park, NC: Burroughs Wellcome Co., 1993.

Alberts, D.S., et al.: Improved therapeutic index of carboplatin plus cyclophosphamide versus cisplatin plus cyclophosphamide: Final report by the Southwest Oncology Group of a phase III randomized trial in stages III and IV ovarian cancer. J. Clin. Oncol. 10:683–685, 1992.

American Medical Association Division of Drugs: AMA Drug Evaluations (15th ed.). New York, John Wiley and Sons, 1993.

Ames, M.M.: Hexamethylmelamine: Pharmacology and mechanism of action. Cancer Treat. Rev. 18(Suppl. A):3–14, 1992.

Anttila, M., et al.: Pharmacokinetics of toremifene. J. Steroid Biochem. 36(3):249–252, 1990.

Berman, E., et al.: Idarubicin in acute leukemia: Results of studies at Memorial Sloan-Kettering Cancer Center. Semin. Oncol. 17(Suppl. 2):30–34, 1989.

Bertino, J.R.: Improving the curability of acute leukemia: Pharmacological approaches. Semin. Hematol. 28(Suppl. 4):9–11, 1991.

Betcher, D.L., and Burnham, N.: Idarubicin. J. Ped. Oncol. Nurs. 7:117–120, 1990.

Betcher, D.L., and Burnham, N.: Melphalan. J. Ped. Oncol. Nurs. 7:35–36, 1990.

Betcher, D.L., and Burnham, N.: Thiotepa. J. Ped. Oncol. Nurs. 8:95–97, 1991.

Beutler, E.: 2-chlorodeoxyadenosine (2-CDA): A potent chemotherapeutic and immuno-suppressive nucleoside. Leukemia and Lymphoma 5:1–8, 1991.

Bishop, J.F., et al.: Carboplatin (paraplatin, JM8) and etoposide (VP-16) as first-line combination chemotherapy for small cell lung cancer. J. Clin. Oncol. 5:1574–1578, 1987.

Blick, M., et al.: Durable complete responses after 2-deoxycoformycin treatment in patients with hairy cell leukemia resistant to interferon alfa. Am. J. Hematol. 33:205–209, 1990.

Broun, E.R., et al.: Long-term outcome of patients with relapsed and refractory germ cell tumors treated with high-dose chemotherapy and autologous bone marrow rescue. Ann. Int. Med. 117:124–128, 1992.

Bruckner, H.W., and Motwani, B.T.: Chemotherapy of advanced cancer of the colon and rectum. Semin. Oncol. 18:443–461, 1991.

Bunn, P.A.: Lung Cancer: Current Understanding of the Biology, Diagnosis, Staging and Treatment. Princeton, NJ, Bristol-Myers Squibb, 1992.

Bunn, P.A., et al.: Carboplatin (JM-8): Current Perspectives and Future Directions. Philadelphia, W.B. Saunders, 1990.

Canadian Pharmaceutical Association. Compendium of Pharmaceuticals and Specialties (27th ed.). Ottawa, Ontario, Canadian Pharmaceutical Association, 1992.

Canellos, P., et al.: Chemotherapy of advanced Hodgkin's disease with MOPP, ABVD, or MOPP alternating with ABVD. N. Engl. J. Med. 327:1478–1484, 1992.

Canetta, R., et al.: Carboplatin: Current status and future prospects. Cancer Treat. Rev. 88(Suppl. B):15,17–32, 1991.

Cheson, B.D.: New chemotherapeutic agents for non-Hodgkin's lymphomas. Hematol./Oncol. Clin. N. Am. 5:1027–1051, 1991.

Collins, P.M.: Diagnosis and treatment of chronic leukemia. Semin. Oncol. Nurs. 6:31–43, 1990.

Cooper, M.R., and Cooper, M.R.: Principles of Medical Oncology. In Holleb, A.I., Fink, D.J., and Murphy, G.P. (eds.): American Cancer Society Textbook of Clinical Oncology. Atlanta, American Cancer Society, 1991.

Crist, W.M., and Krance, R.A.: Acute leukemia in childhood. In Rakel, R.E. (ed.): Conn's Current Therapy (pp. 398–403). Philadelphia, W.B. Saunders, 1993.

Dechant, K.L., et al.: Ifosfamide/Mesna: A review of its antineoplastic activity, pharmacokinetic properties and therapeutic efficacy in cancer. Drugs 42:428–467, 1991.

DeVita, V.T., Jr., and Hubbard, S.M.: Drug Therapy: Hodgkin's Disease. N. Engl. J. Med. 328:560–565, 1993.

Diggs, C.H., et al.: Small cell carcinoma of the lung: Treatment in the community. Cancer 69:2075–2083, 1992.

Doane, L.L., Ratain, M., and Golomb, H.M.: Hairy cell leukemia: Current management. Hematol. Clin. North Am. 4:489–502, 1990.

Doig, B.: Adjuvant therapy in breast cancer. Cancer Nurs. 11(2):118–124, 1988.

Dottino, P.R., et al.: Induction therapy followed by radical surgery in cervical cancer. J. Gynecol. Oncol. 40:7–11, 1991.

Elias, A.D., et al.: High-dose ifosfamide with mesna uroprotection: A Phase I study. J. Clin. Oncol. 8:170–178, 1990.

Estey, E.H., et al.: 2-chlorodeoxyadenosine: A new anticancer agent in lymphoid malignancies. Cancer Bull. 43:253–258, 1991.

Estey, E.H., et al.: Treatment of hairy cell leukemia with 2-chlorodeoxyadenosine (2-CDA). Blood 79:882–887, 1992.

Faulds, D., et al.: Mitoxantrone: A review of its pharmacodynamics and pharmacokinetic properties and therapeutic potential in the chemotherapy of cancer. Drugs 41:400–499, 1991.

Fields, S.M., and Koeller, J.M.: Idarubicin: A second-generation anthracycline. DCIP, Ann. Pharmacotherapy 25:505–517, 1991.

Fisher, B., Constantino, J., and Redmond, C.P.: A randomized clinical trial evaluating tamoxifen in the treatment of patients with node-negative breast cancer who have estrogen-receptor positive tumors. N. Engl. J. Med. 320:479–484, 1989.

Galassi, A.: The next generation: New chemotherapy agents for the 1990's [Review]. Semin. Oncol. Nurs. 8:83–94, 1992.

Gershenson, D.M., Morris, M., and Cangir, A.: Treatment of malignant germ cell tumors of the ovary with bleomycin, etoposide, and cisplatin. J. Clin. Oncol. 8:715–720, 1990.

Goldenberg, S.L., and Bruchovsky, N.: Use of cyproterone acetate in prostate cancer. Urol. Clin. North Am. 18:111–122, 1991.

Goldspiel, B.R., and Kohler, D.R.: Flutamide: An antiandrogen for advanced prostate cancer. DCIP, Ann. Pharmacotherapy 24:616–623, 1990.

Goldspiel, B.R., and Kohler, D.R.: Goserlin acetate implant: A depot luteinizing hormone-releasing hormone analog for advanced prostate cancer. DCIP, Ann. Pharmacotherapy 25:796–804, 1991.

Goodman, M.: Concepts of hormonal manipulation in the treatment of cancer. Oncol. Nurs. Forum 15:639–647, 1988.

Goodman, M.: Adjuvant systemic therapy of stage I and stage II breast cancer. Semin. Oncol. Nurs. 7:75–86, 1991.

Greco, F.A.: *Chronic Oral Etoposide*. Princeton, NJ, Bristol-Myers Squibb, 1991.

Grem, J.L.: Adjuvant chemotherapy of node-positive colon carcinoma with levamisole and 5-fluorouracil. Oncology 5(3):63–73, 1991.

Grem, J.L.: Current treatment approaches in colorectal cancer. Semin. Oncol. 18(Suppl. 1):17–26, 1991.

Gribbins, T.E.: New purine analogues for the treatment of chronic B-cell malignancies. Henry Ford Hosp. Med. J. 39(2):98–102, 1991.

Gullatte, M.M., and Graves, T.: Advances in antineoplastic therapy. Oncol. Nurs. Forum 17:867–876, 1990.

Hamm, J.T., and Allegra, J.C.: New hormonal approaches to the treatment of breast cancer. Crit. Rev. Oncol./Hematol. 11(1):29–41, 1991.

Han, T., and Rai, K.R.: Management of chronic lymphocytic leukemia. Hematol./Oncol. Clin. North Am. 4:431–445, 1990.

Heinzman, K.: High-dose ifosfamise and mesna in the outpatient setting. J. Intravenous Nurs. 15:322–326, 1992.

Held, J. and Volpe, H.: Bladder preserving combined modality therapy for invasive bladder cancer. Oncol. Nurs. Forum 18:1849–1857, 1991.

Higgs, D.J.: The patient with testicular cancer: Nursing management of chemotherapy. Oncol. Nursing Forum 17:243–249, 1990.

Higgs, D., Nagy, C., and Einhorn, L.: Ifosfamide: A clinical review. Semin. Oncol. Nurs. 5(2 [suppl. 1]):70–77, 1989.

Ho, A.D., et al.: Response to pentostatin in hairy cell leukemia refractory to interferon-alpha. J. Clin. Oncol. 7:1533–1538, 1989.

Hochster, H.S., et al.: Activity of fludarabine in previously-treated non-Hodgkin's lymphoma: Results of an Eastern Cooperative Oncology Group study. J. Clin. Oncol. 10:28–32, 1992.

Hood, M.A., and Finley, R.S.: Fludarabine: A review. DCIP, Ann. Pharmacotherapy 25:518–523, 1991.

Horning, S.J.: Non-Hodgkin's lymphomas. In R.E. Rakel (ed.): *Conn's Current Therapy* (pp. 410–415). Philadelphia, W.B. Saunders, 1993.

Ihde, D.C., and Minna, J.D.: Non-small-cell lung cancer Part II: Treatment. Curr. Probl. Cancer 15(3):105–154, 1991.

Jett, J.R., et al.: Treatment of limited-stage small-cell lung cancer with cyclophosphamide, doxorubicin, and vincristine with or without etoposide: A randomized trial of the North Central Cancer Treatment Group. J. Clin. Oncol. *8:*33–38, 1990.

Johnson, D.H., et al.: Current status of etoposide in the management of small cell lung cancer. Cancer *67*(Suppl. 1):231–234, 1991.

Juliusson, G., Elmorn-Resenborg, A., and Lilemark, J.: Response to 2-chloro-deoxyadenosine in patients with B-cell chronic lymphocytic leukemia resistant to fludarabine. N. Engl. J. Med. *327:*1056–1061, 1992.

Kangas, L., Cantell, K., and Schellekens, H.: Additive and synergistic antitumor effects with toremifene and interferons. J. Ster. Biochem. *36:*259–262, 1990.

Kay, A.C., et al.: 2-chlorodeoxyadenosine treatment of low-grade lymphomas. J. Clin. Oncol. *10:*371–377, 1992.

Keating, M.J., et al.: Fludarabine: A new agent with major activity against chronic lympho-cytic leukemia. Blood *74*(1):25, 1989.

Kelson, D., and Atiq, O.T.: Therapy of upper gastrointestinal tract cancers. Curr. Probl. Cancer *15:*239–294, 1991.

Kennealey, G.T., and Furr, B.J.A.: Use of the non-steroidal anti-androgen Casodex in advanced prostatic cancer. Urol. Clin. North Am. *1:*99–110, 1991.

Kilbourn, R.G.: Suramin: New therapeutic concepts for an old drug. Cancer Bull. *43:*265–267, 1991.

Krakoff, I.: Cancer chemotherapeutic and biologic agents. CA: A Cancer Journal for Clini-cians *41:*264–277, 1991.

Krook, J.E., et al.: Comparison of combination chemotherapy programs in advanced ade-nocarcinoma–large cell carcinoma of the lung: A North Central Cancer Treatment Group study. Cancer Treat. Rep. *68:*493–498, 1988.

Kyle, R.A., and Greipp, P.G.: Multiple myeloma. In Rakel, R.E. (ed.): *Conn's Current Therapy* (pp. 419–427). Philadelphia, W.B. Saunders, 1993.

La Rocca, R.V., et al.: Use of Suramin in treatment of prostatic carcinoma refractory to conventional hormonal manipulation. Urol. Clin. North Am. *18*(1):123–130, 1991.

Lasater, S.: Testicular cancer: A nursing perspective of diagnosis and treatment. J. Urol. Nurs. *7:*329–349, 1988.

Legha, S.S., Ring, S., and Papadopoulos, N.: A phase II trial of taxol in metastatic mela-noma. Cancer *65:*2478–2481, 1990.

Levy, W., et al.: Cancer chemotherapy: Chemotherapy agents. Part I (Programmed In-struction). Cancer Nurs. *16*(4):321–336, 1993.

Lobert, S.: Antimitotics in cancer chemotherapy. Cancer Nurs. *15:*22–33, 1992.

Loehrer, P.J., Sr., et al.: A randomized comparison of cisplatin alone or in combination with methotrexate, vinblastine, and doxorubicin in patients with metastatic urothelial carcinoma: A cooperative group study. J. Clin. Oncol. *10:*1066–1073, 1992.

Logothetis, C.J., et al.: Primary chemotherapy for clinical stage II testis tumor cancer. J. Clin. Oncol. *5:*906–911, 1987.

Love, R.R. Tamoxifen therapy in primary breast cancer: Biology, efficacy and side effects. J. Clin. Oncol. *7:*803–815, 1989.

Lowenbraun, S., DeVita, V.T., and Serpick, A.A.: Combination chemotherapy with nitro-gen mustard, vincristine, procarbazine, and prednisone in previously treated patients with Hodgkin's disease. Blood *36:*704, 1970.

Lynch, M.P., and Rutland, T.: Ifosfamide: Patient care management. Cancer Nurs. *16:*362–365, 1993.

MacDonald, J.S.: Adjuvant therapy of colorectal cancer: Where do we stand? Oncology *6:*87–92, 1989.

Markman, M., et al.: Second-line platinum therapy in patients with ovarian cancer previ-ously treated with cisplatin. J. Clin. Oncol. *9:*389–393, 1991.

McGuire, W.P., et al.: Taxol: A unique antineoplastic agent with significant action in advanced epithelial neoplasms. Ann. Int. Med. *111:*273–279, 1989.

McGuire, W.P., and Rowinsky, E.K.: Old drugs revisited, new drugs, experimental approaches in ovarian cancer therapy. Semin. Oncol. *18*:255–269, 1991.

Ozols, R.F., and William, S.D.: Testicular cancer. Curr. Probl. Cancer *13*:285–336, 1989.

Ozols, R.F.: Ovarian cancer: New clinical approaches. Cancer Treat. Rev. *18*(Suppl. A): 77–83, 1991.

Padzur, R., et al.: Phase I trial of taxotere: Five-day schedule. J. Natl. Cancer Inst. *84*:1781–1788, 1992.

Palmer, P., and Meyers, F.: An outpatient approach to the delivery of intensive consolidation therapy to adults with acute lymphoblastic leukemia. Oncol. Nurs. Forum *17*:553–558, 1990.

Pate, R.W.: The role of chemotherapy in the treatment of lung cancer. Nurs. Clin. North Am. *27*:653–661, 1992.

Piro, D., et al.: Lasting remissions in hairy-cell leukemia induced by a single infusion of 2-chlorodeoxyadenosine. N. Engl. J. Med. *322*:1117–1121, 1990.

Pors, H., et al.: Long term remission of multiple brain metastases with tamoxifen. J. Neurooncol. *10*(2):173–177, 1991.

Quint-Kasner, S. et al.: Cancer chemotherapy: Chemotherapy agents. Part II (Programmed Instruction). Cancer Nurs. *16*(5):398–418, 1993.

Quirt, I.C., et al.: Improved survival in patients with poor-prognosis malignant melanoma with adjuvant levamisole, A Phase III study by the National Cancer Institute of Canada Clinical Trials Group. J. Clin. Oncol. *29*:729–735, 1991.

Rich, S.E.: Tamoxifen and breast cancer—from palliation to prevention. Cancer Nurs. *16*(5):341–346, 1993.

Rogers, B.B.: Taxol: A promising new drug of the '90's. Oncol. Nurs. Forum *20*(10):1483–1489, 1993.

Rose, L.J.: Neoadjuvant therapy of non-small cell lung cancer. Semin. Oncol. *18*:536–542, 1991.

Rowinsky, E.K., Cazenave, L.A., and Donehower, L.A.: Taxol: A novel investigational microtubule agent. J. Natl. Cancer Inst. *82*:1247–1259, 1990.

Runowicz, C.D.: Advances in the screening and treatment of ovarian cancer. CA: A Cancer Journal for Clinicians *42*:327–349, 1992.

Santana, V.M., et al.: 2-chlorodeoxyadenosine produces a high rate of complete hematologic remission in relapsed acute myeloid leukemia. J. Clin. Oncol. *10*:364–370, 1992.

Saven, A., et al.: 2-chlorodeoxyadenosine: An active agent in the treatment of cutaneous T-cell lymphoma. Blood *80*:587–592, 1992.

Schein, P.S., Scheffler, B., and McCulloch, W.: The role of hexamethylmelamine in the management of ovarian cancer. Cancer Treat. Rev. *18*(Suppl. A):67–75, 1991.

Schenkenberg, T.D., and Van Hoff, D.D.: Mitoxantrone—a new anticancer drug with significant clinical activity. Ann. Int. Med. *105*:67–81, 1986.

Schnall, S.F., and Macdonald, J.S.: Adjuvant therapy in colorectal carcinoma. Semin. Oncol. *18*:566–570, 1991.

Seidman, A.D., and Scher, H.: The evolving role of chemotherapy for muscle infiltrating bladder cancer. Semin. Oncol. *18*:585–595, 1991.

Sharifi, R., and Soloway, M.: Clinical study of leuprolide depot formation in the treatment of advanced prostate cancer. J. Urol. *143*:68–71, 1990.

Splinter, T., et al. A multi-center phase II trial of cisplatin and oral etoposide (VP-16) in inoperable non-small cell lung cancer. Semin. Oncol. *13*(Suppl. 3):97–103, 1986.

Stone, R.M., and Mayer, R.J.: Treatment of the newly diagnosed adult with de novo acute myeloid leukemia. Hematol./Oncol. Clin. North Am. *7*:47–64, 1993.

Tchekmedyian, N.S., Tait, N., and Abrams, J.: High-dose megestrol acetate in the treatment of advanced breast cancer. Semin. Oncol. *15*(Suppl. 1):44–49, 1988.

Thigpen, J.T., et al.: Chemotherapy in ovarian carcinoma: Present role and future prospects. Semin. Oncol. *16*(Suppl. 6):58–65, 1989.

Thomas, D.B., and Noonan, E.A.: Breast cancer and depot-medroxyprogesterone acetate: A multinational study. Lancet *338*(8771):833–838, 1991.

U.S. Pharmacopeal Convention, Inc.: Drug Information for the Health Care Professional, Vol. 1A, 13th ed. Rockville, MD, The U.S. Pharmacopeal Convention, Inc., 1993.

Valavaara, R., et al.: Safety and efficacy of toremifene in breast cancer patients: A Phase II study. J. Steroid Biochem. *36*(3):229–231, 1990.

Vogler, W.R., et al.: A Phase-three study comparing Daunorubicin and Idarubicin combined with cytosine arabinoside in acute myelogenous leukemia. Semin. Oncol. *17*(Suppl. 2):21–24, 1989.

Weinstein, H.J., et al.: Chemotherapy for acute myelogenous leukemia in children and adults: VAPA update. Blood *6*:315–319, 1983.

Weiss, R.B.: Ifosfamide vs cyclophosphamide in cancer therapy. Oncology *5*(5):67–76, 1991.

Wharton, J.T.: Hexamethylmelamine: Altretamine activity as a single agent in previously untreated advanced ovarian cancer. Cancer Treat. Rev. *18*(Suppl. A):15–21, 1991.

Wiernik, P.H.: New agents in the treatment of acute myeloid leukemia. Semin. Hematol. *28*(Suppl. 4):95–98, 1991.

Wiernik, P.H., et al.: Cytarabine plus idarubicin or daunorubicin, used as induction and consolidation therapy for previously untreated adult patients with acute myeloid leukemia. Blood *79*:313–319, 1992.

Wiernik, P.H., and Dutcher, J.P.: Clinical importance in the treatment of acute myeloid leukemia. Leukemia *6*(Suppl. 1):67–69, 1992.

Yarbro, J.W.: Future potential of adjuvant and neoadjuvant therapy. Semin. Oncol. *18:* 613–619, 1991.

Chapter 4

Biologic Response Modifiers (BRMs)

Constance Engelking, R.N., M.S., O.C.N.
Debra Wujick, R.N., M.S.N., O.C.N.

The use of biological agents re-emerged in the 1980s as a potentially viable treatment modality for patients with selected types of cancer. Originally known as "immunotherapy" because the effects of the biological agents were thought to be limited to the immune response, this treatment strategy is currently referred to as "biotherapy"; and the agents used in biotherapy today are known as "biological response modifiers" (BRMs). Both are labels that more accurately describe the broad physiologic effects of biological agents on either hematopoietic and immunologic host functions or on tumor cell growth, invasion, and metastasis. Though some types of biotherapy are still largely investigational, perceptually it has joined surgery, radiation, and chemotherapy as the fourth mode of anticancer therapy (Suppers and McClamrock, 1985; Abernathy, 1987).

Historical Perspective

The origin of contemporary biotherapy can be traced back to the development of what has been called "classic immunotherapy" (Suppers and McClamrock, 1985). Early in this century, Dr. William Coley administered live bacteria to persons with sarcoma of the head and neck to induce a response to infection in the recipient. Some patients

151

responded, perhaps because the host's response to infection bolstered the body's own natural ability to seek and destroy neoplastic cells. Though the rationale seemed plausible, it was not until the 1960s that interest in researching this treatment strategy became popular. Commonly used bacterial agents included Bacillus Calmette-Guerin (BCG), methanol-extracted residue (MER) of BCG, and *Corynebacterium parvum* (*C. parvum*) (Suppers and McClamrock, 1985).

During that same time, it was recognized and generally accepted that in addition to antibodies (immunoglobulins), key players in humoral immunity, certain other proteins with the capacity to act as immunologic mediators existed. These proteins, known at the time as lymphokines and monokines, were found to differ from antibodies in that they were non–antigen-specific. Like antibodies, however, these proteins did function to mediate the intercellular communication necessary to initiate and sustain host defense responses when challenged by foreign invaders. Because it has been learned that many of these proteins are manufactured by sources external to the lymphoid system, the more general term "cytokine" is now used more often to identify these factors (Herberman, 1989).

But progress in realizing clinical applications of these approaches was slow. The immunotherapeutic approach defined by Coley fell out of favor with clinicians during the mid to late 1970s because of the inability to replicate early therapeutic successes reported in patients with leukemia. One explanation for these failures was the use of impure reagents, which introduced variability in the quality of the products being used (Suppers and McClamrock, 1985; Oldham, 1984). The study of cytokines was hampered by the fact that these naturally occurring protein substances existed in quantities too small to accommodate research and often lasted for only brief periods (Suppers and McClamrock, 1985; Herberman, 1989). Hence, interest in biotherapy waned among clinicians during the 1970s.

Advances during the 1970s and 1980s, including hybridoma technology (Fig. 4–1) and recombinant DNA techniques (Fig. 4–2), have made it possible to produce monoclonal antibodies and a wide range of purified cytokines in quantities large enough to study clinically. Interest and research activity in biotherapy were restimulated during the mid 1980s. To date, several biological agents have received Food and Drug Administration (FDA) approval, including aldesleukin, alpha-interferon, interleukin-2, three hematopoietic growth factors, epoetin alfa (EPO), granulocyte colony-stimulating factor (GCSF), and granulocyte-macrophage colony-stimulating factor (GM-CSF).

Monoclonal antibodies and many more cytokines are currently under investigation. Table 4–1 lists cytokines commonly seen in the clinical area today, along with the various names and acronyms used to identify them and their respective cellular sources.

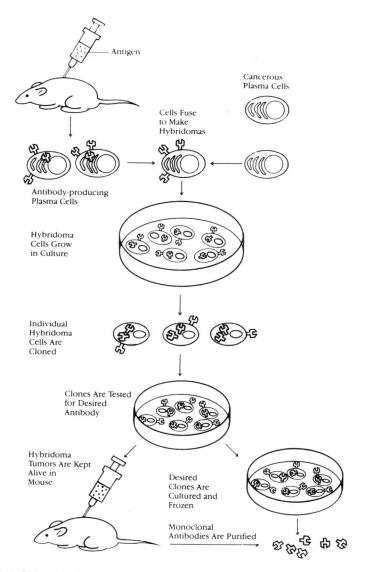

Figure 4–1. Using hybridoma technology to make monoclonal antibodies. (From Schindler, L.W.: *Understanding the Immune System.* Bethesda, MD, National Cancer Institute, 1991, p. 29. Reprinted with permission.)

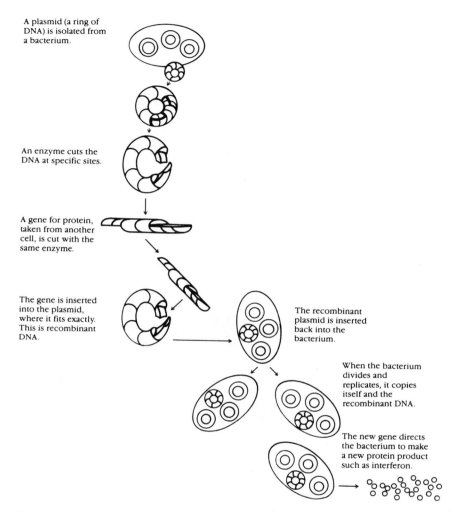

A plasmid (a ring of DNA) is isolated from a bacterium.

An enzyme cuts the DNA at specific sites.

A gene for protein, taken from another cell, is cut with the same enzyme.

The gene is inserted into the plasmid, where it fits exactly. This is recombinant DNA.

The recombinant plasmid is inserted back into the bacterium.

When the bacterium divides and replicates, it copies itself and the recombinant DNA.

The new gene directs the bacterium to make a new protein product such as interferon.

Figure 4–2. Recombinant DNA technology. (From Schindler, L.W.: *Understanding the Immune System*. Bethesda, MD, National Cancer Institute, 1991, p. 32. Reprinted with permission.)

Mechanisms of Action

The rationale for the application of biological agents in cancer treatment is based on the existence of certain relationships and interactions between host and tumor. With the exception of CSFs, BRMs generally have the ability to physiologically alter the immunological host response to the presence of tumor, or to interfere in some way with the tumor cell itself. According to the working definition adopted in 1981 by the National Cancer Institute, BRMs are "those agents or approaches that modify the relationship between tumor and host by modifying the host's biological response to tumor cells with resultant therapeutic effects" (Mihich and Fefer, 1983). Biotherapy is easily distinguished from radiation and chemotherapy, which exert their anticancer effect by interfering with cellular reproduction directly. BRMs (with the exception of a few tumoricidal cytokines) employ the body's own natural defenses to destroy tumor cells indirectly, or serve as adjuncts to chemotherapy and radiation by facilitating regeneration of normal bone marrow elements. Mechanisms of action of BRMs are diverse. Antitumor effects may be the result of interference with the process of cell growth or transformation, alteration of metastatic potential, or activation of effector cells of the immune system when they exhibit tumoricidal activity (Melin and Ozer, 1992, p. 145).

Classification of BRMs

Biological agents can be divided into two major categories of activity, and further subcategorized according to their specific immunologic effects:

I. **Immunomodulating agents.** Alter host immunological responses.
   A. **Immunoaugmenting agents.** Augment the immune response by stimulating cells of the reticuloendothelial system (e.g., monocytes, macrophages) to initiate action against foreign invaders. Examples are:
      1. Bacillus Calmette-Guérin (BCG).
      2. Methanol-extracted residue of BCG (MER).
      3. *Corynebacterium parvum* (*C. parvum*).
      4. Interferons.
   B. **Immunoregulating agents.** Affect developmental or functional balance inherent in the immune response (e.g., T-cell effectors). Enhance or inhibit T- and B-cell production and function. Stimulate secretion of a variety of cytokines. Examples:
      1. Interleukins (ILs).
      2. Interferons (IFNs).
      3. Colony-stimulating factors (CSFs).
         a. Granulocyte colony-stimulating factor (GCSF).
         b. Granulocyte-macrophage colony-stimulating factor (GM-CSF).
         c. Macrophage colony-stimulating factor (MCSF).

    4. Epoetin alfa (EPO).

    5. Tumor necrosis factor (TNF).

  C. **Immunorestorative agents.** Possess no direct cytotoxic effects. Restore or stimulate depressed antigen response and cellular immune function. Examples:

    1. Levamisole (Ergamisole).

    2. Thymosin.

II. **Tumoricidal cytokines.** Exert a direct antitumor effect which is either cytotoxic or cytostatic. May have some immunomodulating properties that are not yet well defined.

  A. **TNF (cachectin).** Induces hemorrhagic necrosis of tumors.

  B. **Lymphotoxin.**

    1. Enhances susceptibility of some tumor cells to the effects of natural killer (NK) cell-regulated lysis.

    2. May also have immunomodulating properties that are not yet well defined.

Although BRMs can be classified according to their primary immunologic properties, it is becoming increasingly apparent that there is significant overlap in the production and effects of these agents. A more detailed discussion of the BRMs follows. The specific immunologic effects and target cells for each of the BRMs appear in Table 4–1.

CSFs play an important regulatory role in hematopoiesis. This dynamic process involves the commitment of bone marrow stem cells to specific cell lines (i.e., erythroid, myeloid, lymphoid, megakaryoid), and the subsequent maturation of cells in each of these lineages into the normal functioning blood elements that are continuously released into the circulating blood cell pool (i.e., erythrocytes, leukocytes, lymphocytes, thrombocytes). This complex phenomenon is described as a hierarchal sequence of events which unfolds in a cascading fashion (Hauber and DiJulio, 1989).

The growth and development of all normal myeloid blood elements are stimulated and regulated by endogenous hormone-like glycoprotein cytokines known as CSFs. CSFs are produced in the bone marrow microenvironment where they remain to exert their regulatory influence on progenitor or precursor cells for specific cell lines in response to either certain events which deplete the marrow of its reserves (e.g., treatment-induced marrow suppression, infection, hemorrhage, stress), or the production of certain mediators of inflammation (e.g., IL-1, IL-6, TNF). Each CSF acts by binding to the specific receptors on the surface of its target cells which trigger cellular gene expression that subsequently results in proliferation, differentiation, or activation depending on the point at which the cell is affected by the CSF (Green, 1991).

CSFs fall into two major categories: (1) those that target their effects to a specific cell line (i.e., single lineage CSF–GCSF), and (2) those that are capable of simultaneous regulation of several cell lines (i.e., multilineage CSF–GM-CSF). The single lineage or unipotent CSFs are considered "terminal stimulators" because their effects are exerted later in the hematopoietic process, after precursor cells have committed to a particular lineage. In contrast, the multilineage CSFs have broader capabilities and effect the process at much earlier stages or "higher up" in the hierarchy. Figure 4–3 illustrates the sites of CSF action. Their names reflect the particular cell lines targeted. For example, the single lineage CSFs are GCSF and MCSF. The best known multilineage CSF is GM-CSF (Green, 1991; Amgen, 1990). Table 4–1 outlines the cellular sources, target cells, and specific biological effects of each of the CSFs.

To date, two of the four identified myeloid CSFs (GCSF and GM-CSF) have FDA approval for clinical use. One erythroid growth factor, recombinant human erythropoietin (Epoetien, EPO), has been used to increase hemoglobin production, initially in patients with end-stage renal disease and later in HIV-infected persons who were receiving AZT therapy. In 1993, EPO was approved for use in the treatment of anemia in patients with cancer.

CSFs have demonstrated, in numerous clinical trials, the capability to reduce the duration of neutropenia and subsequent infectious compli-

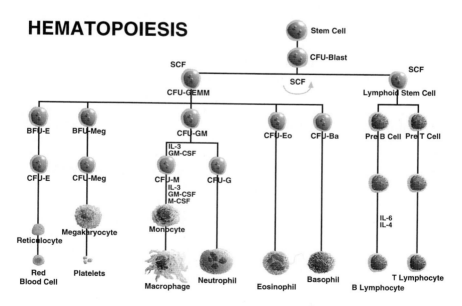

Figure 4–3. Role of colony-stimulating factors in hematopoieses. (Courtesy Amgen, Inc., Thousand Oaks, CA, 1991.)

cations experienced by patients receiving marrow suppressive therapy. This includes dose-intensive conditioning for bone marrow transplantation (BMT). Ultimately, this effect may translate into optimal cancer therapy, reduced length of hospital stay, lower health care costs, and improved quality of life for many patients (Doweiko and Goldberg, 1991; Jassak, 1991; Wujcik, 1992).

The label indications for the two myeloid CSFs are slightly different. GCSF is approved to treat chemotherapy-induced neutropenia, while the more narrow indication for GM-CSF is to treat patients expected to experience protracted neutropenia following autologous or allogeneic BMT. It is also used prior to peripheral stem cell harvesting to stimulate stem cell production, thereby enriching bone marrow harvest. Concern that these CSFs could stimulate the proliferation of leukemic cells in patients with hematologic malignancies has resulted in restricting the label indication for both agents to patients with nonmyeloid malignancies only. Studies are currently underway to investigate the use of CSFs in nonmyeloid malignancies. However, in practice, clinicians are known to use the agents for various indications, interchangeably or concomitantly, in an effort to further refine strategies for the use of CSFs and to identify new research avenues.

The side effects associated with these CSFs are similar to those experienced by patients receiving other biological agents but tend to be relatively mild, ranking between a rating of 1 to 2 in the World Health Organization (WHO) toxicity classification (Appendix G). These include fatigue, fever (though not as high as that seen with IFNs), myalgias, bone pain, flu-like syndrome, and anorexia. Skeletal pain has been observed more frequently with GCSF, while a flu-like syndrome appears to be more common with GM-CSF (Green, 1991; Amgen, 1990).

Although side effects of GCSF and GM-CSF are somewhat different, severity and incidence are generally comparable for similar dosing schedules and routes of administration. Reports of higher toxicity levels with GM-CSF (e.g., capillary leak syndrome) may be related to the published results of early high-dose trials. In addition, the "first dose response syndrome" associated with *Escherichia coli*–derived GM-CSF has not been demonstrated in conjunction with administration of yeast or mammalian-derived products. This syndrome is characterized by a transient cardiopulmonary deterioration including hypotension, facial flushing, dyspnea, and tachycardia (Green, 1991). Specific side effects and nursing interventions for persons receiving CSF appear in Table 4–2.

ILs are a class of cytokines composed of a growing list of proteins that transmit messages between and among leukocytes. (Yasko and Dudjak, 1990). These protein molecules demonstrate a wide range of biological effects which enhance immune responses. The specific immune modulator mechanisms of each are what distinguish one from another and provide the basis for classification according to the numbering system devised at the 1986 Sixth Annual Congress of Immunology (Herberman, 1989). IL-1, for example, plays a key role in the regulatory aspects of the humoral and cellular immune response, as well as in stimulating hematopoiesis. In contrast to these general effects, IL-2 is more specific, promoting the mobilization of lymphocytes with the capacity to destroy tumor cells (i.e., lymphokine activated killer [LAK] cells, NK cells, tumor-infiltrating lymphocytes [TILs]) as well as direct cell-mediated tumor cell destruction. Like IL-1, both IL-2 and IL-6 function as hematopoietic CSFs. IL-7 has been found to support precursor B-cell proliferation and regulate cytotoxic T lymphocytes and LAK cells (Jassak, 1993; Woolery-Antill and Colter, 1993). As research progresses, more ILs continue to be identified.

Because it is still relatively early in the investigative process for many of the ILs, limited data are available about the associated side effects and toxicities. IL-2 is the exception, having been studied extensively before receiving FDA approval in the spring of 1992. Specific side effects and toxicities associated with this agent are summarized in Table 4–3. The full significance of this class of cytokines is yet to be realized. Ongoing research will continue to define their specific functions and role in cancer treatment.

IFNs were discovered in the 1940s when virologists noted that the presence of one viral infection could, if conditions were right, produce protection against other viral infections. In 1957, building on this discovery, Isaacs and Lindenmann isolated the protein substance that appeared to inhibit viral activity in cells exposed to a virus. The protein was named interferon (IFN). The antiviral effect of IFN is twofold. IFN production is stimulated in all nucleated cells by viral exposure. The IFN produced in response to that exposure binds to receptors on the surface of the infected cell and subsequently initiates the manufacture of an enzyme which damages viral DNA. IFN also interferes with intracellular viral replication (Jassak, 1993; Yasko and Dudjak, 1990).

Since it was first discovered, three different types of interferons—alpha (α), beta (β), and gamma (γ)—have been described. In addition to the antiviral property of this family of cytokines, research has revealed that the IFNs also exhibit antiproliferative and immunomodulatory effects in varying degrees. Although the exact mechanism remains unclear, the antiproliferative effects exhibited by IFNs include inhibition of DNA and protein synthesis in tumor cells, and stimulation of human lymphocyte antigen (HLA) and tumor-associated antigen expression on tumor cell surfaces. IFN is also thought to have an inhibiting effect on cell growth by prolonging the duration of phases of the cell cycle. The immunomodulating effects are produced by direct interaction of IFNs with T lymphocytes which, in turn, stimulates the cellular immune response (Jassak, 1993; Yasko and Dudjak, 1990; Woolery-Antill and Colter, 1993).

The primary differences among the three types of IFN appear, at this point, to be the chromosomal location of their encoding genes, their cellular sources, and the degree with which they exert their cellular effects. Interestingly, although alpha and beta IFNs are derived from different sources, the two Type I IFNs are genetically, structurally, and functionally quite similar. In contrast, gamma IFN, referred to as Type II, has demonstrated more pronounced immunomodulatory function and synergy in clinical trials with other cytokines, radiation, and chemotherapy. Table 4–1 summarizes the primary immunologic effects of the IFNs.

There are a range of well-described side effects associated with the IFNs, the most common being flu-like syndrome and pervasive fatigue. Organ system toxicities have been observed as neurological dysfunction (i.e., somnolence, lethargy, confusion, loss of taste and smell, and overall mental slowing), mild to moderate bone marrow suppression, gastrointestinal symptomatology, renal abnormalities (i.e., proteinuria), endocrine malfunction, and skin changes (Yasko and Dudjak, 1990; Quesada et al., 1986; Hahn and Jassak, 1988). Specific effects appear in Table 4–4.

Tumoricidal cytokines are proteins that exert a direct effect on tumor cells by binding with receptors on the cell surface. Two specific proteins with this capability have been isolated to date: (1) tumor necrosis factor (TNF) and (2) lymphotoxin (LT or TNF beta). Although the precise mechanisms of action are still somewhat unclear, TNF may function in several different ways:

1. By causing vascular endothelial damage to capillaries that supply tumor and ultimately causing hemorrhage.
2. By augmenting NK cell cytolytic activity or by increasing the numbers of NK cells, B cells, polymorphonuclear leukocytes (PMNs).
3. By blocking vessels supplying tumor, promoting host inflammatory response, or stimulating macrophage cytotoxicity (Jassak, 1993; Yasko and Dudjak, 1990; Woolery-Antill and Colter, 1993).
4. By inducing release of IL-1 by monocytes and endothelial cells (Jassak, 1990).

Specific cellular sources, target cells, and immunologic properties are outlined in Table 4–1. Associated side effects are listed in Table 4–5.

Monoclonal antibodies (MoAbs) are high molecular weight proteins produced by a clone of cells and are meant to attack one specific antigen (Baird et al., 1991, p. 329). They are used in diagnosing or screening cancers, monitoring disease progression, and as therapeutic agents in the treatment of cancer. There is evidence that MoAbs might interfere with cellular proliferation by one of two mechanisms: (1) blocking receptor access to the required growth factor or (2) inciting the inflammatory response mediated by cells or complement through recognition of the Fc portion of the immunoglobulin molecule (DeVita et al., 1991, p. 603). Side effects with the infusion of murine MoAbs have been tolerable and include fever, chills, flushing, pruritus, urticaria, chest tightness, dyspnea, arthralgia, nausea and vomiting, myalgia, and hypotension (DeVita et al., 1991; Jassak, 1993). Toxicities occur more often with the first one or two treatments, or with rapid infusion rates. Anaphylactoid responses may occur, but are unusual. Results with MoAbs have been somewhat disappointing (Morton and Economou, p. 113). Further investigational studies are currently being conducted to realize the best potential for MoAbs in cancer treatment.

Side Effects and Toxicities

An array of potential acute and chronic side effects and toxicities associated with BRMs are currently being defined. Like those induced by chemotherapeutic agents, the potential side effects associated with the biological agents are systemic and many are universal, occurring generally across the spectrum of agents (though the incidence and severity may differ according to the class of biological agents), while others are unique to a particular agent at a certain dosage level, via specific routes of administration, or in certain combinations. The dosage, treatment schedule, and route of administration appear to significantly influence the incidence and severity of symptoms experienced by patients receiving BRMs.

Unlike chemotherapy, it is characteristic for most side effects to have an immediate onset (occurring within minutes or hours of administration) and to resolve rapidly when the agent is withdrawn. Symptoms associated with CSFs, IFNs, and TNF generally resolve within 24–48 hours of discontinuing therapy, while it may require up to 96 hours for single agent IL-2 (Yasko and Dudjak, 1990).

The two most common symptom complexes experienced by patients undergoing BRM therapy are **flu-like syndrome** and **fatigue. Flu-like syndrome** is the most common side effect associated with BRMs. Hauber (1989) has described flu-like syndrome as a syndrome characterized by a constellation of constitutional symptoms including fever, chills, and rigor that may last up to 60 minutes after treatment; myalgias; arthralgias, dull frontal headaches; and malaise. Upper respiratory symptoms may or may not accompany the syndrome. The pattern of flu-like syndrome varies with different agents.

Fatigue is another common response considered universal across the spectrum of biological agents. Several theories have been offered to explain fatigue and weakness in patients receiving BRMs. Proposed theories involve both central and peripheral mechanisms (Piper et al., 1989). These include subjective conditioned responses, release of substances that stimulate sensation of fatigue by altering neuroendocrine secretion, brain muscle, and enzyme electrical activity or blood–brain barrier permeability, and the cycle in which skeletal muscle wasting necessitates increasing energy expenditure by the patient (St. Pierre et al., 1992).

Detailed data about indications, dosages, routes of administration, and side effects appear in Tables 4–2 through 4–6. Incidence patterns of specific side effects for each of the BRMs are outlined in Table 4–7. Management of side effects associated with BRMs is discussed in Chapters 7–13.

Table 4-1 Cellular Sources, Target Cells, and Immunologic Effects of Commonly Used Cytokines

CYTOKINE (ACRONYM)	CELLULAR SOURCE	TARGET CELLS	IMMUNOLOGIC EFFECTS
Colony-Stimulating Factors (CSFs)			
Granulocyte-macrophage colony-stimulating factor (GM-CSF), **colony-stimulating factor α (CSF α), pluripoietin**	T cells, endothelial cells, fibroblasts, macrophages.	Hematopoietic progenitors, neutrophils, eosinophils, monocytes, macrophages.	Multilineage growth factor; stimulates proliferation/differentiation along granulocyte and macrophage pathways; promotes proliferation of megakaryocyte and erythroid progenitors; enhances ingestion of bacteria and killing of antibody-coated tumor cells; activates/enhances function of mature granulocytes and macrophage/monocytes; stimulates production of TNF and IL-1.
Macrophage colony-stimulating factor (MCSF), **colony-stimulating factor 1 (CSF-1)**	Fibroblasts, monocytes, endothelial cells.	Macrophages and precursors.	Multilineage growth; activating factor for macrophage colonies.
Granulocyte colony-stimulating factor (GCSF)	Macrophages, fibroblasts.	Neutrophilic granulocytes and their precursors.	Single lineage growth factor; stimulates proliferation, differentiation, and maturation of granulocyte progenitor cells; enhances functional activity of mature neutrophils.

(Continued)

163

Table 4–1 Cellular Sources, Target Cells, and Immunologic Effects of Commonly Used Cytokines (Continued)

CYTOKINE (ACRONYM)	CELLULAR SOURCE	TARGET CELLS	IMMUNOLOGIC EFFECTS
Erythropoietin (EPO)	Kidney, liver.	Erythrocyte and megakaryocyte precursors.	Single lineage factor; selectively stimulates the proliferation and differentiation of erythrocytes.
Megakaryocyte colony-stimulating factor (Meg-CSF)	Unknown.	Megakaryocyte precursors.	(Not yet defined.)
Interleukins (ILs)			
Interleukin 1 (IL-1), lymphocyte activating factor (LAF), hematopoietin	Macrophages, endothelial cells, large granular lymphocytes, B cells, fibroblasts, epithelial cells, astrocytes, keratinocytes, osteoblasts.	Thymocytes, neutrophils, hepatocytes, chondrocytes, muscle cells, endothelial cells, epidermal cells, osteocytes, macrophages, T and B cells, fibroblasts.	Activates T cells; mediates inflammation; acute phase response (induces fever, sleep, ACTH release, neutrophilia); cofactor for CSFs; stimulates production of lymphokines, collagen, and collagenases; activates endothelial and macrophage cells to become cytostatic for some tumor cells; induces differentiation of stem cells to develop receptors for CSF or IL-2; induces differentiation of activated B cells in conjunction with IL-6; stimulates proliferation of activated B cells in conjunction with IL-4.

Interleukin 2 (IL-2), **T cell growth factor (TCGF)**	T cells.	T cells, B cells, macrophages.	Growth and differentiation factor for cytotoxic helper and suppressor T cells and NK cells; induces lymphokine production by T cells and monocytes; enhances NK cell activity and induces LAK activity.
Interleukin 3 (IL-3), **multipotential colony-stimulating factor (multi-CSF), burst promoting activity (BP)**	T cells.	Multipotential stem cells, mast cells.	Supports growth of pluripotent stem cells and intermediate myelomonocytic stem cells; growth factor for mast cells.
Interleukin 4 (IL-4), **B cell stimulation factor 1 (BSF-1), T cell growth factor II (TCGF-II)**	T cells.	T cells, B cells, macrophages, hematopoietic progenitors.	Growth factor for resting B cells, mast cells, and resting T cells; increases Class II major histocompatibility complex (MHC) antigen expression on B cells; increases cytotoxicity of killer T cells and macrophages; enhances expression of IgE and Fc receptors.
Interleukin 5 (IL-5), **B cell growth factor II (BCGF-II), eosinophil differentiation factor (EDF)**	T cells (mouse).	Eosinophils, B cells.	Induces differentiation of eosinophils; causes preferential class switch to IgA synthesis and secretion; B cell growth and differentiation factor; causes DNA synthesis and production for IgM and IgE by activated B cells; induces appearance of IL-2 receptors on B cells.

(Continued)

165

Table 4–1 Cellular Sources, Target Cells, and Immunologic Effects of Commonly Used Cytokines *(Continued)*

CYTOKINE (ACRONYM)	CELLULAR SOURCE	TARGET CELLS	IMMUNOLOGIC EFFECTS
Interleukin 6 (IL–6), **interferon** β² **(IFN-β², B-cell stimulation factor 2 (BSF-2)**	Fibroblasts, T cells.	B cells, thymocytes, multipotential stem cells.	Induces differentiation of activated B cells into immunoglobulin-secreting cells; enhances differentiation of killer T cells; supports Class I HLA expression on fibroblasts; induces growth of B cell hybridomas and plasmacytomas; induces acute phase proteins.
Interleukin 7 (IL–7)	Stromal cells.	T cells, B cell precursors, monocytes.	Under certain conditions, induces LAK activity, supports B cell precursors, generates cytotoxic T cells, stimulates cytokine secretion and tumoricidal activity by monocytes.
Tumoricidal cytokines			
Tumor necrosis factor (TNF), cachetin, **tumor necrosis factor** α **(TNFα)**	Macrophages, T cells, thymocytes, B cells, NK cells.	Fibroblasts, macrophages, osteoclasts, neutrophils, eosinophils, endothelial cells, chondrocytes, hepatocytes.	Cytotoxic/cytosystic for some tumor cells; promotes growth of fibroblasts; mediates inflammatory response and septic shock; induces acute phase responses; stimulates production of lymphokines, collagen, and collagenases; activates macrophages, neutrophils, and endothelial cells; causes damage to epithelial cells in capillaries of tumors, resulting in hemorrhagic necrosis of selected tumors; inhibits lipoprotein lipase; synergizes with IL-2 in generation of LAK cells.

Lymphotoxin (LT), **tumor necrosis factor B (TNF-B)**	T cells.	Neutrophils, osteoclasts.	Cytotoxic/cytostatic for some tumor cells; PMN activation; renders some tumor cells more susceptible to NK mediated lysis; in vivo induction of hemorrhagic necrosis of selected tumors.
Interferons (IFNs)			
Interferon alfa (IFN-α) **(leukocyte, Type 1)**	B cells, T cells, macrophages, NK cells, null cells.	B cells, NK cells, T cells, macrophages, monocytes.	Enhances NK cell activity; antiviral; induces Class I MHC surface antigen expression; may induce fever, antiproliferative properties; activates cytotoxic T cells; induces phagocytic activity of macrophages and NK cells.
Interferon beta (IFN-β), β1 **(fibroblast, Type 1)**	Fibroblasts, macrophages, epithelial cells.	B cells, NK cells, T cells, macrophages, monocytes.	(As for IFN Alfa.)
Interferon gamma (IFN-γ), **macrophage activating factor (MAF)**	T cells, NK cells.	NK cells, macrophages, IL-2 receptors, B cells.	Antiviral; induces Class I and Class II MHC antigen expression; induces antimicrobial and tumoricidal activity of macrophages; regulates other lymphokine action; increases NK cell activity; induces production of T-cell suppressor factor; increases Fc factor expression.

Data from Brophy, L., and Trahan Reiger, P.: Implications of biologic response modifier therapy for nursing. In Clark, J.C., and McGee, R.F. (eds.): *Oncology Nursing Society Core Curriculum for Oncology Nursing* (pp. 346–358). Philadelphia, W.B. Saunders, 1992; Herberman, R.B. (ed.): *ImmunoPrimer Series: Part 3—Cytokines*. Emeryville, CA, Cetus Oncology Corporation, 1989; and Smith, D.H.: Use of hematopoietic growth factors for treatment of aplastic anemia. Am. J. Pediatr. Hematol. Oncol. *12*:425–433, 1990.

Table 4-2 Indications, Toxicities, and Nursing Interventions for Colony-Stimulating Factors

Regulate growth of bone marrow stem cells, the precursors of mature blood cells. Regulate proliferation, differentiation, and maturation of hematopoietic progenitor cells. Enhance the functional activity of progeny or descendants of the target cells (i.e., help mature cells work better).

COLONY-STIMULATING FACTOR	DOSE AND MODE OF ADMINISTRATION	INDICATIONS	TOXICITIES	NURSING INTERVENTIONS
Epoetin alfa (Erythropoietin, Epogen, Procrit EPO) AVAILABLE: Vial—2,000, 3,000, 4,000, 10,000 U/cc	For patients on chemotherapy: starting dose 150 U/kg subcutaneously (S.C.) TIW; may be increased up to 300 U/kg TIW.	For treatment of anemias associated with chemotherapy, chronic renal failure, or therapy with AZT in human immunodeficiency virus (HIV)-infected patients.	Hypertension, diarrhea, seizures, thrombotic events, rash.	DO NOT shake vial during preparation. Establish parameters with physician for holding EPO. Monitor baseline hemoglobin, serum iron, total iron-binding capacity (TIBC), transferrin. Administer supplemental iron as ordered. Monitor hematocrit twice weekly, complete blood count (CBC), differential, platelets weekly. Monitor blood pressure and report elevation.

Filgrastim (granulocyte colony-stimulating factor [G-CSF], Neupogen) AVAILABLE: Vial—300 μg in 1 ml; 480 μg in 1.6 ml. COMPATIBILITY: D5/W	S.C. or intravenously (I.V.): 5 μg/kg/d, administered as a single daily dose for up to 2 weeks, or until the absolute neutrophil count (ANC) has reached 10,000/mm³.	Administered to decrease the incidence of infection as manifested by neutropenic fever in patients receiving myelosuppressive antineoplastic chemotherapy for nonmyeloid malignancies.	Bone pain, exacerbation of pre-existing skin diseases such as psoriasis or eczema.	Monitor CBC, platelet count twice weekly. Monitor for side effects such as bone pain, which occur with marrow recovery. Monitor patients with chronic skin diseases for exacerbation of condition. Administer acetaminophen per physician's orders to relieve bone pain. Teach client S.C. injection technique, proper transport and storage of medication, and safe syringe disposal.
Sargramostim (granulocyte-macrophage colony-stimulating factor [GM-CSF] Leukine, Prokine) AVAILABLE: Vial—250 μg, 500 μg. COMPATIBILITY: Saline	I.V.: 250 μg/m²/d for 21 days as a 2–4 hr. infusion beginning 2–4 hr after autologous BMT, and not less than 24 hr after the last dose of chemotherapy and 12 hr after the last dose of radiation.	Administered for acceleration of myeloid recovery in clients with non-Hodgkin's lymphoma, acute lymphoblastic leukemia, Hodgkin's disease undergoing autologous BMT.	Bone pain, skin reaction at injection site, flu-like syndrome, diarrhea, rash, weakness, malaise; with higher doses: capillary leak syndrome (see Chapter 13).	Monitor for side effects. Monitor blood pressure and pulse, and report alterations. Assess CBC, platelets biweekly. Monitor site for phlebitis when administering peripherally. Establish parameters with physician for withholding GM-CSF. Administer acetaminophen per physician's orders to relieve bone pain. With higher doses, monitor fluid balance, assess for indications of fluid retention.

Table 4–3 Indications, Toxicities, and Nursing Interventions for Interleukins

Enhance killer T-cell activity by binding to "high-affinity" receptors on activated T cells. Assist in synthesis and secretion of interferons and other interleukins. Increase production of B lymphocytes, antibodies, NK, and LAK cells.

INTERLEUKIN	MODE(S) OF ADMINISTRATION	INDICATIONS	TOXICITIES	NURSING INTERVENTIONS
Interleukin-1 (α and β— investigational)	I.V. over 30 min. to 2 hr.	Malignant melanoma, carcinoma of the ovary.	Fever, chills, rigors, flu-like syndrome, nausea, vomiting, anorexia, tachycardia, headache, myalgias, hypotension; erythema, phlebitis at injection site; less commonly seen: confusion, irritability, impaired memory, expressive aphasia, sleep disturbances, depression, psychoses, hallucinations; with high dose: capillary leak syndrome (see Chapter 13), edema, arrhythmias, dyspnea, tachypnea, pulmonary edema, cough, nasal congestion.	Must be diluted with human serum albumin after initial reconstitution. Administer IL-1 through central venous catheter. Assess for temperature elevation, other signs of flu-like syndrome. Assess pulse and monitor blood pressure for orthostatic hypotension. Assess for redness or other alterations at injection site.

| Interleukin-2 (IL-2) (Proleukin) | I.V. (bolus or continuous infusion), intraperitoneal, intrahepatic, intrapleural, intraventricular. | Malignant melanoma, metastatic renal cell carcinoma, colorectal adenocarcinoma, carcinoma of the bladder, stomach, ovary, lung, or head and neck; Hodgkin's disease, non-Hodgkin's lymphomas, leptomeningeal cancer. | Capillary leak syndrome, flu-like syndrome (fever, chills, myalgias, headache, malaise) (see Chapter 13); myelosuppression, N, V, A, D, M,* xerostomia, taste alterations; tachycardia (atrial or supraventricular), orthostatic hypotension, confusion, headache, somnolence, irritability, renal, hepatic failure. Altered neutrophil function, progressive anemia, neutropenia, thrombocytopenia. Erythema, dry desquamation, pruritic rash, hypocalcemia, hypomagnesemia. | Assess cardiac status, pulse, irregularities, electrocardiogram (EKG) alterations, daily weight. Monitor blood pressure for orthostatic hypotension. Assess lung sounds and other pulmonary symptoms. Monitor strict I & O, report indications of renal impairment (oliguria, ↑ BUN, ↑ creatinine, proteinuria): Assess for and report indications of hepatic involvement (↑ AST, ALT, LDH, alkaline phosphatase, or bilirubin). Monitor for signs of flu-like syndrome. Administer antipyretic and nonsteroidal anti-inflammatory medication as ordered to control fever. Avoid sources of infection. Perform skin care twice daily with water soluble emollients. |

*N = nausea, V = vomiting, A = anorexia, D = diarrhea, M = myelosuppression.

Table 4–4 Indications, Toxicities, and Nursing Interventions for Interferons

A group of peptides that inhibit viruses and induce various effector cells by damaging viral DNA and interfering with intracellular viral replication. Suppress tumorigenesis and modulate cell-mediated immunity. Stimulate production of other interferons, interleukins, and tumor necrosis factor.

INTERFERON	MODE(S) OF ADMINISTRATION	INDICATIONS	TOXICITIES	NURSING INTERVENTIONS
Interferon alfa (IFN-A, IFN-α, Roferon-A, Intron-A) AVAILABLE: Vial solution—3 million IU/ml, 9 million IU/ml; 18 million IU/ml, 36 million IU/ml; sterile powder for injection—18 million IU with 3 ml diluent.	I.M. S.C. intraperitoneal, intralesional. **For hairy cell leukemia:** Induction—3 million IU daily × 16–24 weeks, maintenance—3 million IU TIW for up to 24 months. Kaposi's sarcoma: I.M. or S.C., induction—36 million IU daily for 10–12 weeks, maintenance—36 million IU TIW.	Hairy cell leukemia, AIDS-related Kaposi's sarcoma, renal cell carcinoma, malignant melanoma. Mycosis fungoides, chronic myelogenous leukemia, non-Hodgkin's lymphomas, cutaneous T-cell lymphomas. (NOTE: Also administered for condyloma acuminata.)	NOTE: Incidence of side effects increases as dose increases. **Flu-like syndrome (headache, arthralgia, fever, chills, fatigue, malaise, myalgias, mild nausea and vomiting), anorexia, xerostomia, taste alterations, weight loss.** Myelosuppression, neutropenia, mild anemia. Partial alopecia (thinning of hair, pruritus, dry skin. Paresthesias, poor concentration, decreased short-term memory, and attention span. Paranoia, psychoses.	Do not shake vial during preparation. Administer antipyretic and antihistamine p.r.n. as ordered. Assess for temperature elevation, chills, other signs of flu-like syndrome. Repeat dose of antihistamine as ordered for chills. Administer acetaminophen q 4 hr p.r.n. as ordered. Avoid sources of infection. Assess urine output and laboratory tests for indications of renal involvement (oliguria, ↑ BUN, ↑ creatinine, or proteinuria) or hepatic involvement (↑ ALT,

AST). Monitor clients with a history of cardiopulmonary disease closely for cardiopulmonary side effects (see Chapter 13). Adjust dose or hold as ordered for dose-limiting side effects (anorexia, fatigue, malaise, neurotoxicity, thrombocytopenia). Encourage patient to increase fluid intake to compensate for losses during fevers. Assess for and have patient report signs of fluid overload (edema, shortness of breath). Teach client S.C. injection technique, proper transport and storage of medication, safe syringe disposal, and measures to take should toxicities occur. Teach patient to pace activities in the presence of fatigue.

β-IV; γ-IM, IV, topical.
Polypeptides produced in response to a variety of stimulating agents. Alter properties of cell surface, suppress tumorigenesis, modulate cell-mediated immunity. Important modifiers of the immune system. Raise amounts of ER in target tissues (Kuppila et al., 1982; Dimitrov et al., 1984).

Table 4–5 Indications, Toxicities, and Nursing Interventions for Tumor Necrosis Factor

Synthesized and secreted mainly from activated macrophages. Binds to receptors on tumor cells and causes damage to tumor capillaries, which might be the mode of tumor destruction. Enhances coagulation and depresses anticoagulation. Augments NK cells, B cells, and PMNs and stimulates IL-1 secretion.

MODE(S) OF ADMINISTRATION	INDICATIONS	TOXICITIES	NURSING INTERVENTIONS
I.V. infusion over minutes to hours, I.M., S.C., intravesical, intracavitary, intra-arterial.	Investigational in a variety of tumor types (metastatic adenocarcinomas of the colon/rectum, liver; bladder carcinomas, non-small cell lung cancer, renal cell cancer, melanoma.	Dose dependent. Flu-like syndrome (fever, chills progressing to rigors, myalgias, arthralgia, headache, mild bone discomfort), N, V, D, A,* orthostatic hypotension, lightheadedness, weight loss. Elevated liver function tests, transient alterations in blood counts. Severe pain at tumor site, erythema at injection site.	Administer antipyretic before TNF and q 4 hr p.r.n. as ordered. Administer premedication for chills if patient has history of chills. Assess for temperature elevation, chills, other signs of flu-like syndrome. Offer heating pads or extra blankets to decrease chilling. Treat chills with meperidine or morphine as ordered. Monitor vital signs frequently during infusion, or for the first 3 hr after S.C. dose if patient is receiving >100 μg/m². Assess blood pressure in sitting, standing, and lying positions to determine normal saline bolus as ordered to treat hypotension. Instruct client to get up slowly and gradually from lying to sitting, or sitting to standing position. For hypotension, administer N.S. bolus as ordered and see Chapter 13 for additional information. Assess for signs of hepatic involvement (↑ serum bilirubin, AST, ALT, LDH, alkaline phosphatase). Monitor coagulation parameters.

*N = nausea, V = vomiting, D = diarrhea, A = anorexia.

Table 4–6 Indications, Toxicities, and Nursing Interventions for Immunorestorative Agents

IMMUNORESTORATIVE AGENT	MODE(S) OF ADMINISTRATION	INDICATIONS	TOXICITIES	NURSING INTERVENTIONS
Levamisole hydrochloride (Ergamisol) AVAILABLE: Tablets—50 mg.	**P.O.:** initial therapy—50 mg q 8 hr for 3 days; **maintenance**—50 mg q 8 hr for 3 days every 2 weeks × 1 year in combination with 5-fluorouracil. **I.V.:** 450 mg/m²/d for 5 days, then every week. (NOTE: Doses and frequency of both medications vary with different regimens.)	Colon carcinoma, Duke's C colon cancer, in conjunction with 5-fluorouracil.	**M, N, S, D,** V, A,* dermatitis, alopecia, taste, alteration, constipation, abdominal pain, fatigue, fever, arthralgia, myalgia, dizziness, headache, somnolence, blurred vision, abnormal tearing of eyes, conjunctivitis. May produce "antabuse-like" side effects when given concomitantly with alcohol.	Monitor CBC, differential, platelets weekly. Report alterations (NOTE: dosage may be discontinued or reduced for platelet count < 3,500/mm³. Instruct patient to refrain from drinking alcoholic beverages while on therapy.

*M = myelosuppression, N = nausea, V = vomiting, D = diarrhea, A = anorexia, S = stomatitis.
NOTE: In combination with 5-fluorourocil, the following toxicities are common (20% or greater): M, N, V, D, S.

Table 4-7 Indications, Toxicities, and Nursing Interventions for Monoclonal Antibodies

Bind to a specific antigen on cell surface. Seek out and bind to tumor cells. Trials investigating use alone (unconjugated) or bound (conjugated) to radioisotopes, toxins, chemotherapeutic agents, and other BRMs. Act as carriers for delivery of tumoricidal agents to cancer cells.

MODE(S) OF ADMINISTRATION	INDICATIONS	TOXICITIES	NURSING INTERVENTIONS
IV: infusion over 30 min. to 2 hr. Intralymphatic.	Investigational for treatment of a variety of tumors (leukemia, lymphoma, metastatic carcinomas of the breast, ovary, prostate, colon/rectum, renal cell carcinoma). Also used to purge bone marrow of T cells to decrease graft versus host disease in allogeneic transplantation.	**Flu-like syndrome (fever, chills, myalgias, headache malaise).** Anaphylaxis, subacute allergic reactions, N, V, D,* hypotension, dyspnea, erythematous rash, urticaria, pruritus. Delayed toxicity (2–4 weeks after therapy)—serum sickness, flu-like symptoms, malaise, arthralgia, urticaria, pruritus, lymphadenopathy, pulmonary edema, renal failure.	Administer MoAbs by infusion pump, never by gravity flow or controller. Administer antipyretic if ordered. Assess for temperature elevation, other signs of flu-like syndrome. Assess for signs of hypersensitivity reaction (HSR)—apprehension, flushing, urticaria or cutaneous wheals, pallor, dyspnea, diaphoresis, cyanosis, hypotension, tachycardia, cardiac arrhythmias. May lead to coma. Keep medications to treat HSR at bedside (see Chapter 13). Assess blood pressure in sitting, standing, and lying positions to determine alterations. Instruct client to get up slowly and gradually from lying to sitting, or sitting to standing position. Instruct client to report signs of delayed serum sickness (see column 3) or alterations in urinary output should they occur 2–4 weeks after therapy.

*N = nausea, V = vomiting, D = diarrhea.

References

Abernathy, E.: Biotherapy: An introductory review. Oncol. Nurs. Forum 14(6)(suppl.): 13–15, 1987.

Amgen, Inc.: *Colony Stimulating Factors: A Review.* Thousand Oaks, CA, Amgen, Inc., 1990.

Brophy, L., and Trahan Reiger, P.: Implications of biologic response modifier therapy for nursing. In Clark, J.C., and McGee, R.F. (eds.): *Oncology Nursing Society Core Curriculum for Oncology Nursing,* 2nd ed. (pp. 346–358). Philadelphia, W.B. Saunders, 1992.

DeVita, V.T., Hellman, S., and Rosenberg, S.A. (eds.): *Biologic Therapy of Cancer.* Philadelphia, J.B. Lippincott, 1991.

Doweiko, J.P., and Goldberg, M.A.: Erythropoietin therapy in cancer patients. Oncology 5(8):31–37, 1991.

Green, M.R.: *The Role of Colony Stimulating Factors in Chemotherapy-induced Neutropenia.* Seattle, Immunex Corporation, 1991.

Hahn, M.B., and Jassak, P.F.: Nursing Management of patients receiving interferon. Semin. Oncol. Nurs. 4(2):95–101, 1988.

Haeuber, D.: Recent advances in the management of biotherapy-related side effects: Flu-like syndrome. Oncol. Nurs. Forum 16(6):35–41, 1989.

Hauber, D., and DiJulio, J.: Hematopoietic colony stimulating factors: An overview. Oncol. Nurs. Forum 16:247–255, 1989.

Herberman, R.B. (ed.): Cytokines. In *ImmunoPrimer Series.* Emeryville, CA, Cetus Corporation, 1989.

Isaacs, A., and Lindenmann, J.: Virus interference I: The interferon. Proc. R. Soc. London 147:258–267, 1957.

Jassak, P.F.: Biotherapy. In Groenwald, S.L., et al. (eds.): *Cancer Nursing: Principles and Practice,* 3rd ed. (pp. 366–392). Boston, Jones and Bartlett, 1993.

Melin, S.A., and Ozer, H.: Biologic response modifiers: Principles of immunotherapy. In Perry, M.C.: *The Chemotherapy Source Book* (pp. 144–164). Baltimore, Williams and Wilkins, 1992.

Mihich, E., and Fefer, A. (eds.): *Biological Response Modifiers: Subcommittee Report, National Cancer Institute.* Bethesda, MD, National Cancer Institute, 1983.

Morton, D.L., and Economou, J.: Cancer immunology and immunotherapy. In Haskell, C.M. (ed.): *Cancer Treatment,* 3rd ed. (pp. 102–119). Philadelphia, W.B. Saunders, 1990.

Oldham, R.K.: Biologicals and biologic response modifiers: Fourth modality of cancer treatment. Cancer Treat. Rep. 68:221–232, 1984.

Piper, B.F., et al.: Recent advances in the management of biotherapy-related side effects: Fatigue. Oncol. Nurs. Forum 16(6):27–34, 1989.

Quesada, J.R., et al.: Clinical toxicity of interferons in cancer patients: A review. J. Clin. Oncol. 4:234–245, 1986.

St. Pierre, B.A., Kasper, C.E., and Lindsey, A.M.: Fatigue mechanisms in patients with cancer: Effects of tumor necrosis factor and exercise on skeletal muscle. Oncol. Nurs. Forum 19:419–425, 1992.

Suppers, V., and McClamrock, E.A.: Biologicals in cancer treatment: Future effects on nursing practice. Oncol. Nurs. Forum 12(3):27–31, 1985.

Woolery-Antil, M., and Colter, C.: Biological response modifier therapy: Symptom management. In Foley, G., Fochtman, D., and Mooney, K.H. (eds.): *Nursing Care of the Child with Cancer,* 2nd ed. (pp. 179–207). Philadelphia, W.B. Saunders, 1993.

Wujick, D.: Overview of colony-stimulating factors: Focus on the neutrophil. In Carroll-Johnson, R.M.: *A Case Management Approach to Patients Receiving G-CSF* (pp. 8–13). Pittsburgh, Oncology Nursing Press, 1992.

Yasko, J., and Dudjak, L. (eds.): *Biologic Response Modifier Therapy: Symptom Management.* Emeryville, CA, Cetus Corporation, 1990.

Recommended Readings

Amgen, Inc.: *Epogen (Epoetin alfa) Recombinant: Product Monograph.* Thousand Oaks, CA, Amgen, Inc., 1989.

Amgen, Inc.: *Neupogen (Filgrastim): Product Monograph.* Thousand Oaks, CA, Amgen, Inc., 1992.

Anderson, K.C., and Braine, H.G.: Specialized cell component therapy. Semin. Oncol. Nurs. 6(2):140–149, 1990.

Atkinson, K., et al: In vivo administration of granulocyte-colony stimulating factor (G-CSF), granulocyte macrophage colony stimulating factor (GM-CSF), interleukin-1 (IL-1) and interleukin-4 (IL-4) alone and in combination, after allogenic murine hematopoietic stem cell transplantation. Blood 77:1376–1382, 1991.

Beauregard-Dillman, J.: Toxicity of monoclonal antibodies. Semin. Oncol. Nurs. 2(4):107–111, 1988.

Benjamin, D., Knobloch, T.J., and Dayton, M.A.: Human B-cell interleukin-10: B-cell lines derived from patients with acquired immunodeficiency syndrome and Burkitt's lymphoma constitutively secrete large quantities of interleukin-10. Blood 80:1289–1298, 1992.

Betcher, D.L., and Burnham, N.: Granulocyte-macrophage colony-stimulating factor. J. Pediatr. Oncol. Nurs., 8:134–135, 1991.

Biggers, P.B.: Administering epoetin alfa: More RBCs with fewer risks. Nursing 19(4):43, 1989.

Bookman, M.A.: Biologic therapy for cancer. Curr. Opinion Oncol. 1:112–118, 1989.

Brogley, J.L., and Sharp, E.J.: Nursing care of patients receiving activated lymphocytes. Oncol. Nurs. Forum 17:187–193, 1990.

Dillman, J.B.: New antineoplastic therapies and inherent risks: Monoclonal antibodies, biological response modifiers and interleukin-2. J. Intravenous Nurs. 12(2):103–113, 1989.

Dudjak, L.A., and Fleck, A.E.: BRMs: New drug therapy comes of age. RN 54(10):42–47, 1991.

Erslev, A.J.: Erythropoietin. N. Engl. J. Med. 324:1339–1344, 1991.

Eschbach, J.W., and Adamson, J.W.: Guidelines for recombinant human erythropoietin therapy. Am. J. Kidney Dis. 16(2, suppl. 1):2–8, 1988.

Faulds, D., and Sorkin, E.M.: Epoetin (recombinant human erythropoietin): A review of its pharmacodynamic and pharmacokinetic properties and therapeutic potential in anaemia and the stimulation of erythropoiesis. Drugs 38:863–899, 1989.

Foon, K.A.: Biotherapy of cancer with interleukin-2, colony-stimulating factors and monoclonal antibodies. Oncol. Nurs. Forum 15(1):13–22, 1988.

Freimann, J.H., and Markowitz, A.B.: Cytokines and chemotherapy: A new approach for solid tumors. Cancer Bull. 43:224–232, 1991.

Frierdich, S.: Back to the future: Biological response modifiers and colony-stimulating factors. J. Pediatr. Oncol. Nurs. 8:72–75, 1991.

Gabrilove, J.L.: Colony-stimulating factors: Clinical Status. In DeVita, V.T., Jr., et al. *Important Advances in Oncology, 1991* (pp. 215–237). Philadelphia, J.B. Lippincott, 1991.

Gunning, R.: Hematopoietic colony-stimulating factors. Oncol. Nurs. Forum 16:247–255, 1989.

Haynes, A.L.: Clinical uses of interferons, interleukins, tumor necrosis factor, monoclonal antibodies, and growth factors in patients with cancer. J. Pediatr. Oncol. Nurs. 7: 54–55, 1990.

Hogan, C.M.: Coping with biotherapy: Physiological and psychological concerns. Oncol. Nurs. Forum 18(1 suppl.):19–23, 1991.

Hollingshead, L.M., and Goa, K.L.: Recombinant granulocyte-colony stimulating factor (rG-CSF): A review of its pharmacological properties and prospective role in neutropenic conditions. Drugs 42:300–330, 1991.

Howard, M., and O'Garra, A.: Biologic properties of interleukin-10. Immunol. Today 13(6):198–200, 1992.

Jackson, B.S., et al.: Long-term biopsychosocial effects of interleukin-2 therapy. Oncol. Nurs. Forum 18:683–690, 1991.

Jordan, J.: Interferon: Clinical uses and nursing implications. J. Intravenous Nurs. 13:388–391, 1990.

Lehmann, S.: Immune function and nutrition. J. Intravenous Nurs. 14:406–420, 1991.

Mayer, D.: Biotherapy: Recent advances and nursing implications. Nurs. Clin. North Am. 25:291–308, 1990.

Melin, S.A., and Ozer, H.: Biologic response modifiers: Principles of immunotherapy. In Perry, M.C. (ed.): The Chemotherapy Source Book (pp. 144–164). Baltimore, Williams & Wilkins, 1992.

Moldawer, N.P., and Figlin, R.A.: Tumor necrosis factor: Current clinical status and implications for nursing management. Semin. Oncol. Nurs. 4(2):120–125, 1988.

Negrin, R.S., and Greenberg, P.: Therapy of hematopoietic disorders with recombinant colony-stimulating factors. Adv. Pharmacol. 23:263–296, 1992.

Oncology Nursing Society: Biological Response Modifiers Guidelines: Recommendations for Nursing Education and Practice. Pittsburgh, Oncology Nursing Society, 1989.

Pazdur, R., et al.: 5-fluorouracil and recombinant interferon alpha-2a: Review of activity and toxicity in advanced colorectal carcinomas. Oncol. Nurs. Forum 18(suppl. 1): 11–17, 1991.

Sell, S.: Basic Immunology: Immune Mechanisms in Health and Disease. New York, Elsevier, 1987.

Smith, D.H.: Use of hematopoietic growth factors for treatment of aplastic anemia. Am. J. Pediatr. Hematol. Oncol. 12:425–433, 1990.

Wyjcik, D.: An odyssey into biologic therapy. Oncol. Nurs. Forum 20(6):879–887, 1993.

Ziegler, L.D., and Murray, J.L.: Monoclonal antibodies in the treatment of malignancy: Rationale for combined treatments with other biological response modifiers. Cancer Bull. 43:240–245, 1991.

Chapter 5

Cancer Drug Development

Jody Gross, R.N., M.S.N., O.C.N.

Selection of Agents

The first step in the development of agents for the treatment of cancer is the screening of potential new drugs in animal tumor models. Substances are selected for screening because their activity or biochemical design indicates that they may kill tumor cells or inhibit their growth, or through a systematic screening of available compounds. The National Cancer Institute (NCI) is a major developer and sponsor of new antineoplastic agents. Each year, the NCI chooses approximately 10,000 substances (from approximately 40,000 available) for screening in the drug development program (Fig. 5–1). This process involves general screening to identify activity, followed by a more thorough study to identify the most promising agents.

Potential antitumor activity is first assessed using mouse P388 leukemia. Approximately 250 of the active compounds identified in this series are then screened in tumor-bearing mice. The panel of tumors currently used in this stage of testing includes L1210 leukemia, B16 melanoma, M5076 mouse tumor, and MX-1, a human mammary xenograft. Drug activity is determined by analyzing mice for reproducible, significant decreases in the size of the tumors, or increases in the life span of the mice.

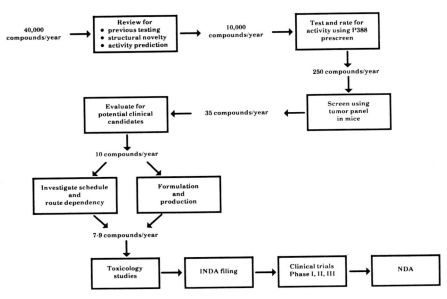

Figure 5–1. National Cancer Institute (NCI) drug development program: Phases of study and new drug research leading to Investigational New Drug Application (INDA). (From Gross, J.: Clinical research in cancer chemotherapy. Oncol. Nurs. Forum 13:59–65, 1986. Reprinted with permission.)

From this series of screening experiments, 10 compounds are chosen as having potential for clinical use.

Determination of Dosage for Use in Humans

Appropriate dosage is determined by drug formulation and production in order to define a clinically feasible dosage form, and testing in experimental tumor systems to define possible dosage schedules.

Toxicology studies are conducted with the seven to nine compounds still remaining, with five to eight drugs ultimately selected for clinical investigation.

Investigational New Drug Application

The manufacturer or sponsor of the drug files an investigational new drug application (INDA) with the Food and Drug Administration (FDA). When IND status is granted, the agent may be administered to humans in specifically defined clinical situations.

After extensive clinical investigation, some drugs that have proven to be useful additions to drugs already in use may be granted a New Drug Application (NDA) by the FDA. At this point the drug can be marketed commercially.

Clinical Investigation

Testing of new drugs for the first time in humans is done routinely in three phases (Table 5–1). Upon successful completion of Phase III studies, the agent becomes commercially available. Chemotherapeutic agents that have been tested already and are commercially available may become part of Phase I, II, or III trials again if they are used in new combinations or administered in new ways.

Phases of Studies

1. Phase I:
   The first phase of testing new antineoplastic agents in humans establishes the maximum tolerated dose (MTD) and the dose-limiting toxicity (DLT) of a drug. The data collected in a Phase I study are analyzed descriptively, since there are no comparisons between groups of patients. Steps in Phase I include:
   a. Determination of initial dose level. This is based upon toxicological information derived from the animal studies conducted in the preclinical investigations. Three patients are entered at the first dose level, the entries occurring about 1 week apart.
   b. Observation of patients for toxicity during a period of therapy, such as two treatment cycles.

Table 5–1   Phases of Clinical Investigation

PHASE	DESCRIPTION
I	Definition of toxicities. Determination of maximum tolerated dose at a given dose and schedule. Investigation of pharmacology.
II	Determination of antitumor activity at a given dose and schedule. Further definition of toxicities.
III	Comparison with other therapies. Recommendations for general use.

Reprinted with permission from Gross, J.: Clinical research in cancer chemotherapy. Oncol. Nurs. Forum *13*:59–65, 1986.

    c. Entry of three additional patients at a pre-established higher dose level, when no irreversible life-threatening or fatal toxicities have occurred.

    d. Determination of MTD: the dose at which toxicities are reversible, treatable, and not life-threatening. This is usually found within five dose escalations, plus or minus three. The expected number of subjects needed for a study of this type is 15 or 20.

    e. Summary of the study findings, including:
      (1) Description of toxicities encountered.
      (2) Severity of toxicities.
      (3) Starting dose for further studies.

Clients entered in these trials already have received treatments and have exhausted current effective cancer therapies. Although agents may have exhibited antitumor activity in preclinical screening, no direct benefit in terms of disease remission can be guaranteed to subjects. Their participation is an indication of their willingness to contribute to the collection of scientific information that may help persons with cancer in the future. Because participants are exposed to greater risk in volunteering to test previously untested or minimally tested drugs, these studies increase the investigator's obligation to successfully complete the trial and proceed to other phases of study. The only reason a Phase I drug is not continued in clinical trials is for unacceptable toxicity or other difficulties encountered in administering the drug to humans.

  2. Phase II:

    a. Begins after Phase I trials have confirmed starting doses and schedules of administration.

    b. Is conducted in order to define the drug's spectrum of activity in humans. This phase usually is studied first in clients with carcinomas of the breast, lung, and colon; lymphoma; leukemia; and melanoma. These represent the leading causes of cancer deaths and lie at opposite extremes in their sensitivity to chemotherapy. Such factors permit study of large numbers of patients in a short period of time and mean that results have an effect on treatment of prevalent cancers. Other tumors may also be studied in Phase II trials if a number of tumor responses were noted in one tumor type in Phase I studies, or the pharmacology of the medication indicates that it may be useful in treating a specific tumor.

    c. Has as its objectives to determine if the new drug is likely to be effective, and if so, to estimate its effectiveness with a certain confidence.

    d. Arrives at initial estimates of the potential number of patients needed for a study. These estimates are based on the premise that the economic and social cost of not identifying an effective drug is greater than the cost of continuing to study an ineffective drug. An estimate is determined by:

(1) Selecting a minimal acceptable response rate. For example, the therapeutic efficacy of pain control with Dilaudid is excellent, so any new analgesic agent would require a high degree of pain relief or an innovative dosage form (such as long-acting morphine) to be considered useful. In colon cancer, for which no truly effective therapy exists, a relatively low response rate in a new drug (about 20 per cent) may still be important.

(2) Estimating the risk of failing to identify an active drug. Typically, this risk, or error rate, is chosen to be 5 per cent or less. If the minimal acceptable response rate is 20 per cent and the true response rate is this low, the probability that the first patient will fail to respond is at least 80 per cent; the probability that two patients will both fail to respond is at least 64 per cent ($0.80 \times 0.80 \times 100$ per cent); and the probability for three patients is 51.2 per cent. These calculations are continued until a 5 per cent probability of failure to respond is reached. In this example, a sample of 14 patients is required to achieve the first objectives of the study. If none of the 14 patients responds, the trial ends with the conclusion that the response rate is less than 20 per cent. If one or more patients respond, then additional patients are studied in order to estimate the true response rate with a certain predetermined confidence. If the standard error of the estimate (inherent variability) is set at 10 per cent, approximately 25 patients are needed to complete the study. Smaller standard errors require more patients (for a standard error of 5 per cent, $N = 100$). For various reasons, such as early discontinuation of treatment or physician or patient decision not to continue, it may be impossible to evaluate some patients for response. In addition, some patients may show no measurable response. To ensure that enough patients have completed the study to allow statistical analysis, a few extra patients usually are entered. As a result, Phase II trials usually involve from 18 to 30 patients.

Most patients treated with drugs in a Phase II trial have received prior treatment, but their disease has progressed or been refractory to

existing standard therapy. In some cancers for which no proven efficacious therapy is available, such as hepatoma or metastatic melanoma,
patients may be offered the opportunity to participate in these studies
as one of the first treatment regimens. As in Phase I trials, the possibility
of risk of the new therapy may outweigh the benefits of a possible
treatment response; on the other hand, a greater chance for therapeutic
benefit exists in this phase. Investigators still have an obligation to complete the trial and analyze the results.

At the completion of Phase II studies, the therapeutic effectiveness
of a drug is determined. This judgment is based on the drug's ability
to decrease the size or growth rate of one or more types of cancer.
For this reason, Phase II trials require that patients have some site of
measurable and quantifiable disease.

Repeated measurements of lesions that are visible by diagnostic imaging or palpable on physical examination are used to determine response. The criteria for response are well established and are described
in Table 5–2.

   3. Phase III:
      a. Is undertaken if response rates in Phase II warrant continued
         clinical trial.
      b. Attempts to determine the usefulness of the drug in the treat-
         ment of disease. This is accomplished through large, random-
         ized trials comparing two or more treatment regimens. The
         new drug may be administered alone, combined with other
         drugs or treatments, or substituted for other drugs or treat-
         ments in standard treatment regimens.

Table 5–2   Criteria for Documentation of Response

DEGREE OF RESPONSE	CRITERIA
Complete response (CR)	Complete disappearance of all known disease for a specified period of time (e.g., 4 weeks, 2 treatment cycles).
Partial response (PR)	50% or greater decrease in size of measurable disease (the sum of the products of the diameters of lesions) and no progression or new disease for a specified time.
Stable disease (SD)	Less than 50% decrease and less than 25% increase in size of measurable disease for a specified time.
Progressive disease (PD)	25% or greater increase in one or more sites of measurable disease or the appearance of new disease.

Reprinted with permission from Gross, J.: Clinical research in cancer chemotherapy. Oncol.
Nurs. Forum *13*:59–65, 1986.

The effectiveness of new drugs or new or changed regimens is compared with the effectiveness of standard drugs or regimens. As in Phase II studies, response is determined using the criteria presented in Table 5–2. Other comparisons that may be made at this stage of investigation include those between two equally effective drugs or regimens, or between different treatment durations of the same drugs or regimens in an attempt to establish less toxic therapy.

Design and sample size considerations for Phase III trials are more complicated than for Phase II trials because the objectives and outcomes of interest are more complicated and can vary considerably from trial to trial. Phase III trials often are large undertakings involving many institutions and hundreds of patients. Cooperation among participating institutions is essential to ensure the quality, accuracy, and comparability of data and measurements. Because these trials are so large, few institutions can complete them alone; a single institution or care provider usually sees too few eligible patients.

Patients who are eligible to participate in these studies have usually received little or no previous therapy. Prior phases of study have indicated that the agent or regimen being tested has some value, and there is every expectation of therapeutic benefit for these patients. Initial Phase III trials are usually conducted in patients with advanced disease, and conclusions from these studies are considered when treating patients with earlier stages of disease. In some instances participation in a Phase III clinical trial may be the best treatment, as there is a strong scientific indication that the study regimen is as good as, if not better than, the standard therapy. It is important to remember that until the trial has been completed, the results analyzed, and (in most instances) the study replicated, the true value of the drug regimen is not known. Often, premature reporting of results or interpretation of data leads to acceptance of therapies without adequate clinical trial, exposing patients to possibly ineffective treatments.

Study Design

Clinical studies all have certain common elements, whether the objective of the research is to evaluate a patient teaching program or to determine the effectiveness of an antiemetic drug or cancer treatment regimen.

The goal of any clinical investigation is to provide the answer to a defined scientific question. In the clinical or laboratory setting this goal is achieved by controlling the conditions of the investigation, in order to ensure that the results of the study are caused by the intervention or variable being investigated (e.g., a new drug) and not by other factors (e.g., sex of patient or stage of disease).

In a laboratory, it is possible to utilize genetically identical animals and establish constant environmental conditions of temperature and humidity, hours of light, and quantity and composition of nutritional and fluid intake. Under these controlled circumstances any difference noted between groups of animals can be attributed to an experimental intervention (e.g., drug, food additive, or negative stimulus) with a great deal of certainty.

Protocols

Standardization and equality are not easily achieved in experiments with humans. For this reason, descriptions of clinical investigations and the instructions for performing these studies are long and detailed. These descriptions and instructions, called *protocols*, include standard sections that explain all aspects of the study.

1. Sections of a protocol include:
   a. Introduction and scientific background.
   b. Objectives.
   c. Selection of patients.
   d. Design of study (including schematic diagram).
   e. Treatment programs.
   f. Procedures in the event of toxicity.
   g. Required clinical and laboratory data.
   h. Criteria for evaluating the effect of treatment.
   i. Statistical considerations.
   j. Informed consent.
   k. Data forms.
   l. References.
   m. Study chairperson, collaborating participants, addresses, and telephone numbers.
2. Protocol sections present:
   a. The objectives of the study.
   b. Available scientific information on the subject, providing the rationale for the particular intervention being studied.
   c. Criteria for including or excluding certain clients, so that participants will be as alike as possible.
   d. Details of the study itself, such as when treatment is administered and at what doses.
   e. Rules for assigning patients to groups so that inevitable dif-

ferences will be spread evenly among groups of participants, and groups will be as alike as possible.

f. Detailed descriptions of the intervention being studied (e.g., drug regimen, patient education, or observation).

g. Parameters used to evaluate the effect of the study intervention (e.g., tumor response, performance on psychological testing, or weight gain).

h. Statistical methods used to measure and analyze these parameters of efficacy.

i. Number of participants required for results to be meaningful.

j. Reference list of relevant literature.

k. Discussion of the ways in which the rights of participants will be protected, and a consent form inviting clients to participate.

Control of study conditions is made possible by adherence to the protocol's comprehensive description of the study. This allows the investigators to collect results that are reliable, easily generalized to larger populations, easily compared with other groups, and easily reproduced in future studies.

Negative results (i.e., a new treatment is not better) are as important as positive results, since ineffective as well as effective interventions and treatments should be identified.

Protection of Human Subjects

Risk/Benefit Ratio.   The risk/benefit ratio of a study is an important consideration. The benefits to the subject of participation and the importance of the scientific information that may be obtained by the study should offset whatever risks may be associated with participation in the investigation. Some studies carry little risk to patients, whereas others carry more. For example, a study whose purpose is a description of current conditions, such as incidence of infection or days of hospitalization, consists primarily of observation and is virtually risk free. In contrast, treatment with new drugs, which may have unknown toxicities and no effect on tumor growth, carries a high degree of risk.

Offsetting the risks of research is the possibility of equal or better therapeutic results when participating in research into new drugs or drug regimens. There is also the benefit to subjects of contributing to the accumulation of new scientific knowledge. For this reason, it is the obligation of every investigator to carefully plan, implement, and complete the research.

Informed Consent.   In addition to the efforts of the investigator to minimize the risks of participation, the rights of subjects in research are protected by providing them with accurate and understandable information. The subject is given both oral and written explanations of:

1. Reasons for the investigation.
2. Procedures utilized, including those for diagnosis and treatment.
3. Alternatives to participate in the study.
4. Risk and benefits of participating.
5. The assurance that questions will be answered at any time and that there will be no adverse effects of refusal to participate.

The elements of informed consent are stipulated by federal regulation and are outlined in Table 5–3.

Institutional Review Boards (IRBs).   All research involving human subjects is reviewed both for scientific validity and for protection of participants. The members of this objective committee are determined by federal regulation and usually include:

1. Physicians and scientists with sufficient expertise to evaluate medical and health-related research.
2. Persons whose primary interests are nonscientific, such as lawyers and clergy.
3. Members of the community who are not affiliated with the institution where the research will be conducted.

An IRB continues to review a research project on at least an annual basis until the study is completed.

Table 5–3   Information Required for Informed Consent

1. Statement regarding study: explanations of purpose duration of participation description of procedure used identification of experimental procedures.	4. Description of maintenance of confidentiality.
	5. Explanation of compensation.
	6. Directions for obtaining further information.
2. Description of risks and benefits.	7. Statement of voluntary participation.
3. Disclosure of alternatives to participation.	

Reprinted with permission from Gross, J.: Clinical research in cancer chemotherapy. Oncol. Nurs. Forum *13:*59–65, 1986.

Nursing Interventions in Clinical Investigations

For a patient to give informed consent to receive treatment for a health-related problem or to participate in a research project, appropriate, understandable, and meaningful information must be made available.

Factors that may interfere with the patient's ability to participate in decisions about his or her treatment include:

1. Age.
2. Lack of understanding of complex treatments.
3. Reluctance to allow knowledgeable health professionals to make decisions.
4. Unclear or inadequate explanations.

Nursing interventions for patients considering participation in clinical research include the following:

1. Serving as advocates for patients who are making decisions during stressful periods, such as time of diagnosis, disease progression, or treatment failure.
2. Interpreting technical explanations of procedures and treatments.
3. Providing printed information and conducting other patient education activities.
4. Communicating unresolved issues to other members of the health care team.
5. Validating patients' perceptions and understanding of the risks, benefits, and goals of research.

Once patients have chosen to participate in a research study, nurses continue to fulfill important roles.

Phase I Studies.   In these studies, nurses are ideally suited to observe the patient for toxicities, record these observations, and develop grading scales for describing toxicities (e.g., nausea and vomiting, fatigue).

Phase II Studies.   The nurse continues to perform the same functions as in Phase I, as well as assisting in careful documentation of response to therapy. Measurements should be taken by the same person, using the same technique, to maintain consistency.

Phase III Studies.   In this stage of investigation, the nurse assumes more data management responsibilities than in Phases I and II. In this role and as coordinator of complex treatment regimens, which differ for each group of patients, the nurse is able to guarantee the accuracy and completeness of data for the most reliable results, thus ensuring that the goals of the study are achieved.

Throughout all phases of study, the nurse continues to serve both as patient advocate and as a liaison between the patient and other health care providers.

Recommended Readings

American Cancer Society: *Clinical Trials for the Treatment of Cancer* (pub. no. 2428). Atlanta, GA, American Cancer Society, 1990.

Antonelli, D.M.: Data management and the cancer treatment protocol. Cancer Nurs. 5:477–479, 1982.

Cassidy, J., and MacFarlane, D.K.: The role of the nurse in clinical cancer research. Cancer Nurs. 14(3):124–131, 1991.

Cheson, B.: Clinical trials programs. Semin. Oncol. Nurs. 7:235–242, 1991.

Conley, B.A., and Van Echo, D.A.: Antineoplastic drug development. In Perry, M.C. (ed.): *The Chemotherapy Source Book* (pp. 15–21). Baltimore, Williams & Wilkins, 1992.

Engelking, C.: Clinical trials: Impact evaluation and implementation considerations. Semin. Oncol. Nurs. 8:148–155, 1992.

Engelking, C.: Facilitating clinical trials: The expanding role of the nurse. Cancer 67(suppl. 6):1793–1797, 1991.

Gordon, V.C., and Wierenga, D.E.: The drug development and approval process. In *New Drug Approvals in 1990*. Washington, DC, Pharmaceutical Manufacturer's Association, 1991.

Grady, C.: Ethical issues in clinical trials. Semin. Oncol. Nurs. 7:288–296, 1991.

Grant, M., Padilla, G., and Ferrell, B.R.: Cancer nursing research. In Groenwald, S.L., et al. (eds.): *Cancer Nursing: Principles and Practice*, 2nd ed. (pp. 1599–1613). Boston, Jones and Bartlett, 1993.

Green, S.B.: Randomized clinical trials: Design and analysis. Semin. Oncol. 8:417–423, 1981.

Gross, J.: Clinical research in cancer chemotherapy. Oncol. Nurs. Forum 13:59–65, 1986.

Gross, S.C., and Garb, S. (eds.): *Cancer Treatment and Research in Humanistic Perspective*. New York, Springer, 1985.

Hazelton, J.: The role of the nurse in Phase I clinical trials. *J. Pediatr. Oncol. Nurs.* 8:43–45, 1991.

Hubbard, S.M.: Cancer treatment research: The role of the nurse in clinical trials of cancer therapy. Nurs. Clin. North Am. 17:763–783, 1982.

Hubbard, S.M.: Principles of clinical research. In Johnson, B.L., and Gross, J. (eds.): *Handbook of Oncology Nursing* (pp. 67–92). Boston, Jones and Bartlett Publishers, 1992.

Hubbard, S.M., and Donehower, M.G.: The nurse in a cancer research setting. Semin. Oncol. 7:9–17, 1980.

Jenkins, J., and Curt, G.: Implementation of clinical trials. In Baird, S.N., et al. (eds.): *Cancer Nursing: A Comprehensive Textbook* (pp. 355–369). Philadelphia, W.B. Saunders, 1991.

Jenkins, J., and Hubbard, S.: History of clinical trials. Semin. Oncol. Nurs. 7:228–234, 1991.

Marcon, S., and Wittes, R.: Clinical development of anticancer drugs: A National Cancer Institute perspective. Cancer Treat. Rep. 68(1):71–85, 1984.

Mayer, D.: Information. In Johnson, B.L., and Gross, J. (eds.): *Handbook of Oncology Nursing* (pp. 115–128). Boston, Jones and Bartlett Publishers, 1992.

McEvoy, M.D., Cannon, L., and MacDermott, M.L.: The professional role for nurses in clinical trials. Semin. Oncol. Nurs. 7:268–274, 1991.

Mili, L.: The community hospital perspective of clinical trials and the role of the nurse educator. Semin. Oncol. Nurs. 7:280–287, 1991.

Melink, T.J., and Whitacre, M.Y.: Planning and implementing clinical trials. Semin. Oncol. Nurs. 7:243–251, 1991.

Miller, A.B., Hoogstraten, B., Staquet, M., and Winkler, A.: Reporting results of cancer treatment. Cancer 47:207–214, 1981.

Nealon, E., Blumberg, B.D., and Brown, B.: What do patients know about clinical trials? Am. J. Nurs. 85:807–810, 1985.

Pocock, S.J.: *Clinical Trials: A Practical Approach.* New York, John Wiley & Sons, 1983.

Reich, S.D.: Clinical trials—a review of terms and principles: Part I. Cancer Nurs. 5:232–233, 1982.

Reich, S.D.: Clinical trials—a review of terms and principles—statistical considerations: Part II. Cancer Nurs. 5:399–402, 1982.

Simon, R.M.: Design and conduct of clinical trials. In DeVita, V.T., Hellman, S., and Rosenberg, S.A. (eds.): *Cancer: Principles and Practice of Oncology,* 3rd ed. (pp. 396–422). Philadelphia, J.B. Lippincott, 1990.

Spilker, B.: *Guide to Clinical Trials.* New York, Raven Press, 1991.

U.S. Code of Federal Regulations, Title 45 CFR 46, Public Welfare: Final regulations amending basic HHS policy for the protection of research subjects. Fed. Reg. 4(16): 8366–8392, January 26, 1981.

U.S. Department of Health, Education and Welfare: *Belmont Report: Ethical Principles and Guidelines for the Protection of Human Subjects of Research.* Washington, DC, Office for Protection from Research Risks, U.S. Department of Health, Education and Welfare, 1979.

U.S. Department of Health and Human Services: *Protection From Research Risks.* Washington, DC, U.S. Department of Health and Human Services, 1979.

Varrichio, C.G., and Jassak, P.F.: Informed consent: An overview. Semin. Oncol. Nurs. 5:95–98, 1989.

Zubrod, C.G.: Origins and development of chemotherapy research at the National Cancer Institute. Cancer Treat. Rep. 68:9–19, 1984.

Chapter 6

Chemoprevention of Cancer

Patricia A. Kramer, R.N., M.S.N., O.C.N.

It is now recognized that the development of cancer is influenced by variables such as genetics, environment, and the immune system. It has been estimated that environmental factors such as diet, use of tobacco, and other lifestyle choices may account for up to 80% of the incidence of cancer. Until recently, research efforts in the field of cancer prevention and control have focused on the identification and elimination of carcinogenic agents (e.g., tobacco). Although these areas continue to be important targets for research, the elimination or avoidance of all carcinogens is neither realistic nor feasible. Other strategies in the field of cancer prevention need to be developed, applied, and promoted if the incidence of cancer is to be reduced significantly.

Carcinogenesis

In recent years, increasing attention has shifted towards the investigation of interrelated causative events in the evolution of human neoplasms. The result has been an increased understanding of the etiology and mechanisms of carcinogenesis. This multistep process involves a dynamic continuum of events leading to the development of a malignancy. The first stage, initiation, involves genetic changes resulting in DNA damage at the cellular level. These cells have the potential to

195

become a neoplastic cell if the mutation is not reversed by cell repair mechanisms prior to cell division. The abnormal, or mutated, cells remain susceptible to the influences of a promoter at any point in time. Promotion, the second stage of carcinogenesis, involves continued stimulation of chemical, physiologic, or biologic carcinogens on the abnormal cells, resulting in their growth and proliferation. The third stage, progression, involves events resulting in additional mutagenic changes and increased malignant behavior (e.g., invasion or metastasis).

This multistep model suggests the possibility of identifying premalignant changes in tissues and subsequently intervening with substances that may reverse or slow down the process leading to frank malignancy. Interventions designed to interfere with carcinogenesis are currently being explored in cancer prevention research.

Strategies in Cancer Prevention Research

Chemoprevention refers to interventions with natural or synthetic substances that demonstrate the potential to prevent, inhibit, or reverse carcinogenesis. The fundamental premise in chemoprevention is that the preinvasive stage of carcinogenesis is not an irreversible process. Epidemiologic, laboratory, and clinical studies support the possibility that chemopreventive agents can inhibit carcinogenesis and, thus, prevent or reverse early premalignant conditions. The proposed relationship between carcinogenesis and chemoprevention is depicted in Figure 6–1.

The Chemoprevention Program, which was established by the National Cancer Institute (NCI) in the 1980s, is designed to identify and evaluate the safety and efficacy of potential cancer-inhibiting compounds. The research process employed by the NCI follows a systematic approach utilizing a variety of methodologies. These include descriptive epidemiology, analytical epidemiology (case-control studies, cohort studies), laboratory studies, and human intervention trials. Epidemiologic and laboratory studies are essential for developing, exploring, and testing hypotheses regarding the etiology of cancer and potential approaches to cancer prevention. Initial interest in a compound as a potential chemopreventive agent generally stems from the results of many laboratory and epidemiologic investigations. Once a compound has been identified as a potential cancer-inhibiting agent, it then must undergo experimental, preclinical evaluation. A variety of animal model systems are used to test agents for efficacy and toxicity. Information obtained from the preclinical studies provides the foundation upon which decisions are made to proceed with the testing of potential chemopreventive agents in humans. Efficacy, toxicity, and ease of adminis-

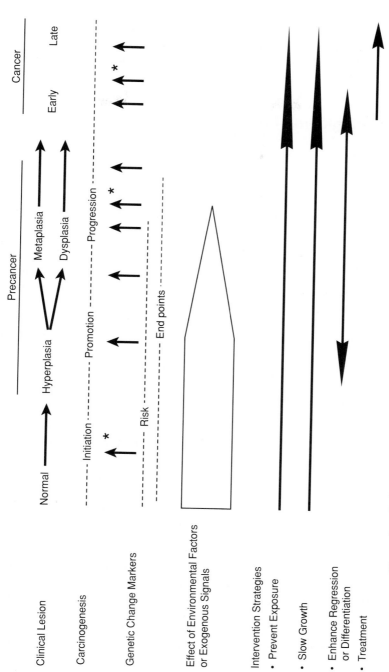

Figure 6–1. Biology and prevention of human preneoplasia. (From Meyskens, F.L., Jr.: Biology and intervention of the premalignant process. Cancer Bull. 43:476, 1991. Copyright 1991 The University of Texas M. D. Anderson Cancer Center, Houston. Reprinted with permission.)

tration of various agents are but a few of the many important factors to be considered prior to the initiation of human trials. A schematic depiction of the NCI's approach to chemoprevention research is presented in Figure 6–2.

Epidemiologic and Laboratory Studies

Laboratory and epidemiologic research findings provide strong evidence that naturally occurring nutrients, synthetic analogues of these nutrients, and a variety of pharmaceuticals and other compounds can markedly influence the growth and development of cancer. Diverse mechanisms of action of potential chemopreventive agents include antioxidant free radical scavengers, inhibitors of cell proliferation, antiinflammatory agents, inducers of cell differentiation, hormone antagonists, and modifiers of oncogene expression.

The most extensively evaluated agents in chemopreventive research are the retinoids (vitamin A and its natural derivatives and synthetic analogues). Vitamin A (or its derivatives) plays a critical role in the normal growth and differentiation of epithelial tissue. In experimental animals, a deficiency of vitamin A is associated with an increased incidence of several types of cancers as well as premalignant changes in some tissues. Examples of synthetic retinoids can be found in Box 6–1.

Research findings from many epidemiologic studies reveal a significant increase in cancer risk associated with a low vitamin A intake. An inverse relationship between low vitamin A intake and the development of lung, upper aerodigestive tract (UADT), colon, and gastric cancers has been identified. Preclinical studies indicate that retinoids inhibit carcinogenesis in a variety of animal model systems, including skin, breast, and bladder. Retinoids have important implications for use in clinical prevention because they can exert their anticarcinogenic effect in cells that have already undergone genetic transformations toward a malignant state.

Beta-carotene, a dietary precursor of vitamin A, also shows promise as a chemopreventive agent. Considerable epidemiologic evidence supports a role for beta-carotene as an inhibitor of epithelial carcinogenesis.

Epidemiologic and laboratory investigations suggest protective roles for a variety of other substances, including vitamin C (ascorbic acid), vitamin E (α-tocopherol), folic acid, selenium, calcium, and NSAIDs.

An inverse association between the ingestion of foods containing vitamin C and the development of cancers of the esophagus, stomach, and colon has been suggested by research findings. Some animal studies support the hypothesis that vitamin E may have protective properties as an antioxidant and free radical scavenger. Selenium, an essential

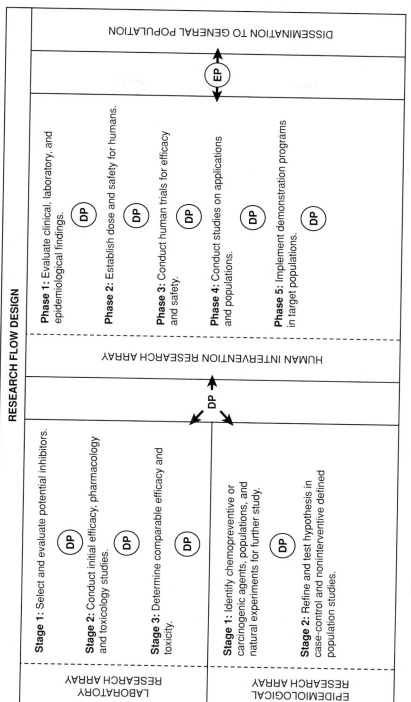

Figure 6–2. Research flow design of NCI Chemoprevention Program. DP, decision point; EP, evaluation point. (From DeVita, V.T., Jr., et al.: *Cancer: Principles and Practice of Oncology*, 4th ed. Philadelphia, J.B. Lippincott, 1993, p. 460. Reprinted with permission.)

> ## Box 6–1
>
> **Retinoids**
>
> Etretinate
> Fenritinide
> Retinol (vitamin A)
> Arotinoid-ethylester
> Tretinoin (all-trans-retinoic acid)
> Isotretinoin (13-*cis*-retinoic acid; acutane)
> All-trans-N-4-hydroxyphenyl retinamide (4-HPR)

---

nutrient, has been shown in more than 70 animal tumor experiments to reduce the incidence of a variety of cancers, and folic acid is being investigated for its role in preventing cervical cancer. The non-steroidal anti-inflammatory drugs (NSAIDs) such as aspirin, indomethacin, piroxicam, and sulindac inhibit the growth of colon tumors in laboratory rodents. Results from recent epidemiologic studies suggest that the regular use of aspirin and other NSAIDs may reduce the risk of fatal colon cancer. Similarly, an inverse association between dietary calcium intake and subsequent colorectal cancer has been identified in other investigations.

Currently, about 100 chemopreventive agents are actively being investigated. The majority of these agents are in the early stages of experimental, preclinical evaluation. A summary of the preclinical data obtained from several of the agents under investigation is outlined in Table 6–1.

Human Intervention Studies

As data from epidemiologic and laboratory studies accumulate, a sound basis is established for testing hypotheses by initiating human trials. Prospective clinical trials generally are accepted as the best method for determining if an agent has chemopreventive activity in humans.

In clinical chemoprevention trials, a target population receives an intervention according to a plan with a specified end point. The population may consist of individuals at high risk because of family history or long-term exposure to a carcinogen (e.g., asbestos, tobacco). Other targeted high-risk individuals would include those with precancerous lesions (e.g., oral leukoplakia), as well as individuals with a personal history of cancer who are currently free of disease but who are at risk for recurrence or new primary lesions.

The use of cancer incidence as a study end point in clinical chemoprevention research necessitates the prolonged duration of prevention trials, which may require a minimum of 5 to 15 years of follow-up. The rationale is simply that the process of carcinogenesis is known to extend over decades for most cancers. It may take several years for any benefit from a potentially preventive agent to become apparent, and that benefit may increase with time. Presently, research is underway to identify reliable *intermediate* end point biomarkers (preinvasive changes in tissues) to facilitate the performance of preventive trials. The careful identification of accurate *intermediate* markers and the role of genetic factors in carcinogenesis could greatly enhance the ability to design effective cancer risk-reduction trials. The presence of specific biomarkers would assist in identifying cancer risk in a study population and would improve the ability to quantify changes in biomarkers resulting from a chemopreventive agent, thus significantly diminishing the length of time needed to conduct these studies.

A particular challenge in chemoprevention research in humans is the task of evaluating acute and chronic toxicity. Unlike acceptable toxicity from a cancer treatment regimen, a cancer prevention intervention must be devoid of notable adverse effects. Toxic effects will decrease compliance and thus the long-term impact of the intervention. Minimal toxicity from long-term administration of a chemopreventive agent is of primary importance. The complex relationship of risks and benefits is a crucial issue that must be addressed and carefully weighed in the performance of human chemoprevention research.

Agents in Chemoprevention

Trials of retinoids in the upper aerodigestive tract (UADT) have indicated that this class of preventive agents has significant activity against oral premalignancy and the development of secondary primary tumors. To date, four positive randomized trials have been reported using three different retinoids. Hong et al. reported the reversal of oral leukoplakia with 13-*cis*-retinoic acid in a randomized, placebo-controlled, phase III trial. Similar findings with vitamin A and 4-hydroxyphenyl retinamide (4-HPR) were reported by Stich and Han, respectively. A randomized adjuvant trial of 13-*cis*-retinoic acid in patients with head and neck cancer demonstrated a significant decrease in the incidence of second primary tumors in this high-risk population. Additional head and neck

Table 6–1 Progress in Chemopreventive Agent Drug Development

AGENT	SOURCE	POSSIBLE MECHANISM OF ACTION	ANIMAL MODEL TEST SYSTEM					PRECLINICAL TOXICOLOGY	PHASE I CLINICAL TRIAL
			SKIN	BREAST	LUNG	COLON	BLADDER		
4-HPR	Synthetic pharmaceutical	Stimulates differentiation	P	P	O	O	P	+	+
Piroxicam	Pharmaceutical	Prostaglandin synthesis inhibitor	O	O	O	P	O	+	+
DFMO	Synthetic pharmaceutical	Ornithine decarboxylase inhibitor, antiproliferative	O	P	P	P	P	+	+
DHEA, DHEA analog(s)	Synthetic pharmaceutical	Glucose-6-phosphate dehydrogenase inhibitor	P	O	O	P	N	+	−
Dithiolthiones	Pharmaceutical	Induces hepatic enzymes that detoxify carcinogens	P	P	P	×	P	+	+
Ellagic acid	Nuts, berries, fruits	Binds benzpyrene	O	P	N	×	P	+	−

Agent	Source	Mechanism							
Molybdate	Mineral, ubiquitous meats, vegetables	Cofactor for xanthine oxidase, maintains differentiation	N	×	P	N	P	+	−
4-HPR-tamoxifen	Combination pharmaceuticals	Stimulates differentiation, binds estrogen receptor	0	P	0	0	0	−	−
4-HPR-selenite-vitamin E	Combination pharmaceutical, mineral, vitamin	Several	N	P	P	×	P	−	−
β-carotene	Green and yellow vegetables	Antioxidant quencher of free radicals	0	0	N	0	N	+	+
β-carotene-vitamin A	Combination green and yellow vegetables—pharmaceuticals	Antioxidant quencher of free radicals, stimulates differentiation	0	0	P	0	0	+	+
Selenite, selenate, selenomethionine	Grains, meat	Component of glutathione peroxidase	N	P	N	N	N	+	−

P, positive; 0, not tested; N, negative; ×, in progress or inconclusive for technical reasons; +, testing satisfactorily completed, in progress, or toxicity evaluation of the agent was not required, because it was generally regarded as safe; —, testing not initiated.

Reprinted with permission from Schatzkin, A., et al.: Research priorities in large bowel cancer prevention. Semin. Oncol. 17:445, 1990.

and lung studies are in progress with retinoids as single agents as well as in combination regimens.

Significant preventive effects with 13-*cis*-retinoic acid also have been noted in patients with xeroderma pigmentosum. A reduction in the incidence of basal cell and squamous cell skin cancers was reported following the administration of 13-*cis*-retinoic acid to this patient population.

Beta-carotene, the next most frequently studied agent, is at an earlier stage of chemopreventive drug development. Data from four clinical trials of beta-carotene have been reported with conflicting results. Although it is an ideal agent for long-term chemoprevention because of its lack of toxicity, the role of beta-carotene in cancer prevention has yet to be defined. Currently, there is clinical interest in a beta-carotene plus retinol combination. Several large-scale chemoprevention trials have been initiated to investigate the role of beta-carotene together with retinol in epithelial carcinogenesis.

Increasing evidence supports a role for tamoxifen as a cancer-inhibiting compound. Data obtained from treatment and adjuvant trials in women with breast cancer indicate that tamoxifen can reduce the incidence of contralateral breast cancer by as much as 50%. The ability of tamoxifen to prevent the development of contralateral breast tumors in premenopausal and postmenopausal women in controlled clinical trials strongly suggests a role for tamoxifen as a potentially effective chemopreventive agent for women at high risk of breast cancer. Adjuvant therapy studies also demonstrate that tamoxifen is well tolerated by most patients and suggest additional health benefits in the form of preservation of bone density and reduction of serum cholesterol. The National Surgical Adjuvant Breast and Bowel Project (NSABP) recently initiated a multi-institutional chemopreventive trial that will evaluate the use of tamoxifen for the prevention of breast cancer in healthy, high-risk women ages 35–69 years. The objectives of this study also include evaluating the cardiovascular and bone effects from tamoxifen in participating women.

Presently, the NCI Chemoprevention Program has more than 20 human intervention trials in progress. These trials are evaluating selective chemopreventive agents with demonstrated potential for inhibiting a variety of common cancers in humans. Studies on the prevention of colon cancer are testing vitamins C and E, beta-carotene, calcium, NSAIDs, and wheat fiber. The prevention of lung and UADT tumors is being studied with various combinations of retinoids, beta-carotene, and vitamin E. Women with cervical dysplasia are being treated with retinoids or folic acid for the prevention of cervical cancer. Four intervention studies are investigating the prevention of skin cancer with retinoids, beta-carotene, and selenium. A summary of the human intervention trials in progress is presented in Table 6–2.

Table 6–2   Chemoprevention Trials in Progress

SITE	TARGET POPULATION	AGENTS
All sites	Healthy male physicians	Beta-carotene, ASA
Bladder	Individuals who are disease-free following resection of TCC	DFMO
Breast	Individuals with a personal history of breast cancer (disease free)	Fenretinide 4-HPR 4-HPR, tamoxifen
	High-risk, healthy women (35–69 yr)	Tamoxifen
Cervix	Individuals with cervical dysplasia	Folic acid Trans-retinoic acid
Colorectal	Individuals with polyposis	Vitamins C, E, fiber Beta-carotene Calcium Sulindac (NSAID) DFMO
Head & neck	Individuals with a personal history of UADTT (free of disease)	13-*cis*-retinoic acid Beta-carotene N-acetylcysteine Beta-carotene, vitamin E Vitamin A and/or N-acetylcysteine
	Individuals with oral leukoplakia	Beta-carotene Vitamin E Retinol, beta-carotene 13-*cis*-retinoic acid
Lung	Smokers	13-*cis*-retinoic acid Beta-carotene, vitamin E
	Individuals with resected NSCLC (free of disease)	Retinyl palmitate Vitamin A and/or N-acetylcysteine
	Tin miners	Beta-carotene, retinol, vitamin E, selenium
	Individuals with occupational exposure to asbestos; smokers	Beta-carotene, retinol
Skin	Individuals with a personal history of squamous/basal cell carcinoma (disease free)	13-*cis*-retinoic acid Beta-carotene Selenium
	Individuals with xeroderma pigmentosum, nevoid, basal cell carcinoma syndrome	13-*cis*-retinoic acid

ASA, acetylsalicylic acid (aspirin); TCC, transitional cell carcinoma; DFMO, 2-difluoromethylornithine; UADTT, upper aerodigestive tract tumor; NSCLC, non-small cell lung cancer; NSAID, non-steroidal anti-inflammatory drug; 4-HPR, 4-hydroxyphenyl retinamide.

Future Directions

The field of cancer prevention and control is at the forefront of exciting new changes, challenges, and breakthroughs. Important strides made in understanding carcinogenesis have created new possibilities for effective prevention. The development of chemopreventive strategies offers hope that cancer deterrence is a realistic prospect. Yet, many questions still need to be addressed and answered. The results of early, promising prevention studies need to be replicated and verified. Large scale, randomized, placebo-controlled, Phase III trials are needed to accurately and precisely define the role of potential cancer-inhibiting compounds. As we continue to learn more about the biology of cancer and gain experience with chemoprevention and the performance of clinical trials, the possibilities for the future of cancer prevention are endless.

References

Bakemeyer, A.H.: The potential role of vitamins A, C, and E and selenium in cancer prevention. Oncol. Nurs. Forum 15:785–791, 1988.

Bernstein, L., Ross, R.K., and Henderson, B.E.: Prospects for primary prevention of breast cancer. Am. J. Epidemiol. 135(2):142–152, 1992.

Castonguay, A.: Methods and strategies in lung cancer control. Cancer Res. 52(Suppl.): 2641s–2651s, 1992.

Clark, L.C., et al.: Design issues in cancer chemoprevention trials using micronutrients: Application to skin cancer. Cancer Bull. 43:519–524, 1991.

Earnest, D.L., et al.: Inhibition of prostaglandin synthesis: Potential for chemoprevention of human colon cancer. Cancer Bull. 43:561–568, 1991.

Garewal, H.S., and Meyskens, F.L., Jr.: Chemoprevention of cancer. In Nixon, D.W. (ed.): Hematol./Oncol. Clin. North Am. 5(1):69–77, 1991.

Garewal, H.S., et al.: Response of oral leukoplakia to beta-carotene. J. Clin. Oncol. 8:1715–1720, 1990.

Garland, C., et al.: Dietary vitamin D and calcium and risk of colorectal cancer: A 19-year prospective study in men. Lancet 2:307–309, 1985.

Goodman, G.E.: The clinical evaluation of cancer chemoprevention agents: Defining and contrasting phase I, II, and III objectives. Cancer Res. 52(Suppl.):2752s–2757s.

Greenwald, P., and Clifford, C.: Principles of cancer prevention: Diet and nutrition. In DeVita, V.T., Jr., Hellman, S., and Rosenberg, S.A. (eds.): Cancer: Principles and Practice of Oncology, 4th ed. (pp. 443–479). Philadelphia, J.B. Lippincott, 1993.

Greenwald, P., Cullen, J.W., and Weed, D.: Introduction: Cancer prevention and control. Semin. Oncol. 17:383–390, 1990.

Han, J., et al.: Evaluation of N-4-(hydroxycarbophenyl) retinamide as a cancer prevention agent and as a cancer chemotherapeutic agent. In Vivo 4:153–160, 1990.

Hong, W.K., et al.: 13-cis-retinoic acid in the treatment of oral leukoplakia. N. Engl. J. Med. 315:1501–1505, 1986.

Hong, W.K., et al.: Prevention of second primary tumors with isotretinoin in squamous cell carcinoma of the head and neck. N. Engl. J. Med. 323:795–801, 1990.

Kelloff, G.J., et al.: Progress in applied chemoprevention research. Semin. Oncol. *17*:438–455, 1990.

Kraemer, K.H., et al.: Prevention of skin cancer in xeroderma pigmentosum with the use of oral isotretinoin. N. Engl. J. Med. *318*:1633–1637, 1988.

Krytopoulos, S.A.: Ascorbic acid and the formation of n-nitrose compounds: Possible role of ascorbic acid in cancer prevention. Am. J. Clin. Nutr. *45*:1344–1350, 1987.

Lippman, S.M., Hong, W.K.: Chemoprevention of aerodigestive tract carcinogenesis. Cancer Bull. *93*:525–533, 1991.

Lippman, S.M., et al.: Biomarkers as intermediate endpoints in chemoprevention trials. J. Natl. Cancer Inst. *82*:555–560, 1990.

Love, R.R.: Antiestrogen chemoprevention of breast cancer: Critical issues and research. Prev. Med. *20*(1):64–78, 1991.

McLarty, J.: An intervention trial in former asbestos workers. Cancer Bull. *43*:538–543, 1991.

Menkes, M.S., et al.: Serum beta-carotene, vitamins A and E, selenium and the risk of lung cancer. N. Engl. J. Med. *15*:1250–1254, 1986.

Meyskens, F.L., Jr.: Biology and intervention of the premalignant process. Cancer Bull. *43*:475–480, 1991.

Meyskens, F.L., Jr.: Coming of age: The chemoprevention of cancer. N. Engl. J. Med. *323*:825–827, 1990.

Moon, T.E.: Statistical considerations for chemoprevention trials. Cancer Bull. *43*:515–518, 1991.

Nayfield, S.G., et al.: Potential role of tamoxifen in prevention of breast cancer. J. Natl. Cancer Inst. *83*:1450–1459, 1991.

Pastorino, U.: Lung cancer chemoprevention: Facts and hopes. Lung Cancer *7*:133–150, 1991.

Ryan, D.H., and Starr, B.M.: Vitamins in prevention and treatment of cancer. Contemp. Oncol. *2*:45–65, 1992.

Sacks, P.G., Hong, W.K., and Hittelman, W.N.: In vitro studies of the premalignant process: Initial culture of oral premalignant lesions. Cancer Bull. *43*:485–489, 1991.

Schatzkin, A., Schiffman, M., and Lanza, E.: Research priorities in large bowel cancer prevention. Semin. Oncol. *17*:425–437, 1990.

Stich, H.F., et al.: Response of oral leukoplakias to the administration of vitamin A. Cancer Lett. *40*:93–101, 1988.

Thun, M.J., Namboodiri, M.M., and Heath, C.W., Jr.: Aspirin use and reduced risk of fatal colon cancer. N. Engl J. Med. *325*:1593–1596, 1991.

Veronesi, U., and Costa, A.: Breast cancer chemoprevention. Cancer Treat. Res. *60*:357–367, 1992.

Vogel, V.G.: Prevention of breast cancer with tamoxifen. Cancer Bull. *43*:569–573, 1991.

Wattenberg, L.W., et al.: *Cancer Chemoprevention.* Boca Raton, FL, CRC Press, 1992.

Wattenberg, L.W.: Inhibition of carcinogenesis by minor dietary constituents. Cancer Res. *52*(suppl.):2085s–2091s, 1992.

Weinstein, I.B.: Cancer prevention: Recent progress and future opportunities. Cancer Res. *51*(18, suppl.):5080s–5085s, 1991.

Nursing Management of Problems Associated with Chemotherapy and Biotherapy

Chemotherapeutic and biologic agents are effective in the treatment of cancer in part because of the effects they have on the dividing cell. During therapy, normal cells as well as tumor cells are affected by these agents. Tumor cells divide rapidly in the body. Other cells with high turnover rates include those of the bone marrow, oral and gastrointestinal linings, and integumentary system (skin, hair, and nails), which are frequently proliferating to renew supplies.

Many antineoplastic agents affect the most rapidly dividing cells, causing the common toxicities of myelosuppression, nausea and vomiting, anorexia, diarrhea, alopecia, and skin and nail changes. Organ system toxicity due to cancer therapy occurs with less frequency in the reproductive, renal, cardiac, neurological, and hepatic systems, and in the eye and ear.

Some chemotherapeutic agents cause alterations in the fluid and electrolyte balance in the body. Biologic agents may cause fevers, chills, and rigors. A small number in each category may cause psychological alterations, such as anxiety and depression. These and other effects of antineoplastic agents and biologic response modifiers are summarized in the tables that follow.

(*Text continued on page 220*)
209

Summary of Toxicities of Antineoplastic Agents

GENERIC NAME (BRAND NAME)	VESICANT	NAUSEA AND VOMITING	ANOREXIA	DIARRHEA	STOMATITIS	ALOPECIA	MYELOSUPPRESSION
Aldesleukin (Proleukin, Interleukin-2, IL-2)		×	×	×	×		×
Altretamine (Hexalen)		×	×				×
Amsacrine (AMSA-PD, M-AMSA)	V	×			×		×
Asparaginase (Elspar, Kidrolase, L-ASP)		×					Mild
Bleomycin (Blenoxane)		×			×	Rare	Rare
Busulfan, busulphan (Myleran)		Mild	×			×	×
Carboplatin (Paraplatin)		×					×
Carmustine (BiCNU, BCNU)		×					×
Chlorambucil (Leukeran)		Mild	Mild				×
Cisplatin (Platinol, CIS, DDP)		×	×				×
Cladribine (Leustatin, 2-CDA)		×	×	×			×
Cyclophosphamide (Cytoxan, Endoxan, Neosar, Procytox)		×	×	×		×	×

PULMONARY	RENAL	HEPATIC	NEUROLOGICAL	REPRODUCTIVE	OTHER
	×	×			Fever, chills, rigors, pruritis, bone pain, urticaria. Altered mental status, impaired thyroid function, capillary leak syndrome.
			×	×	Fatigue, skin rash, agitation, confusion, dizziness, vertigo, ataxia, mood disorders. May develop postural hypotension when administered with MAO inhibitors.
			×	×	Pain and local phlebitis at infusion site if not adequately diluted, cardiotoxicity when administered to the client with low serum potassium. Pruritus, rash, and discoloration of skin and urine.
	×	×	×		Hyperpigmentation along vein, hyperglycemia, depression of clotting factors, fatigue, confusion, agitation, somnolence, personality changes, anaphylaxis.
×	×	×		×	Rash, photosensitivity, hyperpigmentation, fever, flulike syndrome, anaphylaxis.
×		×	×	×	Hyperpigmentation, cataract formation, hyperuricemia.
	×	×	×		Hypocalcemia, hypomagnesemia, hyponatremia, ototoxicity. Cardiotoxicity (rare).
×	×	×			Burning at infusion site and facial flushing if infused rapidly.
Rare		Rare	×	×	Dermatitis, urticaria.
	×		×		Ototoxicity, hyperuricemia, anaphylaxis, hypermagnesemia, hypocalcemia, hypokalemia, hypophosphatemia.
×	×		×		Rash, malaise, myalgia, arthralgia. **WITH HIGH DOSES:** Irreversible paraparesis/quadraparesis, acute nephrotoxicity.
Rare	×	Rare		×	Hemorrhagic cystitis, hyperpigmentation, cardiac toxicity (at high dose only), hyponatremia. May potentiate cardiotoxic effects of daunorubicin, doxorubicin.

(Continued)

Summary of Toxicities of Antineoplastic Agents (Continued)

GENERIC NAME (BRAND NAME)	VESICANT	NAUSEA AND VOMITING	ANOREXIA	DIARRHEA	STOMATITIS	ALOPECIA	MYELOSUPPRESSION
Cytarabine (Cytosar-U, Cytosan, Tarabine, Ara-C)		×	×	×	×		×
Dacarbazine (DTIC, DTIC-Dome)	I	×	×	Rare		Rare	×
Dactinomycin (Cosmegen, Actinomycin-D)	V	×	×	×	×	×	×
Daunorubicin HCl (Cerubidine)	V	×			×	×	×
Doxorubicin HCl (Adriamycin RDF)	V	×			×	×	×
Epirubicin HCl (Pharmorubicin)	V	×		×	×	×	×
Etoposide (VePesid, VP-16-213)		×	×	×		×	×
Filgrastim (Neupogen, G-CSF)							
5-Fluorouracil (5-FU, Adrucil, Efudex, Fluoroplex)		×	×	×	×	×	×
Floxuridine (FUDR)		×	×	×	×	×	×
Fludarabine (Fludara)		×	×	×	×		×
Hydroxyurea (Hydrea, OH-urea)		Mild	×	×	Rare	Rare	×
Idarubicin (Idamycin)	V	×		×	×	×	×

PULMONARY	RENAL	HEPATIC	NEUROLOGICAL	REPRODUCTIVE	OTHER
×	×	×	×	×	Thrombophlebitis at infusion site, Ara-C syndrome (see Table 3–3), anaphylaxis, pancreatitis, fever, rash, conjunctivitis.
		Rare	×		Facial flushing, pain at infusion site, paresthesias, erythema, urticaria, photosensitivity, flulike syndrome.
				×	Rash, hyperpigmentation, photosensitivity, radiation recall, thrombophlebitis, hypocalcemia, coagulation disorders.
		×	×	×	Rash, chills, fever, cardiotoxicity, hyperuricemia, radiation recall.
				×	Radiation recall, flulike syndrome, photosensitivity, cardiotoxicity (cumulative, orange/reddish urine × 24 hr), hyperuricemia, urticaria, flare along vein track, hyperpigmentation.
			Headache	×	Radiation recall, urticaria, streaking along vein, phlebitis at infusion site, fever, cardiotoxicity.
			×	×	Orthostatic hypotension if infused too rapidly, muscle cramps, anaphylaxis.
					Bone pain, rash, fever, splenomegaly, pain at injection site.
				×	Photosensitivity, dermatitis, increased lacrimation, blurred vision, ataxia, slurred speech.
					Dermatitis, rash, esophagopharyngitis, abdominal cramps, gastritis, malaise.
×	×		×		Fever, chills, myalgia, fatigue, rash, dysuria, edema, tumor lysis syndrome.
	×			×	Reversible renal tubular dysfunction, facial erythema.
			×	×	Cardiotoxicity, urticaria, rash, local reaction at injection site, abdominal cramps, peripheral neuropathy.

(Continued)

Summary of Toxicities of Antineoplastic Agents (Continued)

GENERIC NAME (BRAND NAME)	VESICANT	NAUSEA AND VOMITING	ANOREXIA	DIARRHEA	STOMATITIS	ALOPECIA	MYELOSUPPRESSION
Ifosfamide (Ifex)		×	×		×	×	
Alfa Interferon (α IFN, Intron-A, Roferon-A)		N, Vr (mild)		Mild		× (partial)	
Interleukin-2 (see aldesleukin)							
Levamisole (Ergamisol)		×	×	×	Rare		Rare
Lomustine (CeeNU, CCNU)		×	×		Rare	Rare	×
Mechloreth-amine (Mustargen, HN²)	V	×	×	×		×	×
Melphalan (Alkeran)		Rare				×	×
Mercaptopurine (Purinethol, 6-MP)		×	×		×		×
Methotrexate (Folex, Mexate)		×	×	×	×	×	×
Mitomycin (Mutamycin, Mitomycin-C)	V	×	×	×	×	×	×
Mitotane (Lysodren)		×	×	×			
Mitoxantrone (Novantrone)	I	×			×	×	×
Monoclonal antibodies							

PULMONARY	RENAL	HEPATIC	NEUROLOGICAL	REPRODUCTIVE	OTHER
	×		×		Hematuria, cystitis, fatigue, weakness, hallucinations.
	×	×	×		Fever, chills, rigors, myalgia, fatigue, arthralgia, headache, mild pruritis, decreased concentration, depression, somnolence, ataxia, hypotension, taste alterations.
		Rare	×		Dermatitis, flulike syndrome, arthralgia, myalgia, taste alterations, headache, somnolence.
Rare	×	Rare		×	
		Rare	×	×	Hyperuricemia, thrombophlebitis at infusion site, metallic taste, ototoxicity.
Rare			Headache	×	Maculopapular rash, urticaria.
	Mild	×			Hyperuricemia, cholestatic jaundice.
Rare	×	×	×	×	Photosensitivity, flulike syndrome, transient paresis, blurred vision, taste alterations.
Rare	×			×	Dermatitis, pruritus, phlebitis, fever, malaise, blurred vision.
	×		×		Rash, visual blurring, diplopia, retinopathy, hematuria, hemorrhagic cystitis, hypertension, orthostatic hypotension.
×	Rare	Rare		×	Cardiotoxicity, blue-green urine, bluish discoloration of vein, and sclerae during therapy.
		Rare	×		Urticaria, pruritis, fever, chills, rigors, myalgia, fatigue, arthralgia, anaphylaxis (rare).

(Continued)

Summary of Toxicities of Antineoplastic Agents (Continued)

GENERIC NAME (BRAND NAME)	VESICANT	NAUSEA AND VOMITING	ANOREXIA	DIARRHEA	STOMATITIS	ALOPECIA	MYELOSUPPRESSION
Paclitaxel (Taxol)		×		×	×	×	×
Pentostatin (Nipent)		×		×			Mild
Plicamycin (Mithracin)	I	×	×	×	×		
Procarbazine (Matulane, Natulan)		×	×	×	Rare	×	×
Sargramostim (Leukine, Prokine)							
Streptozocin (Zanosar)		×		×	Rare	×	×
Teniposide (Vumon)		×	×	×	Rare	×	×
Thioguanine (Lanvis, 6-TG)		×	×	×	×		×
Thiophosphoramide (Thiotepa)		×	×				×
Tumor necrosis factor							
Vinblastine (Velban, Velbe)	V	×	×	×	×	×	×
Vincristine (Oncovin, Vincasar)	V	×	×			×	Mild
Vindesine (Eldisine)	V	×	×	×	×	×	×

V = vesicant, I = irritant, N = nausea only, Vr = vomiting rare.

PULMONARY	RENAL	HEPATIC	NEUROLOGICAL	REPRODUCTIVE	OTHER
×	×	×	×		Local erythema along vein, urticaria, pruritis, peripheral neuropathy, fatigue, headache, taste alterations.
		×	×	×	Rash, pruritis, fever, confusion, fatigue, pain.
	Mild			×	Fever, hypocalcemia, coagulation disorder, hypokalemia, hypophosphatemia.
Rare		×	×	×	Dermatitis, hyperpigmentation, fever, diaphoresis, myalgia, arthralgia.
×					Fever, malaise, rash, edema, pericardial effusion.
	×	×			Decreased glucose tolerance, hypoglycemia, glycosuria.
	Rare	Rare	Rare		Hypotension may occur with rapid administration.
	×			×	Hyperuricemia.
				×	Local pain at infusion site, dizziness, headache, allergic reaction (rare).
×					Irritation at injection site, myalgia, headache, bone pain, fever, chills, rigor, transient elevations in hepatic enzymes.
			×	×	Constipation, paresthesias, loss of deep tendon reflexes, mental depression, headache.
			×	×	Constipation, increased excretion of antidiuretic hormone, peripheral neuropathy (motor weakness, loss of deep tendon reflexes, jaw pain).
			×	×	Constipation, increased excretion of antidiuretic hormone.

Side Effects Associated with Hormonal Therapy

GENERIC NAME (BRAND NAME)	EDEMA OR FLUID RETENTION	WEIGHT GAIN	APPETITE	SALT/WATER RETENTION	NAUSEA, VOMITING	HOT FLASHES	VAGINAL BLEEDING	MENSTRUAL IRREGULARITY	HEADACHE
Aminoglutethimide (Cytadren)			↓		+				
Cyproterone acetate (Androcur)	+								+
Estrogen	+			+	+ +		+	+	+
Flutamide (Eulexin)					+	+			+
Fluoymesterone Android F, Halotestin)	+	+	↑	+				+	+
Goserlin acetate implant (Zoladex)			↓			+			
Leuprolide (Lupron, Lupron depot)			↓		+	+			+
Megestrol acetate (Megace, Pallace)		+ +	↑	+		+	+		
Prednisone		+	↑	+					
Tamoxifen citrate (Nolvadex)	+	+			+	+ +	+	+	+

GYNECOMASTIA	LETHARGY	ALTERED LIBIDO	ERECTILE IMPOTENCE	TUMOR FLARE	HYPERCALCEMIA	ADDITIONAL TOXICITIES AND COMMENTS
	+					Skin rash common. Hypotension may occur. Thrombocytopenia. Liver function tests may be elevated. Suppresses adrenal function in 3–5 days. Drowsiness, ataxia. Lethargy (more common in elderly). Consider drug withdrawal if rash persists for more than 5–8 days during therapy. Avoid taking antacid within 2 hr of taking enteric coated tablet.
						Mood changes, gastrointestinal disturbance. Use with caution in person with liver dysfunction.
+ +						Abdominal pain. Take with food to minimize nausea. May be poorly metabolized in patients with liver dysfunction. Vaginal candidiasis may occur. Gingivitis may occur—encourage good oral hygiene. Thrombophlebitis may occur.
+		+	+			Sexual dysfunction, lethargy, insomnia, diarrhea, ↑ pain at tumor site and bone pain for first 30 days, CHF.
						Voice alterations (may not improve after drug is discontinued). Acne, alopecia (virulism).
		+	+	+	+	Hot flashes, sexual dysfunction, lethargy, ↑ pain at tumor site and bone pain for first 30 days.
		↓	+	+		Constipation, dizziness, breast tenderness, diarrhea. Urine may become amber or green-yellow.
				+		Relatively nontoxic. DVT, alopecia may occur. Therapeutic effect seen after 2 mo.
						Cushingoid symptoms may occur. Gastrointestinal upset common. Increased appetite. Anxiety, irritability, depression may be minimized by tapering dose over 3–4 days.
				+	+	Tumor flare, especially increase in bone pain for first 3–7 days after therapy begins. May take as adjuvant therapy for 3–5 yr. Monitor calcium level. Advise use of nonhormonal contraception.

+ = occurrence common with mild intensity, + + = occurrence more frequent and usually more intense, ↑ = increased frequency or intensity, ↓ = decreased frequency or intensity.

Adapted with permission from Goodman, M.: Concepts of hormonal manipulation in the treatment of cancer. Oncol. Nurs. Forum 15:639–647, 1988.

The World Health Organization (WHO) toxicity grading scales, or those developed by cooperative oncology study groups, can be used as a standard for assessment and quantification of toxicities. A grading scale for mucositis/stomatitis can be found in Chapter 10 and a grading scale for hypersensitivity reactions in Chapter 13. The WHO grading scales for all system toxicities can be found in Appendix G.

Toxicities, or side effects, of antineoplastic agents may be classified as acute, chronic, or delayed. As more persons survive cancer and go on to live following completion of therapy, we are becoming more aware of late effects of chemotherapy, which are addressed in Chapter 12.

This section includes information that will help the nurse understand and recognize effects of chemotherapy and/or biotherapy on the physiological and psychological status of the patient, and develop appropriate goals and interventions for clients receiving chemotherapy and/or biotherapy. Most information is presented as a plan for care so that it may be adapted for use in your hospital or agency. Care plans adhere to the 1986 ANA/ONS Guidelines for Nursing Practice and the 1991 NANDA nursing diagnoses.

This book was written for the nurse who is familiar with all phases of the nursing process. Nursing assessment directs the formulation of nursing diagnoses; patient outcomes and nursing interventions emanate from the assessment. It is therefore assumed that a complete nursing assessment will precede each nursing diagnosis.

Recommended Readings

American Nurses' Association and Oncology Nursing Society: *Standards of Oncology Nursing Practice.* Kansas City, MO, American Nurses' Association, 1987.

Burke, M.B., Wilkes, G.M., and Ingwersen, K.: *Chemotherapy Care Plans: Designs for Nursing Care.* Boston, Jones and Bartlett, 1992.

Carpenito, L.: *Handbook of Nursing Diagnosis,* 4th ed. Philadelphia, J.B. Lippincott, 1991.

Carpenito, L.: *Nursing Diagnosis: Application to Clinical Practice,* 3rd ed. Philadelphia, J.B. Lippincott, 1989.

Daeffler, R.J., and Petrosino, B.M.: *Manual of Oncology Nursing Practice Nursing Diagnoses and Care.* Rockville, MD, Aspen, 1990.

Doenges, M.E., Moorhouse, M.F., and Geissler, A.C.: *Nursing Care Plans: Standards for Planning Patient Care,* 3rd ed. Philadelphia, F.A. Davis, 1993.

Goodman, M.: Managing the side effects of chemotherapy. Semin. Oncol. Nurs. 5(2, suppl. 1):29–52, 1989.

Gordon, M.: *Manual of Nursing Diagnosis, 1990–1991.* St. Louis, Mosby–Year Book, 1991.

Gulanick, M., Knoll, M., and Wilson, C.R.: *Nursing Care Plans for Newborns and Children.* St. Louis, Mosby–Year Book, 1992.

Kim, M.J., McFarland, G.K., and McLane, A.M.: *Pocket Guide to Nursing Diagnosis.* St. Louis, Mosby–Year Book, 1991.

Lilley, L.L.: Side effects associated with pediatric chemotherapy: Management and patient issues. Pediatr. Nurs. 16:252–257, 1990.

Chapter 7

Hematopoietic Alterations Associated with Chemotherapy and Biotherapy

Linda Tenenbaum, R.N., M.S.N., O.C.N.
Debi Leshin, R.N., B.S.N., O.C.N.

Normal Cell Maturation

Hematopoiesis is the development of mature blood cells from the **pluripotent stem cells,** or precursor cells in bone marrow. As cells develop through blast and less mature phases, maturation and differentiation results and, finally, mature cells are released into the bloodstream. The process of cell maturation is dependent in part on the body's natural production of biologic response modifiers, which are covered in more detail in Chapter 4. Figure 4–3 depicts the role of individual factors in hematopoiesis.

Myelosuppression

Myelosuppression is a common and often dose-limiting effect of most antineoplastic agents. The degree of myelosuppression will vary with the agent and dose. Other factors that may influence myelosuppression are age (younger patients are more tolerant of a given dose than the elderly); amount of bone marrow reserve; degree of compromise by prior chemotherapy and/or radiation therapy; nutritional status (myelosuppression is more pronounced with a negative nitrogen balance and

223

its associated weight loss); and ability of the hepatic and renal systems to metabolize and/or excrete the compounds (Dewys, et al., 1980; Creaven and Mihich, 1977).

Myelosuppression has a greater effect on the bone marrow than it does on the peripheral blood count. When the stem cell is affected, all cell lines will be suppressed. This occurs frequently with nitrosoureas. Other antineoplastic agents affect the cell cycle at specific phases (see Chapter 1).

The normal white blood cell (WBC) count is 4000–10,000 leukocytes/ mm^3. **Leukopenia,** which is a reduction in the number of total circulating WBCs (granulocytes, lymphocytes, and monocytes) below 4000/ mm^3, is a common side effect of most chemotherapy agents. L-asparaginase, bleomycin, cisplatin, methotrexate (with leucovorin rescue), and streptozocin have mild myelosuppressive activity.

The time at which chemotherapy exerts its maximum effect on the bone marrow and the blood count reaches its lowest point is referred to as the *nadir*. This varies with individual agents, but usually occurs 7–14 days after administration of the medication. Nadirs for leukocytes, platelets, and erythrocytes may be the same with one agent, or may show slight variation. WBC and thrombocyte nadirs of antineoplastic agents appear in Table 7–1.

Granulocytopenia, or deficiency of granulocytes (neutrophils, basophils, and eosinophils), is a major consequence of the myelosuppressive effect of antineoplastic agents. Granulocytes are our first line of defense against infection. Neutrophils, the most numerous of granulocytes, play an important role as phagocytes against foreign microorganisms. Box 7–1 indicates the formula for calculation of the absolute neutrophil count (ANC). With **neutropenia** (circulating neutrophils < 1000/mm^3), the risk of infection increases. Neutropenia is often associated with a high mortality rate, secondary to systemic bacterial and fungal infections, in the immunocompromised patient. Over time, a patient with an ANC less than 500/mm^3 will develop a significant infection that requires aggressive management (Brandt, 1990). Neutropenia has been cited as a major cause of infection-related deaths in the patient with cancer (Rostad, 1991; Brandt, 1990). The risk of infection increases if the duration of neutropenia is prolonged. Inadequate WBCs of any type may aggravate an existing or developing infectious process.

Nursing interventions to prevent infection must be taken in the immunocompromised patient. Anti-infective (antibiotic, antifungal, and/ or antiviral) agents may be administered prophylactically or specific to the sensitivity of the cultured organism(s).

Thrombocytopenia is a decrease in the number of circulating platelets below 75,000/mm^3. The patient with thrombocytopenia must be observed closely for evidence of superficial or internal bleeding. The risk of mild bleeding episodes is present when the platelet count drops below 50,000/mm^3; spontaneous bleeds or major bleeding episodes may occur when the count is below 20,000/mm^3. Administration of platelet concentrate may be indicated.

The patient who receives chemotherapy in an outpatient clinic or physician's office must be taught to observe for evidence of bleeding and report significant findings to the physician or nurse. All persons with low platelet counts must be taught to avoid trauma or injury. Drugs which may result in prolonged bleeding must be avoided or, if prescribed, used with caution when a low platelet count exists. This includes some prescription drugs and many over-the-counter medications that contain acetylsalicylic acid (aspirin) and other forms of salicylates or salicylamides, or non-steroidal anti-inflammatory drugs (NSAIDs). Medications in these groups are listed in Table 7–2.

Anemia results when the number of circulating erythrocytes (red blood cells [RBCs]) decreases, as indicated by decreased hemoglobin and hematocrit levels. It is present in patients with cancer (more often as a result of the disease process), but may be related to or aggravated by the myelosuppressive effect of chemotherapy or biotherapy on the developing RBC.

A plan of care for the patient with altered hematopoietic status can be found in Table 7–3.

Recent Advances in the Management of the Patient with Altered Hematopoietic Status

In past years, researchers have identified lymphokines and growth factors that are capable of stimulating cell growth and antibody production. These are discussed in detail in Chapter 4.

Erythropoietin

Erythropoietin, a naturally occurring growth factor, stimulates erythrocyte production in response to the body's need. The primary site of production is in the kidneys. A recombinant form of erythropoietin (epoetin alfa, Epogen, Procrit, EPO) has been used in the management of anemia associated with renal failure for many years. Epoetin alfa was approved in 1993 for use in persons with a low erythrocyte count caused by cancer, or to treat the myelosuppressive effects of antineoplastic drugs and/or radiation therapy.

(*Text continued on page 237*)

Table 7–1 Myelosuppressive Effects of Antineoplastic Agents

MEDICATION	ROUTE	DOSE	FREQUENCY	NEUTROPENIA	WBC NADIR (DAYS)	WBC RECOVERY (DAYS)	THROMBO-CYTOPENIA	COMMENTS
Altretamine	I.V.	8–12 mg/kg	Daily × 21 days	Mild to moderate	21–28	42	Mild to moderate	
Amsacrine	I.V.	120 mg/m^2	Daily × 5 days	Moderate	11–14	17–25	Moderate	
Bleomycin	I.V.	10 U/m^2	q week	Rare	10	14	Rare	Marrow-sparing
Busulfan	P.O.	2–6 mg/m^2	Daily	Marked	11–30	25–54	Marked	Cumulative
Carboplatin	I.V.	300 mg/m^2	Daily × 5 days	Marked	21	28	Marked	Increased with poor renal function or prior cisplatin therapy
Carmustine	I.V.	200–225 mg/m^2	q 6 weeks	Marked	28–42	42–56	Marked	Cumulative
Chlorambucil	P.O.	1–3 mg/m^2	Daily	Moderate	21–28	42–56	Moderate	Cumulative
Cisplatin	I.V.	50–100 mg/m^2	q 3–4 weeks	Moderate	18–23	21–39	Moderate	
Cladribine (Leustatin, 2-CDA)	I.V.	0.09 mg/kg	Daily × 7 days	Mild to moderate	11	42–56	Moderate	
Cyclophosphamide	I.V.	100 mg/m^2	Daily × 5 days	Moderate	8–14	18–25	Mild	Platelet-sparing

Drug	Route	Dose	Schedule		7–9 and 15–24	9–12 and 25–34		
Cytarabine	I.V.	100 mg/m²	Daily × 7 days	Marked	7–9 and 15–24	9–12 and 25–34	Marked	Biphasic with second nadir deeper than first
Dacarbazine	I.V.	200	Daily × 5 days	Mild	21–28	28–35	Mild	
Dactinomycin	I.V.	0.6 mg/m²	Daily × 5 days	Marked	14–21	22–25	Marked	
Daunorubicin	I.V.	30 mg/m²	Daily × 3 q 3 weeks	Marked	10–14	21–28	Marked	
Doxorubicin	I.V.	75 mg/m²	q 3 weeks	Marked	10–14	21	Marked	
Etoposide	I.V.	80 mg/m²	× 2 days q 2 weeks	Moderate	7–14	16–20	Mild	
Fludarabine	I.V.	25 mg/m²	Daily × 5 days	Moderate to severe	3–25		Moderate to severe	May be cumulative
5-Fluorouracil	I.V.	800–1200 mg/m²	Daily × 5 days q 3–4 weeks	Mild	7–14	20–30	Mild	WBC nadir may be delayed as late as 20th day
Hydroxyurea	P.O.	1000 mg/m²	qd	Marked	7	14–21	Moderate	
Idarubicin	I.V.	12 mg/m²	Daily × 3 days	Moderate to severe	10–14	21–23	Moderate to severe	
Ifosfamide	I.V.	1800–2400 mg/m²	qd × 5 days	Moderate	10	18	Moderate	Platelet-sparing
Lomustine	P.O.	100–150 mg/m²	q 6 weeks	Marked	40–50	60	Marked	Cumulative, thrombocytopenia more common than leukopenia
Mechlorethamine	I.V.	0.4 mg/kg	q 4 weeks	Moderate to marked	6–8	16–28	Moderate to marked	

(Continued)

Table 7–1 Myelosuppressive Effects of Antineoplastic Agents (Continued)

MEDICATION	ROUTE	DOSE	FREQUENCY	NEUTROPENIA	WBC NADIR (DAYS)	WBC RECOVERY (DAYS)	THROMBO-CYTOPENIA	COMMENTS
Melphalan	P.O.	16 mg/m²	q 2–4 weeks	Moderate to marked	14–21	28–35	Moderate to marked	Cumulative, thrombocytopenia more common than leukopenia
	I.V.	4 mg/m²						
6-Mercaptopurine	P.O.	100 mg/m²	qd × 5 days	Moderate to marked	7	14–21	Moderate to marked	
Methotrexate	I.V.	25 mg/m²	b.i.w.	Moderate to marked	7–14	14–21	Moderate to marked	
Methotrexate (high-dose)	I.V.	>500 mg/m²	q 3 weeks	Mild	7–14	14–21	Mild	
Mitomycin-C	I.V.	2.0 mg/m²	qd × 3 weeks q 3 weeks	Rare	28–42	42–70	Rare	Cumulative, (especially platelets) and prolonged (may occur as late as 8 weeks after therapy)
Mitoxantrone	I.V.	14 mg/m²	q 3 weeks	Moderate	10–14	21	Moderate	
Taxol	I.V.	200 mg/m²	qd × 5 days	Marked	8–15	21	Marked	
Pentostatin	I.V.	4 mg/m²	q other week	Mild	10	14	Mild	Usually occurs during first few courses of treatment

Plicamycin	I.V.	1.75 mg/m²	qod to toxicity	Mild	14	21	Marked	May cause prolonged prothrombin time, depression of clotting factors II, V, VII, and X
Procarbazine	P.O.	100 mg/m²	qd × 14 days	Moderate	25–36	35–50+	Moderate	Prolonged and delayed
Streptozocin	I.V.	500	qd × 5 days, q 3–4 weeks	Mild	10–14	14–21	Mild	
6-Thioguanine	I.V.	100 mg/m²	qd × 5 days	Moderate to marked	14–28	28–35	Moderate to marked	
Vinblastine	I.V.	2.0 mg/m²	q week	Marked	5–10	7–14	Marked	Leukopenia mild during maintenance therapy
Vincristine	I.V.	1.0 mg/m²	q week	Mild	4–5	7–10	Mild	
Vindesine	I.V.	3–4 mg/m²	q 7–10 days	Dose-related	3–6	7–10	None or mild	May develop elevated platelet count, thrombocytopenia more common in persons with prior bone marrow irradiation or other oncolytic drugs.

Data from DeVita, V.T., Jr., Hellman, S., and Rosenberg, S.A. (eds.): *Cancer: Principles and Practice of Oncology*, 3rd ed. (pp. 354–355) Philadelphia, J.B. Lippincott, 1989; Goodman, M.: *Cancer Chemotherapy and Care*, 2nd ed. Princeton NJ, Bristol-Myers Oncology Division, 1992; Haskell, C.M. (ed.): *Cancer Treatment*, 3rd ed. Philadelphia, W.B. Saunders, 1990; See-Lasley, K., and Ignoffo, R.J.: *Manual of Oncology Therapeutics*. St. Louis, C.V. Mosby, 1981; and product literature.

The precise time and course of myelosuppression may vary with the dose, route, and schedule of drug administration as well as the patient's hematopoietic reserve.

Box 7–1

Formula for Calculating the Absolute Neutrophil Count

Segmented neutrophils _____ %
  + Band neutrophils _____ %
  = Total neutrophils _____ %
  × White blood cell count (WBC) _____ cells/mm^3
  = Absolute neutrophil count (ANC) _____ cells/mm^3

Example:

Segmented neutrophils (%)	.55
+ Band neutrophils (%)	.05
= Total neutrophils (%)	.60
× WBC (cells/mm^3)	5000
= ANC (cells/mm^3)	3000

From Amgen, Inc.: *Blood Values Record.* Thousand Oaks, CA, Amgen, Inc., 1993; and Otto, S.E.: *Oncology Nursing.* St. Louis, Mosby–Year Book, 1991. Reprinted with permission.

Table 7–2 Medications to Avoid When Taking Myelosuppressive Agents

A

ABC Compound
Acucron tablets
Advil ibuprofen caplets
Advil ibuprofen tablets
Alkabutazolidin
Alkabutazone
Alka-Phenylbutazone
Alpha-Phed
Alpha-Phed capsules
Alka-Seltzer
Alka-Seltzer Extra Strength
Alka-Seltzer Plus cold tablets
Amigesic
Amersol
Anacin capsules, tablets
Anacin maximum-strength
Ancasal
Anodynos tablets
APAP fortified tablets

Apa-San tablets
Apo-Asen compound capsules
Apo-Phenylbutazone
Argesic-SA
Arthra-G tablets
Arthralgen tablets
Arthrin tablets
Arthritis strength Bayer aspirin
Arthritis pain formula (Anacin)
Arthritis strength BC powder
Arthritis strength Tribuffered Bufferin
Arthropan liquid
A.S.A. caplets
A.S.A. enseals
A.S.A. pulvules
A.S.A. tablets
Ascriptin A/D tablets
Ascriptin extra-strength tablets
Ascriptin tablets
Ascriptin with codeine tablets
Aspergum

Table 7–2 Medications to Avoid When Taking
Myelosuppressive Agents (Continued)

Aspergum junior
Aspirin suppositories
Aspirin tablets
Aspirin with codeine phosphate
Asproject
Axotal tablets
Azolid

B

B-A-C tablets
B-A-C #3 with codeine
Bayer aspirin tablets
Bayer children's chewable ASA
Bayer children's cold tablets
Bayer timed-release aspirin tablets
BC powder
BC tablets
Buff-a-Comp tablets
Buffaprin tablets
Buffered Aspirin
Bufferin arthritis-strength
Bufferin extra-strength analgesic tablets
Bufferin tablets
Buffets II
Buffinol tablets
Buf-tabs
Butabarbital compound tablets
Butal
Butal compound tablets
Butazolidin

C

C 2
C 2 buffered
C 2 with codeine
C 2 buffered with codeine
CAMA arthritis-strength tablets
Cenaid tablets
Choline magnesium trisalicylate
Codolan
COPE tablets
Corilyn infant liquid drops
Coryphen
Cosprin 650
CP-2 tablets

D

Damason-P
Darvon with aspirin
Darvon-N with aspirin
Dasikon capsules
Dasin capsules
Dia-Gesic tablets
Diflunisal
Dinol tablets
Disalcid capsules
Disalcid tablets
Doan's pills
Dolene compound-65 capsules
Dolobid tablets
Dolprin #3 tablets
Drinophen capsules
Duoprin-S syrup
Duradyne tablets
Durasal
Dynosal tablets

E

Easprin
Ecotrin maximum-strength tablets
Ecotrin tablets
Efficin
Emagrin tablets
Empirin tablets
Empirin with codeine tablets
Encaprin capsules
Entrophen
Epromate
Equagesic tablets
Equazine-M tablets
Excedrin extra-strength tablets
Excedrin tablets
Extra Strength Tribuffered Bufferin
caplets, tablets

F

Feldene
Fendol tablets
Fiogesic tablets
Fiorgen PF tablets

(Continued)

Table 7–2 Medications to Avoid When Taking
Myelosuppressive Agents (Continued)

Fiorinal capsules
Fiorinal
Fiorinal with codeine capsules
Fiorinal-C
4-way cold tablets
Froben
Froben-SR

G

Gaysal-S tablets
Gemnisyn tablets
Genprin
Gensan

H

Haltran ibuprofen tablets
Hista-Compound #5 tablets
Histadyl and A.S.A. pulvules

I

Idarac
Indocid
Indocin
Intrabutazone
Isollyl Improved capsules
Isollyl Improved tablets

K

Kolephrin capsules
Korigesic tablets

L

Lanorinal capsules
Lanorinal tablets
Lortab ASA tablets

M

Magan capsules
Magan tablets
Magnaprin
Magnaprin Arthritis Strength caplets
Magsal tablets

Major-cin tablets
Marnal capsules
Marnal tablets
Maximum strength Bayer aspirin
Maximum strength Midol
Measurin
Medipren with ibuprofen tablets
Mejoral with aspirin tablets
Meprogesic Q tablets
Methocarbamol with aspirin
Micranin tablets
Midol 200 tablets
Midol PMS
Mobidin
Mobifles
Motrin
Motrin JM
Myochrysine

N

Nalfon
Naprosyn
Naxen
Neo-cylate tablets
Neo-Zoline
Norgesic tablets
Norgesic Forte tablets
Novasen
Norwich Aspirin
Norwich extra-strength aspirin
Novobutazone
Nuprin analgesic tablets

O

Os-Cal-Gesic tablets
Orudis
Oravil
Osteolate
Oxycodone with ASA tablets

P

Pabalate tablets
Pabalate-SF
P-A-C new revised formula

Table 7–2 Medications to Avoid When Taking
Myelosuppressive Agents (Continued)

Pain Reliever tablets
Pampirin-IB
Percodan tablets
Pepto-Bismol liquid
Pepto-Bismol tablets
Percodan tablets
Percodan-demi tablets
Persistin tablets
Phenetron Compound tablets
PMS-ASA
Ponstan
Presalin tablets
Propoxyphene compound capsules
Protension tablets

R

Rexolate
Rhinex D-Lay tablets
Rhinocaps capsules
Rhinogesic tablets
Rid-a-pain compound capsules
Riphen-10
Robaxisol tablets

S

St. Joseph Aspirin for children
St. Joseph cold tablets for children
S-A-C tablets
Salatin tablets
Saleto tablets
Saleto-D capsules
Salflex
Salemeph
Sal-infant tablets
Salocol tablets
Salphenyl capsules
Salsalate
Salsitab
Sino-Comp tablets
Sine-Off
Sinulin tablets
SK-oxycodone with ASA tablets
SK-65 compound capsules
Sodium salicylate tablets
Sodium thiosalicylate
Soma compound tablets
Soma compound with codeine

Supac
Supasa
Suspac tablets
Synalgos
Synalgos-DC capsules

T

Talwin compound tablets
Tenol-Plus tablets
Tenstan tablets
Tisma tablets
Tranquigesic tablets
Trendar tablets
Trigesic tablets
Trilisalicylate
Trilisate liquid
Trilisate tablets
Triaphen-10
Tricosal
Tri-pain
Tusal
Tussirex liquid
Tussirex syrup
217 Tablets
217 Strong Tablets
222 Tablets
282 Tablets
282 MEP
292 Tablets

U

Uromide tablets
Ursinus Inlay tablets

V

Valesin
Vanquish capsules
Verin tablets

W

Wesprin buffered aspirin

Z

ZORprin capsules

Table 7–3 Plan of Care for the Patient Experiencing Hematopoietic Alterations

PATIENT PROBLEM	EXPECTED OUTCOMES	STANDARD OF PRACTICE
Knowledge deficit related to potential myelosuppression • neutropenia • thrombocytopenia • anemia	The patient/significant other will: State potential manifestations of infection. Discuss signs and symptoms indicative of bleeding. Describe three signs and symptoms associated with anemia. Describe signs and symptoms to be reported to health care personnel. List measures to be taken to manage exacerbation of hematologic-related symptoms.	1. Assess level of knowledge. 2. Instruct patient/significant other about signs and symptoms associated with myelosuppression (e.g., temperature elevation, petechiae, fatigue). 3. Provide written learning aids to reinforce teaching. 4. Provide time and climate to allow for questions, discussion, feedback, and demonstration as needed. 5. Assist patient/significant other in coping process by providing emotional support.
Potential for infection related to neutropenia	The patient will remain free of infection: WBC within normal limits; no evidence of local or systemic infection. The patient/significant other will demonstrate proper handwashing techniques and other measures to prevent transmission of infection.	1. Monitor temperature at least q 4 hr and report elevation >38.6°C. 2. Administer antibiotic and/or antipyretic medication as ordered. 3. Monitor granulocyte count as indicated and report abnormal values. 4. Monitor WBC count and differential and report abnormal values.

5. Monitor WBC nadir of antineoplastic agents (see Table 7–1).
6. Institute neutropenic precautions if ANC <1000/mm^3.
   - Place patient in private room if possible, or in room with noninfected patient.
   - Maintain asepsis.
   - Instruct patient on personal hygiene measures.
   - Avoid invasive procedures.
   - Maintain a protected environment (no fresh fruits or flowers, no standing water).
   - Limit contact with persons with a cold or other infection.
   - Maintain a low bacteria diet (no fresh fruits or uncooked vegetables).
   - Consult with physician on use of leukocyte filter for administration of blood products.
   - Offer emotional support for the isolation the patient may feel due to neutropenic precautions.

(Continued)

235

Table 7–3 Plan of Care for the Patient Experiencing Hematopoietic Alterations (Continued)

PATIENT PROBLEM	EXPECTED OUTCOMES	STANDARD OF PRACTICE

Potential alteration in health maintenance related to thrombocytopenia	The patient/significant other will:
	Demonstrate the knowledge to prevent or manage problems associated with a low platelet count.
	State four signs and symptoms indicative of bleeding.
	State medications to avoid that may interfere with platelet aggregation (see Table 7–2).
	The patient will be free of bleeding.
		1. Monitor platelet count and other coagulation tests and report abnormal values.
		2. Assess vital signs q 4 hr.
		3. Test stools, urine, emesis for occult blood as ordered, and report positive results.
		4. Maintain thrombocytopenic precautions:
		  a. Use soft toothbrush or Toothette.
		  b. Avoid dental trauma (e.g., flossing, hard foods).
		  c. Instruct client in safe personal hygiene (use electric razor, avoid cutting nails).
		  d. Avoid invasive procedures (e.g., rectal temperature, I.M. injection).
		  e. Administer stool softener to avoid straining.
		  f. Maintain a safe environment to avoid falls or trauma.
		5. Administer platelet transfusion if ordered.
		6. Obtain post-transfusion platelet count.
		7. Avoid aspirin, salicylates, and non-steroidal anti-inflammatory medications (see Table 7–2), unless specifically ordered by physician.

Alteration in tissue perfusion related to anemia	The patient will: Maintain adequate oxygenation of tissue. Be able to perform activities of daily living. Hemoglobin and hematocrit will be within normal limits, or physician will be notified.	

Colony Stimulating Factors (CSFs)

Immunomodulators such as colony stimulating factors (CSFs) (hematopoietic growth factors) aid in the cell maturation process. Small amounts are produced naturally in the body, and recombinant forms are now available. The major clinical application for CSFs in the client receiving chemotherapy is restoration of hematopoiesis by preventing or accelerating recovery from chemotherapy-related myelosuppression (Gabrilove, 1988). The relationship of CSFs to hematopoietic development is shown in Figure 4–3. Recombinant CSFs that are now commercially available include:

Granulocyte colony stimulating factor (G-CSF) (Filgrastim, Neupogen) supports growth of granulocyte colonies and has been administered to reduce severity and duration of chemotherapy-induced neutropenia in nonmyeloid malignancies (Bronchud, et al., 1987; Gabrilove and Golde, 1993). In other studies, the incidence and severity of mucositis was noted as well (Gabrilove, et al., 1988).

Granulocyte macrophage colony stimulating factor (GM-CSF) (sargramostim, Leukine, Prokine) is administered to persons undergoing bone marrow transplantation for nonmyeloid malignancies to help them overcome the myelosuppressive effects of high doses of cytotoxic agents. The primary action is stimulation of WBCs (neutrophils, eosinophils, and basophils), with less impact on maturation of erythrocytes and platelets.

Chemoprotective Agents

Intravenous (I.V.) infusion of amifostine (WR-2721, Ethyol), an organic thiophosphate, is currently undergoing clinical investigation. The drug has shown action in reducing the incidence and severity of the hematologic toxicity of some alkylating agents and platinum-containing compounds (Schucter and Glick, 1993). Unlike CSFs, the mechanism of action of this agent is protection rather than stimulation (Schucter and Glick, 1993).

References

Brandt, B.: A nursing protocol for the patient with neutropenia. Oncol. Nurs. Forum *17*(1, Suppl.):9–15, 1990.

Bronchud, M.H., et al.: Phase I/II study of recombinant human granulocyte colony-stimulating factor in patients receiving intensive chemotherapy for small cell lung cancer. Br. J. Cancer *56*:809–813, 1987.

Creaven, P.J., and Mihich, E.: The clinical toxicity of anticancer drugs and its prediction. Semin. Oncol. 4:147–163, 1977.

Dewys, W.B., et al.: Prognostic effect of weight loss prior to chemotherapy in cancer patients. Am. J. Med. 69:491–497, 1980.

Gabrilove, J.L., and Golde, D.W.: Hematopoietic growth factors. In DeVita, V.T., Jr., Hellman, S., and Rosenberg, S.A. (eds.): Cancer: Principles and Practices of Oncology, 4th ed. (pp. 2275–2291). Philadelphia, J.B. Lippincott, 1993.

Gabrilove, J.L., et al.: Effect of granulocyte-colony stimulating factor on neutropenia and associated morbidity due to chemotherapy for transitional-cell carcinoma of the urothelium. N. Engl. J. Med. 318:1414–1422, 1988.

Rostad, M.E.: Current strategies for managing myelosuppression in patients with cancer. Oncol. Nurs. Forum 18:7–15, 1991.

Schucter, L.M., and Glick, J.H.: The current status of WR-2721 (Amifostine): A chemotherapy and radiation therapy protector. In DeVita, V.T., Jr., Hellman, S., and Rosenberg, S.A. (eds.): Biologic Therapy of Cancer Updates 3:1–10, 1993.

Recommended Readings

Alkire, K., and Collingwood, J.: Physiology of blood and bone marrow. Semin. Oncol. Nurs. 6:99–108, 1990.

Antman, K.D., et al.: Effect of recombinant human granulocyte-macrophage colony stimulating factor on chemotherapy-induced myelosuppression. N. Engl. J. Med. 319:593–598, 1988.

Baronowski, L.: Current trends in blood component therapy: The evolution of a safer, more effective product. J. Intravenous Nurs. 15:136–149, 1992.

Bartlett, J.G.: 1991–1992 Pocketbook of Infectious Disease Therapy. Baltimore, Williams and Wilkins, 1991.

Brogley, J.L., and Sharp, E.J.: Nursing care of patients receiving activated lymphocytes. Oncol. Nurs. Forum 17:187–193, 1990.

Camp-Sorrell, D.: Chemotherapy: toxicity management. In Groenwald, S.L., et al. (eds.): Cancer Nursing: Principles and Practice, 2nd ed. (pp. 337–339). Boston, Jones and Bartlett, 1993.

Champlin, R.E.: Therapeutic use of hematopoietic growth factors for patients receiving high-dose chemotherapy and bone marrow transplantation. Cancer Bull. 43:197–207, 1991.

Coleman, N., Bump, E., and Kramer, R.: Chemical modifiers of cancer treatment. J. Clin. Oncol. 6:709–733, 1988.

Cunningham, R.: Infection prophylaxis for the patient with cancer. Oncol. Nurs. Forum 17(Suppl.):16–19, 1990.

Dessypris, E.N., and Krantz, S.B.: Erythropoietin: Regulation of erythropoiesis and clinical use. Adv. Pharmacol. 21:127–147, 1990.

Doz, F., et al.: Experimental basis for increasing the therapeutic index of carboplatin in brain tumor therapy by pretreatment with WR compounds. Cancer Chemother. Pharmacol. 28:308–310, 1991.

Erikson, J.: Blood support for the myelosuppressed patient. Semin. Oncol. Nurs. 6:61–66, 1990.

Etinger, A.R.: Chemotherapy. In Foley, G., Fochman, D., and Mooney, K.H. (eds.): Nursing Care of the Child With Cancer. Philadelphia, W.B. Saunders (in press).

Fazio, M.T., and Glaspy, J.A.: The impact of granulocyte-colony stimulating factors on the quality of life in patients with severe chronic neutropenia. Oncol. Nurs. Forum 18:1411–1414, 1991.

Feigin, R.D., and Cherry, J.D. (eds): *Textbook of Pediatric Infectious Diseases*, 3rd ed. Philadelphia, W.B. Saunders, 1992.

Freedman, S., et al.: Nursing considerations in the administration of blood component therapy. Semin. Oncol. Nurs. 6:155–162, 1990.

Fuller, A.K.: Platelet transfusion therapy for thrombocytopenia. Semin. Oncol. Nurs. 6:123–128, 1990.

Gawlikowski, J.: White cells at war. Am. J. Nurs. 91(3):44–51, 1991.

Glaspy, J.A., and Ambersley, J.M.: Promise of colony-stimulating factors in clinical practice. Oncol. Nurs. Forum 17(suppl. 1):20–24, 1990.

Haeuber, D., and DiJulio, J.E.: Hematopoietic colony stimulating factors: An overview. Oncol. Nurs. Forum 16:247–255, 1989.

Haeuber, D.: Future strategies in the control of myelosuppression: The use of colony-stimulating factors. Oncol. Nurs. Forum 18(Suppl.):16–21, 1991.

Ho, W.G., and Winston, D.J.: Infection and transfusion therapy in acute leukemia. Clin. Haematol. 15:873–904, 1986.

Hoagland, H.C.: Hematologic complications of cancer therapy. In Perry, M.C. (ed.): *The Chemotherapy Source Book* (pp. 498–507). Baltimore, Williams & Wilkins, 1992.

Hughes, C.B.: Interpreting the white blood count in the cancer chemotherapy patient: Nursing responsibilities. J. Natl IV Therapy Assoc. 8:280–282, 1985.

Hughes, W.T.: New drugs for infections in patients with cancer. Cancer 70:950–965, 1992.

Jassak, P.F.: Biotherapy. In Groenwald, S.L., et al. (eds.): *Cancer Nursing: Principles and Practice*, 2nd ed. (pp. 366–392). Boston, Jones and Bartlett, 1993.

Karp, J.E., et al.: Management of infectious complications of acute leukemia and antileukemic therapy. Oncology 4(7):45–54, 1990.

Maxwell, M.B., and Maher, K.E.: Chemotherapy-induced myelosuppression. Semin. Oncol. Nurs. 8:113–123, 1992.

McConnell, E.A.: Leukocyte studies: What the counts can tell you. Nursing 16(3):42–43, 1986.

Metcalf, D., and Morstyn, G.: Colony-stimulating factors: General biology. In DeVita, V.T., Jr., Hellman, S., and Rosenberg, S.A. (eds.): *Biologic Therapy of Cancer* (pp. 417–444). Philadelphia, J.B. Lippincott, 1991.

Miller, C.B., et al.: Phase I-II trial of erythropoietin in the treatment of cisplatin-associated anemia. J. Natl Cancer Inst. 84(2):98–103, 1992.

Muggia, F., et al.: WR-2721 (WR) pretreatment protects against the bone marrow toxicity of carboplatin (CB) and cisplatin (CP). Proc. Am. Soc. Clin. Oncol. 10:116, 1991.

Nadhan-Raj, S.: Hematopoietic growth factors in chemotherapy-induced myelosuppression. Cancer Bull. 43:208–223, 1991.

Oniboni, A.C.: Infection in the neutropenic patient. Semin. Oncol. Nurs. 6:50–60, 1990.

Parsons, L., and Klopovich, P.M.: Immune globulin therapy. Semin. Oncol. Nurs. 6:136–139, 1990.

Pavel, J.N.: Red blood cell transfusions for anemia. Semin. Oncol. Nurs. 6:117–122, 1990.

Pizzo, P.A., et al.: Infections in the cancer patient. In DeVita, V.T., Hellman, S., and Rosenberg, S.A. (eds.): *Cancer: Principles and Practices of Oncology*, 4th ed. (pp. 2292–2337). Philadelphia, J.B. Lippincott, 1993.

Rutherford, C.: Erythropoietin: A new frontier. J. Intravenous Nurs. 14(3):163–165, 1991.

Summers, S.H., Smith, D.M., and Agranenko, V.A. (eds.): *Transfusion Therapy: Guidelines for Practice*. Arlington, VA, American Association of Blood Banks, 1991.

Chapter 8

Gastrointestinal System Alterations

Linda Tenenbaum, R.N., M.S.N., O.C.N.
Debi Leshin, R.N., B.S.N., O.C.N.

The effects of chemotherapeutic agents and biological response modifiers on the gastrointestinal system are physiological and psychological in nature. Gastrointestinal toxicities can be graded using the World Health Organization (WHO) grading scale, which can be found in Appendix G.

Nausea and Vomiting

Nausea and vomiting are early manifestations of toxicity of antineoplastic therapy (Mitchell, 1992) and are the side effects most feared by patients receiving chemotherapy (Coates, 1983). The emetic potential of antineoplastic medications varies with medication and dosage, as indicated in Table 8–1.

Nausea is a subjective sensation that often leads to the urge to vomit. Vomiting (emesis) is expulsion of stomach contents, and is objective. Nausea usually precedes vomiting, but is a distinctly separate phenomenon.

Emesis is induced *in vivo* by interaction of antineoplastic agents with receptors at one or more of three anatomic regions: the **chemotherapy trigger zone,** in the fourth ventricle of the brain; the pharynx and gastrointestinal tract; and the cerebral cortex. Afferent impulses from these regions are integrated at the true vomiting center in the medulla. When the emesis threshold is exceeded, the act of vomiting is initiated through medullary control centers and somatic and visceral efferent nerves (Haskell, 1990, p. 28). Neurotransmitters, such as dopamine, serotonin, and histamine, may mediate physiologic stimulation of the vomiting center.

Nausea and/or vomiting may also occur as a result of the disease process, electrolyte imbalances, or gastrointestinal (GI) obstruction, or may be related to other therapies (e.g., radiation therapy, pain medications, bone marrow transplantation).

Patterns of chemotherapy-induced emesis include acute, delayed, and anticipatory.

Acute emesis is the most common form of chemotherapy-related nausea and vomiting. The onset may take place minutes after the medication is administered, but usually occurs 2 to 6 hours after administration. It usually lasts up to 24 hours after chemotherapy administration.

Delayed nausea and vomiting develops after the first 24 hours following chemotherapy administration. Its pathophysiology is unclear, but may be the result of residual drug or metabolites. It is more common in persons treated with high-dose cisplatin (total greater than 100 mg/m^2), or in persons who experience nausea on the day of chemotherapy administration (Gralla, 1993, p. 2340).

Anticipatory nausea and vomiting (ANV) is reported to occur in up to one-third of patients receiving chemotherapy (Duigon, 1986; Morrow, 1988) and is proposed to be a learned or conditioned response, i.e., any sight, sound, taste, or odor related to the treatment, such as the sight of the hospital, clinic, or nurse, the odor of alcohol swabs, or the color red (for a person taking doxorubicin). These sensory cues then become conditioned stimuli that may elicit nausea and vomiting even in the absence of chemotherapeutic drug administration.

Anticipatory nausea and vomiting may occur at any time after the initial chemotherapy dose has been administered, usually after three to four treatments. It is most likely the result of stimuli to the emetic zone in the cerebral cortex, and is more commonly seen in persons who previously received drugs with high emetogenic potential. Patients who experience four or more of the following characteristics have been reported to be at risk to develop ANV (Morrow, 1984; Morrow, 1989):

1. Age younger than 50 years.
2. Nausea and/or vomiting after last chemotherapy session.
3. Posttreatment nausea described as "moderate, severe, or intolerable."
4. Posttreatment vomiting described as "moderate, severe, or intolerable."
5. Feeling warm or hot all over after last chemotherapy session.

6. Susceptibility to motion sickness.
7. Sweating after last chemotherapy session.
8. Generalized weakness after last chemotherapy session.

Dr. William Redd, an Attending Psychologist at Memorial Sloan-Kettering Cancer Center in New York, stated:

> Anticipatory side effects can develop rapidly, often appearing after only one infusion and escalating in severity during subsequent treatments. Patients beginning treatment are typically apprehensive; most have heard stories about the horrors of chemotherapy. Interestingly, most patients find the first infusion to be much easier than they had expected. As treatment continues, however, patients begin to notice anticipatory side effects. They are at first confused and wonder why they feel uneasy as they prepare for treatment. . . . With repeated treatments, the problem becomes worse. . . . Unfortunately, many patients do not understand why they are acting in what, to them, seems a bizarre manner. (Redd, 1988, p. 11)

Management

Measures that have been successful in allaying or alleviating nausea and vomiting associated with chemotherapy include pharmacological and nonpharmacological interventions such as the administration of antiemetics individually (Table 8–2) or, more commonly, in combinations (Table 8–3 and Figure 8–1). Most antiemetics inhibit the chemoreceptor trigger zone (CTZ) in the medulla. Antiemetics used in the management of chemotherapy-related nausea and vomiting fall within five major categories:

1. **Butyrophenones** act by suppressing the CTZ, blocking dopamine-mediated stimuli, decreasing vestibular stimuli, reducing agitation and restlessness, and producing sedation. Examples include droperidol (Inapsine) and haloperidol (Haldol).

2. **Cannabinoids** (dronabinol [Marinol]) are better tolerated and more effective in younger than older patients. They are sometimes effective in persons who have been refractory to standard antiemetics (Lucas, 1980). The mechanism of action is not fully understood.

3. **Phenothiazines** act by suppressing or blocking input to the CTZ, blocking dopamine-mediated stimuli, depressing the emetic center, and inhibiting vagal stimulation to the GI tract. Examples include prochlorperazine (Compazine), perphenazine (Trilafon), and triethyperazine (Norzine, Torecan).

4. **Serotonin antagonists** act by selectively blocking HT^3 receptors in the medulla and GI tract. Examples are ondansetron (Zofran) and granisetron (Kytril). Other medications in this category are currently undergoing clinical investigation.

5. **Substituted benzamides** act by suppressing the CTZ, blocking do-

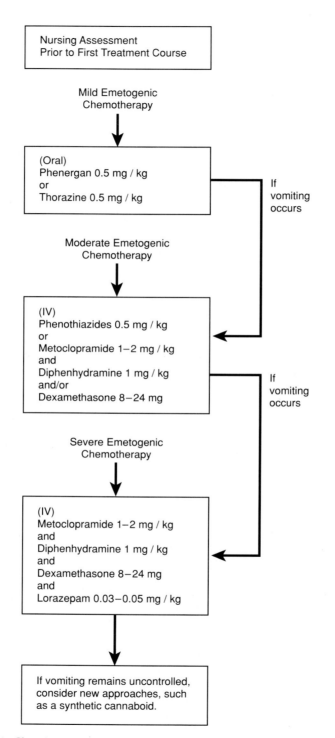

Figure 8–1. Choosing antiemetics for children. (From Hockenberry-Eaton, M., and Benner, A.: Patterns of nausea and vomiting in children: Nursing assessment and intervention. Oncol. Nurs. Forum 17:579, 1990. Reprinted with permission.)

pamine-mediated stimuli, and accelerating gastric emptying. Examples include metoclopramide (Reglan) and trimethobenzamide (Tigan).

Other medications, known as adjunctive medications, may be included in an antiemetic regimen. These include:

1. **Antihistamines** (diphenhydramine HCl [Benadryl]) prevent or ameliorate extrapyramidal side effects of phenothiazines and other antiemetics.

2. **Benzodiazepines** (diazepam [Valium] and lorazepam [Ativan]) function as anxiolytic (reduce anxiety) and amnesiac agents.

3. **Corticosteroids** (dexamethasone [Decadron] and methylprednisolone [Solu-Medrol] are administered as part of many antiemetic regimens. The exact mechanism of action in chemotherapy-related nausea and vomiting is unclear.

Some antiemetic regimens include the administration of a sedative or hypnotic (e.g., lorazepam) prior to chemotherapy. This allows the client to sleep through the peak hours of nausea and vomiting, and may make the chemotherapy experience more tolerable to the patient.

Ondansetron, a serotonin antagonist, has demonstrated the ability to reduce the frequency and severity of nausea and vomiting when administered prior to and following highly emetogenic agents such as cisplatin (Cebeddu et al., 1990; Marty et al., 1990; Hainsworth et al., 1991). Some studies indicate effectiveness with other antineoplastic drugs and combinations in adults (Bonneterre et al., 1990; Chaffee and Tankanow, 1991) and children (Blumer et al., 1990; Pinkerton et al., 1990; Carden et al., 1990). Granisetron (Kytril) was released from clinical trial as this book went to press, thus limited information about it is contained in this book. Other serotonin antagonists, including dolasetron, are presently in clinical trial. Other serotonin antagonists are presently being studied in clinical trials.

Nonpharmacologic interventions used to treat the nausea and vomiting associated with chemotherapy include:

1. **Behavioral therapy.** The goal of behavioral therapies is to relax the patient and block sensations of nausea. This may be accomplished by use of guided imagery, progressive muscle relaxation, or hypnosis.

2. **Systematic desensitization** is used in an effort to desensitize a person to particular objects or situations of which he or she is fearful. It is accomplished by teaching the client relaxation techniques and progressive muscle relaxation and having the client practice relaxation while systematically visualizing the increasingly aversive scenes.

3. **Distraction** is used in an attempt to block the patient's perception of the nausea by active involvement in a challenging task. It has been effective in adults and children. Modes of distraction include involving the patient in a video game, music therapy, watching television, listening to the radio or tapes, or any activity which holds the patient's interest and attention.

Other Factors Affecting Nutritional Status

Appetite Alterations

Anorexia is a side effect of some chemotherapeutic or biologic agents, or the cancer itself, and may occur along with nausea and vomiting. The oral pain and discomfort that accompany mucositis and/or infections of the oral mucosa may make the patient reluctant to eat, and add to the direct effects of the medications (Sonis, 1993, p. 2386).

Anorexia may compromise immune status and/or may progress to cachexia and depletion of protein stores as cancer advances. Anorexia or nausea and vomiting may have psychological (i.e., body image alterations, fear of eating) as well as physical consequences (i.e., pain, nutritional deficiency). A nutritional history and assessment (Figure 8–2) should be done early in the course of therapy so that specific needs can be identified.

If the patient cannot consume adequate calories, oral nutritional supplements (Table 8–4) may be added to the diet. Corticosteroids, which are part of many combination chemotherapy regimens, may increase the appetitite. Progestational agents, such as medroxyprogesterone acetate (Provera) and megestrol acetate (Megace), and other hormonal agents are being investigated in the management of cancer and acquired immunodeficiency syndrome (AIDS)-related cachexia (Loprinzi et al., 1990).

When oral intake is not tolerated or retained, the client may require tube feeding (e.g., nasogastric [NG] tube, gastrostomy, jejunostomy) or total parenteral nutrition (TPN) (e.g., hyperalimentation) to maintain nutritional requirements.

Taste alterations may occur with some cytotoxic and biologic agents, including cisplatin, interferons, levamisole, mechlorethamine, and paclitaxel. Taste may also be affected as the result of oral surgery, radiation therapy, tumor growth, mucositis, or infection in the oral cavity. Chemotherapy-induced taste alterations include increased threshold for sweets, lowered threshold for tart foods, metallic taste, or aversion for meats or other foods eaten during treatment.

Table 8–5 details a plan of care for the client anticipating or experiencing nausea, vomiting, anorexia, or taste alterations related to cancer chemotherapy or biotherapy. For a list of some medications used in the management of GI side effects of interferon and interleukin therapy, see Box 8–1.

For the patient receiving chemotherapy and/or biological response modifiers, early assessment, symptom management, and maintenance of adequate nutritional status present a challenge to the nurse, dietitician, and other members of the health care team.

NUTRITIONAL ASSESSMENT FORM
FOR THE CANCER PATIENT

Patient name _____ Date _____ ID number _____

HISTORY

General

How is the patient's appetite at present? How does it compare with the patient's appetite in the past?

_____

What has the patient eaten during the last 24 hours?

_____

_____

Ask the patient to keep a food diary of everything eaten during the next 3 days. Nutrition management decisions can be based on this information about amount and type of food intake.
Does this patient take nutritional supplements? If so, what kind? _____

Medical

Has there been a loss of body weight? If so, how much weight has been lost? Was the loss gradual or rapid? Over how long a period?

_____

Are there oral/dental problems that interfere with chewing and eating? _____

Are there cancer-related organic conditions (especially pain in the mouth, pharynx, or abdomen; mucositis; dysphagia; diarrhea or constipation; nausea or vomiting) that might interfere with eating?

_____

Are there treatable signs/symptoms that interfere with food intake or nutrient absorption (GI pain, nausea, vomiting, diarrhea, constipation)?

_____

_____

Does the patient report certain changes in taste, food aversions, or nausea that can be associated with chemotherapy or radiotherapy?

_____

Does the patient have a history of malabsorption? _____

Psychosocial

Are there any nonmedical problems that might account for diminished food intake? These may include: insufficient funds to buy food, lack of transportation to or from stores, eating alone, and/or inability to prepare meals.

_____

Follow-Up (date) _____

(date) _____

(date) _____

(date) _____

(date) _____

This information should be obtained during the routine history and physical examinations. This form can be reused during each patient visit so that parameters can be monitored over time. The physician should address any existing medical or psychosocial problems that negatively affect the patient's appetite or food intake. Patients who are nutritionally at risk should receive nutritional counseling from a dietitian or nutritionist.

Figure 8–2. A guide to the nutritional assessment of the patient with cancer. (From Irwin, M.M.: *A Guide to the Nutritional Assessment of the Cancer Patient: Review and Assessment Form.* Princeton, NJ, Bristol-Myers Squibb Oncology Division, 1992. Reprinted with permission.)

PHYSICAL EXAMINATION

Date _____ _____ _____ _____ _____ _____

Body weight _____ _____ _____ _____ _____ _____

Muscle weakness _____

Muscle wasting _____

Findings suggestive of specific nutrient deficiencies _____

LABORATORY PARAMETERS

Date _____ _____ _____ _____ _____ _____

Total lymphocyte count _____ _____ _____ _____ _____ _____

Serum proteins _____ _____ _____ _____ _____ _____

  Albumin _____ _____ _____ _____ _____ _____

  Prealbumin _____ _____ _____ _____ _____ _____

  Transferrin _____ _____ _____ _____ _____ _____

Blood levels of specific trace elements, vitamins, minerals (when appropriate)

_____ _____ _____ _____ _____ _____

_____ _____ _____ _____ _____ _____

_____ _____ _____ _____ _____ _____

ANTHROPOMETRIC PARAMETERS

Date _____ _____ _____ _____ _____ _____

Body Fat

  Triceps skin fold _____ _____ _____ _____ _____ _____

Skeletal Muscle

  Midarm muscle circumference _____ _____ _____ _____ _____ _____

  Percentage of usual body weight _____ _____ _____ _____ _____ _____

  Percentage of ideal body weight _____ _____ _____ _____ _____ _____

Figure 8–2   (Continued)

Box 8–1

Medications Used in the Management of Gastrointestinal Side Effects of Interferon and Interleukin Therapy

Medication	Route, Dose, Frequency
For nausea	See Tables 8–2 and 8–3.
For gastric upset:	
Simethicone	P.O.: 20 mg q 3–4 hr p.r.n.
Aluminum hydroxide	P.O.: 200 mg q 3–4 hr p.r.n.
Magnesium hydroxide	P.O.: 200 mg q 3–4 hr p.r.n.
For gastritis:	
Rantidine HCl	I.V.: 50 mg q 8 hr p.r.n.
For diarrhea:	
Loperamide	P.O.: 2 mg q 3 hr p.r.n.
Atropine sulfate	P.O.: 25 μg q 3–4 hr p.r.n.
Codeine sulfate	P.O.: 30–60 mg q 3–4 hr p.r.n.

Adapted from DeVita, V.T., Jr., Hellman, S., and Rosenberg, S.A. (eds): *Biologic Therapy of Cancer* (p. 162). Philadelphia, J.B. Lippincott, 1991. Reprinted with permission.

Alterations in Elimination

Chemotherapeutic agents may alter bowel function in one of two ways. **Constipation** may occur in direct response to a tumor located in the large intestine or pelvic region. It may be a side effect of Vinca (plant) alkaloids or ondansetron. Other causes of constipation in the patient with cancer include opioid analgesics, oral or parenteral iron preparations, antidepressants, aluminum antacids, antiparkinsonian agents, spinal cord compression, dehydration, immobility, hypercalcemia, and hypokalemia.

All patients with potential or actual lower GI hypomotility must have the abdomen and bowel sounds assessed, and require adequate teaching and proper medical and nursing intervention. An individualized program for bowel control can usually provide effective relief and prevention of cancer-related constipation. This may be accomplished with the use of dietary alterations, bulk stimulants, lubricants, or laxatives. If constipation is not prevented or treated, it can progress to obstipation and paralytic ileus.

Diarrhea is a more common side effect than constipation. It may be the result of chemotherapy- or biotherapy-induced destruction of the GI epithelium. It is frequently associated with antimetabolites and is the dose-limiting side effect of 5-fluorouracil, especially in combination with leucovorin (Levy, 1991, p. 415). An intestinal tumor, radiation therapy to the abdominal region, and many antibiotic agents may also be the cause of diarrhea in a patient being treated for cancer. Diarrhea may lead to dehydration and may be fatal if allowed to continue for several days.

Agents used in the management of diarrhea include anticholinergics (belladonna, atropine sulfate) and opiates (diphenoxylate, loperamide, paregoric). Octreotide (Sandostatin) is an antisecretory agent that had demonstrated the ability to control diarrhea by inhibiting GI hormones and prolonging GI transit time (Gaginella, 1990; Kennedy et al., 1990). In clinical trials, subcutaneous doses of octreotide (0.1 mg b.i.d.) have been effective in controlling chemotherapy-related diarrhea (Cascino et al., 1993).

A plan of care for the client experiencing alterations in elimination may be found in Table 8–6.

Electrolyte alterations may occur with GI toxicities of antineoplastic agents. Excess vomiting may result in the loss of electrolytes and **metabolic alkalosis.** Conversely, the loss of fluid from the lower GI tract in the form of diarrhea may cause electrolyte imbalances and **metabolic acidosis.** These alterations are discussed further in Chapter 13.

Table 8–1 Classification of Single Chemotherapeutic Agents According to Emetogenic Potential

CLASS 5 (HIGH EMETIC POTENTIAL [>90%])	CLASS 4 (MODERATELY HIGH EMETIC POTENTIAL [60–90%])	CLASS 3 (MODERATE EMETIC POTENTIAL [30–60%])	CLASS 2 (MODERATELY LOW EMETIC POTENTIAL [10–30%])	CLASS 1 (LOW EMETIC POTENTIAL [<10%])
Carmustine ≥200 mg	Carboplatin	Altretamine	Bleomycin	Aminoglutethamide
Cisplatin ≥75 mg	Carmustine <200 mg	Asparaginase	Cladarabine	Androgens
Cyclophosphamide >1 g	Cisplatin <75 mg	Daunorubicin 30–60 mg	Cytarabine ≤20 mg	Aminoglutethamide
Cytarabine >1 g	Cyclophosphamide 1 g	Doxorubicin 20–75 mg	Doxorubicin ≤20 mg	Antiandrogens
Dacarbazine ≥500 mg	Cytarabine 250 mg–1 g	Fludarabine	Etoposide	Busulfan
Lomustine ≥60 mg	Dacarbazine <500 mg	5-Fluorouracil ≥1000 mg	Fluorouracil <1000 mg	Chlorambucil
Mechlorethamine	Doxorubicin ≥75 mg	Ifosfamide	Hydroxyurea	Corticosteroids
Pentostatin	Idarubicin	Mitoxantrone	Melphalan	Cyclophosphamide (oral)
Streptozocin	Methotrexate >250 mg	Pentostatin	Mercaptopurine	Estramustine
	Mitomycin		Methotrexate <100 mg	Estrogens
				Goserlin
	Mitoxantrone consolidation (12 mg/m^2 daily × 2)		Mitomycin	Levamisole
	Plicamycin		Vinblastine	Leuprolide
	Teniposide			Progestins
				Thioguanine
				Thiotepa
				Vincristine

Data from Chaffee and Tankanow, 1991, p. 434; Graves, 1990, p. S52; Lindley, Bernard, and Fields, 1989; Nicholson and Leonard, 1992, p. 320; Pisters and Kris, 1992, p. 100; product literature; and personal communication with Medical Information Offices of pharmaceutical companies.

Table 8-2 Pharmacologic Management of Chemotherapy- or Biotherapy-Induced Nausea and Vomiting

MEDICATION	DOSAGE ROUTE AND RANGE	TOXICITIES AND NURSING INTERVENTIONS
Dexamethasone (Dalalone, Decadron, Hexadrol)	P.O., I.V.: 4–20 mg as a single dose, or q 4–6 hr.*† P.O.: 10–40 mg q 3 hr.‡ I.V.: 10–25 mg before chemotherapy, repeat p.r.n. q 4–6 hr × 4.§ I.V.: 8–20 mg q 3 hr.‡ I.V.: 10–20 mg × 1 dose.†	Lethargy, weakness, anxiety, insomnia, mood changes, hyperglycemia. Perirectal burning may occur with rapid I.V. bolus. Administer slow I.V. push. Assess blood glucose and neurological status.
Diazepam (Valium)	P.O.: 2–4 mg q 4–6 hr.‖ I.V.: 2–10 mg q 4–6 hr p.r.n.‖	Amnesia, sedation, confusion, ataxia. May add to central nervous system effects of other drugs (e.g., phenothiazines, narcotics, antidepressants, barbiturates, MAO inhibitors). Use with caution in elderly patients and patients with hepatic or renal disorders. Administer I.M. dose deep I.M. Administer I.V. injection slowly, over at least 1 minute for each 5 ml.
Diphenhydramine HCl (Benadryl)	P.O., I.M., I.V.: 25–50 mg q 6–8 hr.¶ I.M., I.V.: 12.5–50 mg q 3–4 hr.‖	Drowsiness, sedation, dry mouth.
Dronabinol (Marinol, THC)	P.O.: 5–10 mg q 4 hr.‖ P.O.: 5 mg/m² 1–3 hr prechemotherapy, and q 2–4 hr p.r.n. (maximum 4–6 doses/day).§ P.O.: 10 mg q 3–4 hr.# P.O.: 5–10 mg q 3–4 hr.† P.O.: 2.5–5 mg q 3–6 hr.**	Tachycardia, postural hypotension, ataxia, visual hallucinations, memory loss, dysphoria, anxiety, drowsiness, dizziness, xerostomia, paresthesia, hypotension, impaired coordination, irritability. Better tolerated and more effective in younger rather than older patients.

Drug	Dose/Route	Side Effects/Nursing Considerations
		Assess for toxicities. Instruct patient not to drive or perform critical tasks. Assess B/P for postural hypotension. Teach patient to arise slowly and gradually.
Droperidol (Inapsine)	I.V.: 0.5–2 mg q 4 hr.* I.V.: 4 mg q 2 hr × 4.§ I.V.: 1 mg q 4–6 hr p.r.n.¶ I.V.: 2.5 mg q 3 hr.‡	Tachycardia, hypotension OR hypertension, restlessness, dizziness, drowsiness, sedation, mental depression, hallucinations. Extrapyramidal symptoms, akathesias, dyskinesia, laryngospasm. Instruct patient not to drive or perform critical tasks. Assess B/P for alterations.
Granisetron (Kytril)	I.V.: 10 μg administered over 5 minutes.**	Constipation, headache, dizziness.
Haloperidol (Haldol)	P.O., I.V.: 1–2 mg q 3–6 hr.¶ P.O., I.M.: 0.5–1 mg q 8 hr.# I.V.: 1–3 mg q 2–6 hr × 3–5 doses.† I.V.: 1–3 mg q 2–4 hr × 2 or 3 doses.**	Same as droperidol.
Lorazepam (Ativan)	P.O., S.L.: 1–3 mg q 3–4 hr.‖ P.O.: 0.5 mg q 3–4 hr p.r.n.¶ P.O., I.M., I.V.: 1–2 mg q 4–6 hr.# I.V.: 1.0–1.5 mg/m² as a single dose, or q 6 hr.†	Pain or burning at injection site, drowsiness (higher in patients older than age 50 years), amnesia, hypotension. Use with caution in patients with hepatic, respiratory, or renal dysfunction. Monitor V/S and report alterations.
Methylprednisolone (Solu-Medrol)	I.V.: 250–500 mg as a single dose, or q 4–6 hr p.r.n.* 125–250 mg q 4–6 hr × 4 doses.	Sodium and fluid retention, increased appetite, psychic stimulation, osteoporosis, delayed wound healing, decreased antibody formation, and increased risk of infection. May cause loss of contraceptive action in female, or adverse sperm effect in male.

(Continued)

Table 8–2 Pharmacologic Management of Chemotherapy-
or Biotherapy-Induced Nausea and Vomiting (Continued)

MEDICATION	DOSAGE ROUTE AND RANGE	TOXICITIES AND NURSING INTERVENTIONS
Metoclopramide (Reglan)	For medications with high emetogenic potential: I.V.: 1–3 mg/kg q 2 hr.*** I.V.: 1–3 mg/kg q 2 hr × 3–5 doses.† For medications with less emetogenic potential: P.O.: 1 mg/kg q 4–6 hr. P.O.: 1–3 mg/kg q 2–4 hr.*	Extrapyramidal symptoms, sedation, diarrhea.
Nabilone (Cesamet)	P.O.: 2 mg q 6–12 hr.*	Drowsiness, vertigo, psychological high, euphoria, hallucinations, dry mouth, ataxia, blurred vision, anorexia, headache, orthostatic hypotension. With high dose, may experience respiratory depression. Instruct patient not to drive or perform critical tasks. Assess B/P for postural hypotension. Teach patient to arise slowly and gradually.
Ondansetron HCl (Zofran)	**With highly emetogenic agents:** I.V.: single dose of 32 mg, administer over 15 min.†† I.V.: 0.15 mg/kg 30 min before chemotherapy; repeat q 4 hr × 2, or until N/V subside.** **With moderately emetogenic agents:** P.O.: **(adult or child >12 years old):** 8 mg 30 min before therapy; repeat at 4 and 8 hr after chemotherapy, and t.i.d. p.r.n. for 1–2 additional days.** **Child 4–12 years old:** 4 mg; same schedule as adult doses.**	Diarrhea, constipation (less common than diarrhea), headache, transient elevation of hepatic enzymes (ALT, AST), tachycardia, angina, EKG alterations, hypokalemia, transient blurred vision. (NOTE: With severe hepatic insufficiency, maximum total daily dose should not exceed 8 mg.)

Prochlorperazine (Compazine, Stemetril)	P.O., I.M., I.V.: 10 mg.‖ P.O.: 5–10 mg q 2–4 hr.* P.O.: 10–20 mg q 4 hr.‡ P.O.: 10–20 mg q 3–6 hr.† P.O.: (spansule) 30 mg q 12 hr.‡ P.O.: (spansule) 15 mg b.i.d. (increase to 20 mg b.i.d. in resistant cases).** I.M., I.V.: 10–20 mg q 3–6 hr.* P.R.: 25 mg q 3–6 hr p.r.n.*¶ P.R.: 25 mg q 4–6 hr p.r.n.† P.R.: 25 mg b.i.d.** P.O., I.M., P.R., I.V.: 25 mg q 6 hr.#	Drowsiness, dizziness, hypotension, blurred vision, extrapyramidal symptoms, cholestatic jaundice, leukopenia, amenorrhea. With I.V. or I.M. dose: Irritation to surrounding tissue. Administer I.V. dose over 15–30 minutes. Administer I.M. dose deep I.M. by Z-track method. Assess B/P for postural hypotension. Teach patient to arise slowly and gradually.
Promethazine (Phenergan)	P.O., I.M., I.V., P.R.: 25 mg.‖ P.R.: 50 mg q 3–4 hr p.r.n.¶	Drowsiness, sedation, leukopenia, agranulocytosis, GI irritation, dry mouth, nausea, diarrhea, hallucinations, disorientation, urinary frequency or retention. Administer with food or milk to lessen GI upset. Assess urinary output.
Triethyperazine (Norzine, Torecan)	P.O., I.M., I.V., P.R.: 10 mg q 3–4 hr.‖ P.O.: 10–20 mg q 4 hr.‡ I.M.: 10 mg q 4 hr.‡ P.R.: 10 mg q 4–6 hr.‡	Same as prochlorperazine.

References: * Gralla, R., 1993, p. 2342; † Pisters, K.M.W., et al., 1992, p. 101; ‡ Fischer, D., and Knobf, M.T., 1989, pp. 506–507; § Haskell, C.M., 1990, p. 29; ‖ Camp-Sorrell, D., 1993, p. 347; ¶ Lotze, M.T., and Rosenberg, S.A., 1991, p. 162; # Mitchell, E.P., 1992, p. 625; ** Product literature; †† Brown, G.W., et al., 1992, p. 274; Laszlo, J., 1985, p. 864.

Table 8-3 Combination Antiemetic Regimens

MEDICATIONS	ROUTE	DOSE	FREQUENCY
For inpatient receiving highly emetogenic drug (e.g., cisplatin ≥70 mg/m²; cyclophosphamide 750 mg/m²; carboplatin; dacarbazine):			
Metoclopramide (Reglan)	I.V.	3 mg/kg	20 min prior to chemotherapy, and 90 minutes after chemotherapy
Dexamethasone (Decadron)	I.V.	20 mg over 5 min	20 min prior to chemotherapy
Lorazepam (Ativan)	I.V.	1.5 mg/m²	30 min prior to chemotherapy
Ref.: Gralla, 1993, p. 2343.			
Ondansetron (Zofran)	I.V. infusion over 15 min	0.15 mg/kg	30 min before initial chemotherapy dose and q 4 hr × 3 doses
Dexamethasone (Decadron)	I.V.	20 mg	5 min prior to chemotherapy
Ref.: Hesketh et al., 1993.			
Granisetron (Kytril)	I.V.	10 μg/kg	Over 5 min immediately
Dexamethasone (Decadron)	I.V.	10 mg	Prior to chemotherapy
Ref.: Goodman, M., 1994.			
Ondansetron (Zofran)	I.V. infusion over 45 min	32 mg	Single dose 30 min before initial chemotherapy
Dexamethasone (Decadron)	I.V.	20 mg	
At hour of sleep:			
Prochlorperazine SR (Compazine Spansule, Stemetril)	P.O.	15–30 mg	H.S.
Lorazepam (Ativan)	P.O.	1–2 mg	H.S.
Diphenhydramine (Benadryl)	P.O.	25–50 mg	H.S.
Ref.: Goodman, 1994.			
Metoclopramide (Reglan)	I.V.	3 mg/kg	30 min before and 90 min after chemotherapy
Diphenhydramine (Benadryl)	I.V.	40 mg	45 min before chemotherapy
Dexamethasone (Decadron)	I.V.	20 mg	As above
Ref.: Kris, 1987, p. 2816.			

Table 8-3 Combination Antiemetic Regimens (Continued)

MEDICATIONS	ROUTE	DOSE	FREQUENCY
For inpatient receiving moderately emetogenic drug (e.g., cisplatin 40–70 mg/m^2; cyclophosphamide ≤600 mg/m^2; doxorubicin; ifosfamide):			
Metoclopramide (Reglan)	I.V.	2 mg/kg	20 min prior to chemotherapy and 90 min after chemotherapy
Dexamethasone (Decadron)	I.V.	20 mg	For 5 min period 20 min prior to chemotherapy
Diphenhydramine (Benadryl)	I.V.	50 mg	30 min prior to chemotherapy
Ref.: Gralla, 1993, p. 2343.			
Metoclopramide (Reglan)	I.V.	2 mg/kg	20 min prior to chemotherapy
		2 mg/kg	12 hr after cyclophosphamide
Dexamethasone (Decadron)	I.V.	20 mg	40 min prior to chemotherapy
Lorazepam (Ativan)	I.V.	1.5 mg/m^2 (maximum 3 mg)	35 min prior to chemotherapy
Ref.: Pisters and Kris, 1992, p. 101.			
For inpatient receiving drugs with moderate or low emetogenic potential:			
Dronabinol (Marinol)	P.O.	10 mg	q 6 hr beginning 24 hr before chemotherapy
Prochlorperazine (Compazine, Stemetril)	P.O.	10 mg	As above
Continue combination until 24 hr after the last dose of chemotherapy.			
Ref.: Lane et al., 1991, p. 354.			
Prochlorperazine SR* capsules (Compazine-Spansule)	P.O.	30 mg	t.i.d. day 1
		30 mg	b.i.d. day 1
		15 mg	b.i.d. day 3–6
Dexamethasone (Decadron)	I.V.	10 mg	Daily × 5, **or:**
	P.O.	8 mg	b.i.d. days 1, 2, 3
	P.O.	4 mg	b.i.d. days 4, 5
Ref.: Strum et al., 1985.			

(Continued)

Table 8-3 Combination Antiemetic Regimens (Continued)

MEDICATIONS	ROUTE	DOSE	FREQUENCY
Diphenhydramine (Benadryl)	P.O.	50 mg	1 hr prior to cisplatin
Lorazepam (Ativan)	P.O.	0.5 mg/m^2	1 hr prior to cisplatin
Metoclopramide	I.V.*	2 mg/kg	1 hr prior to cisplatin
Droperidol	I.M.	1 mg	15 min prior to cisplatin, and q 6 hr p.r.n.

Ref.: Sridhar et al., 1992, p. 193.

Lorazepam (Ativan) or	I.V.	1.5 mg/m^2	45 min before chemotherapy
Diphenhydramine (Benadryl)	I.V.	40 mg	45 min before chemotherapy
Metoclopramide (Reglan)	I.V. over 30 min	3 mg/kg	30 min before and 90 min after chemotherapy
Dexamethasone	I.V.	20 mg	As above

Ref.: Haskell, 1990, p. 29.

Lorazepam (Ativan) or	I.V.	1.5 mg/m^2	35 min before chemotherapy
Diphenhydramine (Benadryl) and	I.V.	50 mg	35 min before and 90 min after chemotherapy
Metoclopramide (Reglan)	I.V. over 30 min	3 mg/kg	30 min before and 90 min after chemotherapy

Ref.: Tyson et al., 1987.

Home management of delayed emesis:

Metoclopramide (Reglan)	P.O.	0.5 mg/kg	q.i.d. days 1, 2 after chemotherapy
		20–40 mg	p.r.n. only days 3, 4
Dexamethasone (Decadron)	P.O.	8 mg	b.i.d. days 1, 2 after chemotherapy
		4 mg	b.i.d. days 3, 4 after chemotherapy

Ref.: Tyson et al., 1987.

Table 8-3 Combination Antiemetic Regimens (Continued)

MEDICATIONS	ROUTE	DOSE	FREQUENCY
Low-dose cisplatin (<20 mg/m^2):			
Prochlorperazine SR* (Compazine Spansule)	P.O.	30 mg	q 8–12 hr × 1–2 days, then q 12 hr p.r.n.
If unable to tolerate P.O. dose:	P.R. (suppository)	25 mg	q 6 hr p.r.n.
and:			
Diphenhydramine (Benadryl)	P.O.	25–50 mg	q 4–6 hr p.r.n.
Ref.: von Enck, 1992.			
Moderate-dose cisplatin (50–70 mg/m^2):			
Prochlorperazine SR* (Compazine Spansule)	P.O.	30 mg 15 mg	q 8 hr day 1; q 12 hr days 2 and 3; 12 hr days 4–6
If unable to tolerate P.O. dose:			
Compazine	Suppository	25 mg	q 6 hr p.r.n.
Diphenhydramine (Benadryl)	P.O.	<35 years old: 25–50 mg	q 6 hr
		>35 years old: 25–50 mg	q 12 hr p.r.n.
Ref.: von Enck, 1992.			
High-dose cisplatin (>100 mg/m^2):			
Prochlorperazine SR (Compazine Spansule)	P.O.	30 mg 15 mg	q 8 hr day 1 q 12 hr days 2 and 3 q 12 hr days 4–6
If unable to tolerate P.O. dose:			
Compazine	P.R. (suppository)	25 mg	q 6 hr p.r.n.
Dexamethasone (Decadron)	P.O.	8 mg 4 mg	q 8 hr day 1 q 12 hr days 2 and 3 q 12 hr days 3–6
Diphenhydramine (Benadryl)	P.O.	<35 years old: 25–50 mg	q 6 hr
		>35 years old: 25–50 mg	q 12 hr p.r.n.
Ref.: von Enck, 1992.			

*Administer in 75 ml 5% dextrose in water over 15 minutes.

Table 8–4 Nutritional Supplements for the Client with Cancer

PRODUCT (MANUFACTURER)	PROTEIN, gm/240 ml (8 oz)	CALORIES PER 240 ml (8 oz)	DESCRIPTION
Lactose-free Products			
Citrisource (Sandoz)	8.8	180	Clear liquid in 237 ml. Brik-pak. Flavor: orange.
Citrotein (Sandoz)	10.5	170*	Low residue, lactose-free powder. Flavors: orange, grape, fruit punch. Dilute with 8 oz of water.
Compleat Modified (Sandoz)	10.7	265	Unflavored. Administer via enteral feeding tube.
Ensure (Ross)	8.8	250	Low-residue liquid. Flavors: vanilla, chocolate, strawberry, coffee, eggnog, black walnut.
Ensure-HN (Ross)	10.5	250	Low-residue liquid. Flavors: vanilla, chocolate.
Ensure Plus (Ross)	13.0	355	High-calorie, high-nitrogen liquid. Flavors: vanilla, chocolate, strawberry, eggnog. Administer P.O. or via enteral feeding tube.
Ensure Plus-HN (Ross)	14.8	355	Low-residue liquid. Flavors: vanilla, chocolate.
Ensure with fiber (Ross)	9.4	260	High in dietary fiber (3.3 gm/8 fl oz). Flavors: vanilla, chocolate. Administer P.O. or via enteral feeding tube.
Fibersource (Sandoz)	10.8	300	Flavor: mild vanilla. Administer P.O. or via enteral feeding tube.
Fiberlan (Elan)	12.0	288	Fiber-containing isotonic. Unflavored. Administer via enteral feeding tube.
Fibersource HN (Sandoz)	13.3	300	High-nitrogen plus fiber. Flavor: mild vanilla. Administer P.O. or via enteral feeding tube.
Forta (Ross)	5.0	85*	Flavors: orange, fruit punch. Mix ¼ cup (0.8 oz) powder with water. For higher calories, mix with juice. Serving size, 5 oz.
Impact (Sandoz)	14.0	250	Unflavored. Administer via enteral feeding tube.
Impact with fiber (Sandoz)	14.0	250	Unflavored. Administer via enteral feeding tube.
Introlan (Elan)	5.5	127.2	Isotonic, half-strength. Unflavored. Administer via enteral feeding tube.

Table 8–4 Nutritional Supplements for the Client with Cancer (Continued)

PRODUCT (MANUFACTURER)	PROTEIN, gm/240 ml (8 oz)	CALORIES PER 240 ml (8 oz)	DESCRIPTION
Isocal (Mead-Johnson)	8.1	250	Unflavored. Administer via enteral feeding tube.
Isocal HCN (Mead-Johnson)	17.4	470	Unflavored. Administer via enteral feeding tube. For persons on fluid restriction.
Isocal HN (Mead-Johnson)	10.4	250	High-nitrogen. Unflavored. Administer via enteral feeding tube. For persons on fluid restriction.
Isolan (Elan)	9.6	254	Isotonic. Unflavored. Administer via enteral feeding tube.
Isosource (Sandoz)	10.8	300	Flavor: mild vanilla. Administer via enteral feeding tube.
Isosource HN (Sandoz)	13.3	300	Flavor: mild vanilla. Administer via enteral feeding tube.
Isotein-HN (Sandoz)	20	350*	Packets (2.9 oz). Flavor: vanilla. Dilute with 8 oz of water.
Nitrolan (Elan)	14.4	297.6	High protein, isotonic. Unflavored. Administer via enteral feeding tube.
Nutren 1.0 with fiber (Clintec)	40	237	Flavors: vanilla, chocolate, unflavored. 14 gm/L of fiber added to increase absorption. Less sweet taste for improved oral compliance.
Nutren 1.5 (Clintec)	60	355	Flavors: vanilla, chocolate, unflavored. Less sweet taste for improved oral compliance.
Nutren 2.0 (Clintec)	80	473	Flavor: vanilla. Less sweet taste for improved oral compliance.
Nutrilan (Elan)	9.1	254	Isotonic oral supplement. Flavors: vanilla, chocolate, strawberry.
Osmolite (Ross)	8.8	250	Unflavored. May add Vari-flavor flavor packs (pecan, strawberry, cherry, lemon, or orange).
Osmolite HN (Ross)	10.5	250	High-nitrogen, isotonic, low-residue fluid. Unflavored, mild. Administer P.O. or via enteral feeding tube.

(Continued)

Table 8–4 Nutritional Supplements for the Client with Cancer (Continued)

PRODUCT (MANUFACTURER)	PROTEIN, gm/240 ml (8 oz)	CALORIES PER 240 ml (8 oz)	DESCRIPTION
Pediasure (Ross)	7.1	237	For child age 1–6 yr. Flavor: vanilla. Administer via enteral feeding tube.
Resource (Sandoz)	8.8	250	Flavors: vanilla, chocolate, strawberry.
Resource Plus (Sandoz)	13.0	355	Flavors: vanilla, chocolate, strawberry.
Sustacal HC (Mead-Johnson)	14.4	360	Flavors: vanilla, chocolate, eggnog.
Sustacal Powder (Mead-Johnson)	12.5	200*	Flavors: vanilla, chocolate.
Sustacal with Fiber (Mead-Johnson)	10.8	250	Flavors: vanilla, chocolate, strawberry.
Sustacal 8.8 (Mead-Johnson)	8.8	250	Flavors: vanilla, chocolate.
Ultracal (Mead-Johnson)	10.4	250	Bland taste. Administer P.O. or via enteral feeding tube.
Ultralan (Elan)	14.4	360	High calorie, high protein. Unflavored. Administer via enteral feeding tube.
Milk-based Beverages			
Carnation Diet Instant Breakfast (Clintec)	12.0	190† 220‡	Flavors: vanilla, chocolate, strawberry, chocolate malt. Add to milk.
Carnation Instant Breakfast (Clintec)	12.0	250† 280‡	Flavors: vanilla, chocolate, strawberry, chocolate malt. Add to milk.
Forta Shake (Ross)	17	230† 290‡	Powder. Instant milkshake mix. Flavors: vanilla, chocolate, eggnog.
Meritene Powder (Sandoz)	18.0	215† 275‡	Powder—mix with milk. Flavors: vanilla, chocolate, milk chocolate, eggnog, plain.
Sustacal Powder (Mead-Johnson)	12.5	290† 350‡	Flavors: vanilla, chocolate.

Table 8–4 Nutritional Supplements for the Client
with Cancer (Continued)

PRODUCT (MANUFACTURER)	PROTEIN, gm/240 ml (8 oz)	CALORIES PER 240 ml (8 oz)	DESCRIPTION
Puddings (Note: serving size, 5 oz)			
Ensure Pudding (Ross)	6.8§	250§	Flavors: vanilla, chocolate, butterscotch, tapioca.
Sustacal pudding (Mead-Johnson)	6.8§	240§	Flavors: vanilla, chocolate, butterscotch.
Carbohydrate Modular Components			
Moducal (Mead-Johnson)	0	380	Nearly tasteless. Add to foods, beverages, or tube-feeding formulas. Can be used in cooking or baking.
Polycose liquid (Ross)	0	480	As above.
Polycose powder (Ross)	0	380	As above.
Protein Modular Components			
Casec (Mead-Johnson)	0.8/g (4.1‖)	17‖	Almost tasteless. Mix with cereals, beverages, liquid nutritionals, tube feedings, and other foods.
ProMod Powder (Ross)	0.75/g (5¶)	28¶	Concentrated protein supplement. Add to beverages, foods, or tube feedings to increase protein content.

Calories: whole milk—150; 2% milk—120; skim milk—90.
*When diluted in 8 oz (240 ml) of water.
†When diluted in 8 oz (240 ml) of skim milk.
‡When diluted in 8 oz (240 ml) of whole milk.
§Per 5-oz serving.
‖Per packed level tablespoon (4.7 gm).
¶Per scoop provided with cannister of power.

Table 8–5 Plan of Care for the Patient with Potential or Actual Alteration in Nutritional Status

PATIENT PROBLEM	EXPECTED OUTCOMES	STANDARD OF PRACTICE
Knowledge deficit related to potential nutritional alterations of chemotherapy/biotherapy • anorexia • nausea • emesis.	The patient/significant other will: Identify emetogenic potential of chemotherapeutic agents. Discuss measures utilized to manage nausea, vomiting, and/or anorexia. State daily nutritional requirements. Identify/demonstrate measures to prevent nutritional deficit.	1. Assess level of knowledge. 2. Instruct patient/significant other about emetogenic potential of specific antineoplastic agent(s) and dose(s) that he/she will receive (see Table 8–2). 3. Provide written learning aids to reinforce teaching. 4. Provide time and climate to allow for questions, discussion, and feedback as needed. 5. Assist patient/significant other in coping process by providing emotional support.
Alteration in nutritional status: less than body requirement related to nausea and/or vomiting	The patient will: Experience minimal or no nausea or vomiting. Maintain weight within 5% of baseline. List foods and fluids that provide optimal comfort during periods of nausea. Describe and avoid foods that potentiate nausea. State additional interventions that may minimize nausea.	1. Assess client's nutritional status, including height and weight, eating habits, skin turgor, serum albumin, total lymphocyte count. 2. Administer antiemetic medication(s) as ordered. 3. Use general behavioral techniques, such as relaxation therapy, visual imagery, distraction, to help reduce nausea and vomiting. 4. In inpatient setting: Monitor I & O, daily weight. 5. Avoid the following foods: highly sweetened, greasy or fried, heavily spiced, or foods with strong odors. 6. Minimize stimuli (sights, sounds, odors) that may stimulate nausea and vomiting. 7. Provide fresh air to minimize odors when possible. 8. Identify and utilize nursing interventions that have relieved nausea during prior illness or stress. 9. Provide frequent oral hygiene. 10. When administering oral fluids, offer cool (not cold) fluids. 11. Encourage small, frequent meals. 12. Encourage family to provide favored foods, as tolerated. 13. Include nutritional supplements in diet, if necessary. 14. Arrange for dietary consultation if necessary.

| Potential fluid volume deficit related to vomiting | Patient/significant other states three clinical signs associated with fluid volume deficit.
The patient will maintain fluid intake of at least 2000 cc/day unless contraindicated.
Patient will comply with prescribed antiemetic regimen based on stated personal desire to eliminate or reduce episodes of emesis. | 1. Assess client's hydration status, including height and weight, vital signs, skin turgor, condition of mucous membranes, baseline laboratory values (e.g., serum electrolytes, urine specific gravity).
2. Monitor I & O if in hospital, or teach patient to record I & O if at home.
3. Monitor weight and V/S daily.
4. Monitor laboratory values daily or as ordered.
5. Administer I.V. replacement fluids and electrolytes if indicated.
6. Provide frequent oral hygiene.
7. Assess neurologic and cardiac status.
8. Should emesis occur, monitor and record frequency of episodes and amount and character of vomitus.
9. Assess need for dietary consultation if indicated. |
| Alteration in nutrition, less than body requirements related to anorexia and/or taste alterations. | The patient will:
Maintain weight within 5% of baseline.
Be able to perform activities of daily living.
Implement measures that promote appetite.
Select dietary alternatives to provide sufficient nutrients when customary foods are not well tolerated.
Have laboratory values that reflect adequate nutritional status (e.g., total protein, serum albumin). | 1. Assess client's nutritional status, including height and weight, anthropometric measurements, laboratory values (e.g., serum albumin, total lymphocyte count).
2. Implement measures to improve nutritional status:
a. Eat 6 frequent, small, attractive meals/day including foods from all food groups.
b. Concentrate on foods high in protein and calories, unless contraindicated.
c. Avoid drinking fluids with meals, but encourage them between meals.
d. Encourage nutritional supplements.
e. Provide oral hygiene prior to meals and snacks.
3. Monitor weight and V/S daily.
4. Monitor laboratory values daily or as ordered.
5. Administer medications to stimulate appetite as ordered (e.g., progestational agents, corticosteroids).
6. Encourage family to bring favored foods if possible, taking into account cultural, social, and ethnic preferences. |

Table 8–6 Plan of Care for the Patient with Alterations in Gastrointestinal Elimination

PATIENT PROBLEM	EXPECTED OUTCOMES	STANDARD OF PRACTICE
Knowledge deficit related to potential alterations in elimination caused by chemotherapy/biotherapy • constipation • diarrhea	The patient/significant other will: Identify chemotherapeutic agents and other factors that may cause diarrhea or constipation. Discuss measures utilized to prevent and/or manage diarrhea or constipation. State daily nutritional and fluid requirements. Maintain his or her normal pattern of elimination.	1. Assess level of knowledge. 2. Instruct patient/significant other about specific antineoplastic agents that may cause constipation or diarrhea. 3. Provide written learning aids to reinforce teaching. 4. Provide time and climate to allow for questions, discussion, and feedback as needed. 5. Assist patient/significant other in coping process by providing emotional support.
Potential for constipation	The patient/significant other will: Name cytotoxic and other agents that he/she is currently receiving that are commonly associated with constipation.* Describe signs and symptoms of constipation. List foods that are high in residue, and state how he/she will incorporate these foods into the diet. Consume at least 2000 cc of fluid daily unless contraindicated. Participate in activity daily within physical limitations.	1. Assess knowledge of cytotoxic agents that may cause constipation. 2. Assess elimination pattern, including past history and present pattern (e.g., use of laxatives, cathartics, enemas). 3. Assess bowel sounds q shift (for hospitalized patient), or with each home or clinic visit. 4. Evaluate present pain control regimen. 5. Encourage increased intake of foods high in fiber and bulk (e.g., raw fruits and vegetables, whole-grain cereals and breads). 6. Encourage fluid intake of 2000–3000 ml/day, unless contraindicated. 7. Encourage intake of prune juice, warm fluids. 8. Administer stool softener, bulk-forming laxative daily as ordered. 9. Encourage physical exercise and ambulation as tolerated. 10. Assure privacy when patient is using bedpan, commode, or toilet.

| Potential for diarrhea | The patient/significant other will: Name cytotoxic agents that he/she is currently receiving that are commonly associated with diarrhea. Describe signs and symptoms of diarrhea and dehydration. List foods that are high in residue and should be avoided. State four low-residue foods and how these will be incorporated into the diet. Consume at least 2000 cc of fluid daily unless contraindicated. | 1. Assess character, amount, and frequency of stools and bowel sounds q shift (for hospitalized patient), or with each home or clinic visit. 2. Monitor weight, I & O, and electrolyte balance and report alterations. 3. Assess for signs or symptoms of dehydration (e.g., poor skin turgor, dry mucous membranes). 4. Administer antidiarrheal agents as ordered. 5. Adjust diet as appropriate. a. Eat foods low in residue, high in protein and calories. b. Avoid beverages containing caffeine (coffee, chocolate, tea, colas). c. Encourage increased fluid intake unless contraindicated. d. Eat small, frequent meals. e. Avoid foods that are extremely hot or cold. 6. Administer I.V. fluids as ordered. 7. Initiate perianal care measures after each loose bowel movement. |

---

*NOTE: Vinca alkaloids, narcotic analgesics, granisetron, or ondansetron may be the cause of constipation in the patient with cancer.

References

Blumer, J.L., et al.: Evaluation of pharmacokinetics, safety, efficacy of ondansetron in children receiving chemotherapy. Proc. ASCO 9:1284, 1990.

Bonneterre, J., et al.: A randomized double-blind comparison of ondansetron and metoclopramide in the prophylaxis of emesis induced by cyclophosphamide, fluorouracil, and doxorubicin or epirubicin therapy. J. Clin. Oncol. 8:1063–1069, 1990.

Brown, G.W., et al.: The effectiveness of a single intravenous dose of ondansetron. Oncology 49:273–278, 1992.

Camp-Sorrell, D.: Chemotherapy: Toxicity management. In Groenwald, S.L., et al. (eds.): Cancer Nursing: Principles and Practice, 3rd ed. (pp. 331–365). Boston, Jones and Bartlett Publishers, 1993.

Carden, P.A., et al.: Prevention of cyclophosphamide/cytarabine-induced emesis with ondansetron in children with leukemia. J. Clin. Oncol. 8:1531–1535, 1990.

Cascino, S., et al.: Octreotide versus Loperamide in the treatment of fluorouracil-induced diarrhea: A randomized trial. J. Clin. Oncol. 11:148–151, 1993.

Cebeddu, L.X., et al.: Efficacy of ondansetron (GR38032F) and the role of serotonin in cisplatin-induced nausea and vomiting. N. Engl. J. Med. 22:810–816, 1990.

Chaffee, B.J., and Tankanow, R.M.: Ondansetron: The first of a new class of antiemetic agents. Clin. Pharm. 10:430–446, 1991.

Clintec Nutrition Company: Enteral Product Reference. Deerfield, IL, Clintec Nutrition Company, 1992.

Coates, A., et al.: On the receiving end: Patient perception of the side effects of cancer chemotherapy. Eur. J. Cancer Clin. Oncol. 19:203–208, 1983.

Duigon, A.: Anticipatory nausea and vomiting associated with cancer chemotherapy. Oncol. Nurs. Forum 13(1):35–40, 1986.

Essesse, G., et al.: Effective control of cisplatin (DDP)-induced acute and delayed emesis with ondansetron (OND) and dexamethasone (DEX): A follow-up report. Proc. Am. Soc. Clin. Oncol. Abstract 1586, 1993.

Fischer, D.S., and Knobf, M.T.: The Cancer Chemotherapy Handbook, 3rd ed. (pp. 495–547). St. Louis, Mosby–Year Book, 1989.

Gaginella, T.S., et al.: Treatment of endocrine and non-endocrine secretory diarrheal states with Sandostatin. Metabolism 39(Suppl. 2):172–175, 1990.

Goodman, M.: Rush-Presbyterian St. Lukes Medical Center, Chicago, 1994 (unpublished).

Gralla, R.J.: Antiemetic drugs for chemotherapeutic support. Cancer 70(4,Suppl.):1003–1006, 1992.

Gralla, R.: Antiemetic therapy. In DeVita, V.T., Jr., Hellman, S., Rosenberg, S.A. (eds.): Cancer: Principles and Practices of Oncology, 4th ed. (pp. 2338–2348). Philadelphia, J.B. Lippincott, 1993.

Graves, T.: Ondansetron: A new entity in emesis control. DCIP 24(11) (Suppl.):S51–S54, 1990.

Hainsworth, J., et al.: A single blind comparison of intravenous ondansetron, a selective serotonin antagonist, with intravenous metoclopramide in the prevention of nausea and vomiting associated with high-dose cisplatin chemotherapy. J. Clin. Oncol. 9:721–728, 1991.

Haskell, C.M.: Principles and practice of cancer chemotherapy. In Haskell, C.M. (ed.): Cancer Treatment, 3rd ed. (pp. 21–43). Philadelphia, W.B. Saunders, 1990.

Hesketh, P.J., et al.: A randomized, double-blind comparison of intravenous ondansetron alone and in combination with intravenous dexamethasone in the prevention of nausea and vomiting associated with high dose cisplatin. Proc. Am. Soc. Clin. Oncol. Abstract 1491, 1993.

Irwin, M.M.: *A Guide to the Nutritional Assessment of the Cancer Patient: Review and Assessment Form.* Princeton, NJ, Bristol-Myers Oncology Division, 1992.

Kennedy, P., et al.: Sandostatin therapy for chemotherapy and radiotherapy-related diarrhea. Proc. Am. Soc. Clin. Oncol. 9:34, 1990.

Krasnow, S.H.: New directions in managing chemotherapy-related emesis. Oncology 5(9 [Suppl.]):19–24, 1991.

Kris, M.J., et al.: Antiemetic control and prevention of side effects of anticancer therapy with lorazepam and diphenhydramine when used in combination with metoclopramide plus dexamethasone: A double-blind, randomized trial. Cancer 60:2816–2822, 1987.

Lane, M., et al.: Dronabinol and prochlorperazine in combination for treatment of cancer chemotherapy-induced nausea and vomiting. J. Pain Symptom Management 6:352–359, 1991.

Levy, M.H.: Constipation and diarrhea in cancer patients. Cancer Bull. 43:412–422, 1991.

Lin, E.M.: Nutritional support: Making the difficult decisions. Cancer Nurs. 14:236–242, 1991.

Lindley, C.M., Bernard, S., and Fields, S.M.: Incidence and duration of chemotherapy-induced nausea and vomiting in the outpatient oncology population. J. Clin. Oncol. 7:1142–1149, 1989.

Loprinzi, C.L., et al.: A controlled trial of megestrol acetate for the treatment of cancer anorexia-cachexia. J. Natl Cancer Inst. 82:1127–1132, 1990.

Lotze, M.T., and Rosenberg, S.A.: Interleukin-2: Clinical applications. In DeVita, V.T., Jr., Hellman, S., and Rosenberg, S.A. (eds.): *Biologic Therapy of Cancer* (pp. 159–177). Philadelphia, J.B. Lippincott, 1991.

Lucas, V.S., and Lazlo, J.: Delta-9-tetrahydrocannabinol for refractory vomiting induced by cancer chemotherapy. JAMA 243:1241–1243, 1980.

Marty, M., et al.: Comparison of the 5-hydroxytryptamine 3 (serotonin) antagonist ondansetron (GR38032F) with high dose metoclopramide in the control of cisplatin-induced emesis. N. Engl. J. Med. 322:816–821, 1990.

Mead Johnson Nutritional Division: *Mead Johnson Enteral Nutritional Products Handbook.* Evansville, IN, Mead Johnson Nutritional Division, 1993.

Mitchell, E.P.: Gastrointestinal toxicity of chemotherapeutic agents. Semin. Oncol. 19:566–579, 1992.

Morrow, G.R.: Chemotherapy-related nausea and vomiting: Etiology, and management. CA: A Cancer Journal for Clinicians 39:89–104, 1989.

Morrow, G.R.: Clinical characteristics associated with the development of anticipatory nausea and vomiting in cancer patients undergoing chemotherapy treatment. J. Clin. Oncol. 2:1170–1176, 1984.

Nicholson, M., and Leonard, R.C.F.: Adverse effects of cancer chemotherapy: An overview of techniques for avoidance/minimisation. Drug Saf. 7:316–322, 1992.

Pinkerton, C.R., et al.: 5-HT₃ antagonist ondansetron: An effective outpatient antiemetic in cancer treatment of refractory Hodgkin's disease. Arch. Dis. Child. 65:822–825, 1990.

Pisters, K.M.W., and Kris, M.G.: Management of nausea and vomiting caused by anticancer drugs: State of the art. Oncology 6:99–104, 1992.

Redd, W.H.: Behavioral approaches to treatment-related distress. In *Psychosocial Issues and Cancer* (pp. 10–16). Atlanta, American Cancer Society, 1988.

Ross Laboratories: *Ross Laboratories Product Handbook.* Columbus, OH, Ross Laboratories, 1992.

Sandoz Nutrition: *Sandoz Nutrition Enteral Products and Services Guide.* Minneapolis, MN, Sandoz Nutrition, Clinical Products Division, 1992.

Sonis, S.: Oral complications of cancer therapy. In DeVita, V.T., Jr., Hellman, S., Rosenberg, S.A. (eds.): *Cancer: Principles and Practices of Oncology*, 4th ed. (pp. 2385–2394). Philadelphia, J.B. Lippincott, 1993.

Sridhar, K.S., et al.: Five-drug antiemetic combination for cisplatin therapy. Cancer Invest. 10(3):191–199, 1992.

Strum, S.B., McDermed, J.E., and Liponi, D.F.: High-dose intravenous metoclopramide versus combination high-dose metoclopramide and dexamethasone in preventing cisplatin-induced nausea and emesis: A single-blind crossover comparison of antiemetic efficacy. J. Clin. Oncol. 3:245–251, 1985.

Tchekmedyian, N.S., et al.: Megestrol acetate in cancer anorexia and weight loss. Cancer 69:1268–1274, 1992.

Tyson, L.B., et al.: Double-blind, randomized trial for the control of delayed emesis: Comparison of placebo vs. dexamethasone vs. metoclopramide plus dexamethasone. Proc. Am. Soc. Clin. Oncol. 6(abstr):267, 1987.

Von Enck, D.Z.: Management of chemotherapy-induced nausea and vomiting: An update. In *Challenges in Treatment and Management—Proceedings of the Sixth National Conference on Cancer Nursing* (pp. 33–45). Atlanta, American Cancer Society, 1992.

Recommended Readings

Addelman, M., Erlichman, C., Fine, S., et al.: Phase I/II trial of granisetron: A novel 5-hydrotryptamine antagonist for the prevention of chemotherapy-induced nausea and vomiting. J. Clin. Oncol. 8(2):337–341, 1990.

Alba, E., et al.: Anticipatory nausea and vomiting: Prevalence and predictors in chemotherapy patients. Cancer Nurs. 12:236–242, 1989.

Allan, S.G.: Antiemetics. Gastroenterol. Clin. North Am. 21:597–611, 1992.

Angel, F.: An overview of ondansetron for chemotherapy-induced nausea and emesis. J. Intravenous Nurs. 16:84–89, 1993.

Avants, S.K., and Margolin, A.: Psychological and behavioral approaches to symptom management in the cancer patient. In Hubbard, S.M., Greene, P., and Knobf, M.T.: *Current Issues in Cancer Nursing Practice* (pp. 1–11). Philadelphia, J.B. Lippincott, 1990.

Basch, A.: Changes in elimination. Semin. Oncol. Nurs. 3:287–292, 1987.

Berg, S.: Dexamethasone's new use in cancer treatment. J. Assoc. Pediatr. Nurs. 2(2): 46–48, 1985.

Betcher, D.L., and Burnham, N.: Ondansetron. J. Pediatr. Oncol. Nurs. 8:183–185, 1991.

Bloch, A.S.: *Nutritional Management of the Cancer Patient*. Rockville, MD, Aspen Publishers, 1990.

Brown, G.W., et al.: The effectiveness of a single intravenous dose of ondansetron. Oncology 49:273–278, 1992.

Burish, T.G., et al.: Conditioned side effects induced by cancer chemotherapy: Prevention through behavioral treatment. J. Consult. Clin. Psychol. 55:42–47, 1987.

Canty, R.M., Ziegler, P., and Spaulding, M.B.: Lorazepam as a premedication for chemotherapy. J. Natl Intravenous Therapy Assoc. 10:285–289, 1987.

Carey, M.P., and Burish, T.G.: Providing relaxation training to cancer chemotherapy patients: A comparison of three delivery techniques. J. Consult. Clin. Psychol. 55:732–737, 1987.

Cheblowski, R.T.: Nutritional support of the medical oncology patient. Hematol. Oncol. Clin. North Am. 5:147–160, 1991.

Chevallier, B.: The control of acute cisplatin-induced emesis—a comparative study of granisetron and a combination regimen of high-dose metoclopramide and dexamethasone. Granisetron Study Group. Br. J. Cancer 68(1):176–180, 1993.

Clark, R.A., et al.: Antiemetic therapy: Management of chemotherapy-induced nausea and vomiting. Semin. Oncol. Nurs. 5(2 [Suppl. 1]):53–57, 1989.

Cotanch, P., and Strum, S.: Progressive muscle relaxation as antiemetic therapy for cancer patients. Oncol. Nurs. Forum 14(1):33–37, 1987.

Coons, H.L., et al.: Anticipatory nausea and emotional distress in patients receiving cisplatin-based therapy. Oncol. Nurs. Forum 14:31–33, 1987.

Curtas, S., Chapman, G., and Meguid, M.M.: Evaluation of nutritional status. Nurs. Clin. North Am. 24:301–313, 1989.

de Wet, M., Falkson, G., and Rappaport, B.L.: Repeated use of granisetron in patients receiving cytostatic agents. Cancer 71(12):4043–4049, 1993.

Dolgin, M.J., et al.: Behavioral distress in pediatric patients with cancer receiving chemotherapy. Pediatrics 84:103–109, 1989.

Edelstein, S.: Nutritional assessment in cancer cachexia. Pediatr. Nurs. 17:237–240, 1991.

Egan, A.P., Taggart, J.R., and Bender, C.M.: Management of chemotherapy-related nausea and vomiting using a serotonin antagonist: Summaries of eight clinical trials completed between 1988 and 1991. Oncol. Nurs. Forum 19:791–795, 1992.

Fraschini, G. et al.: Evaluation of three oral dosages of ondansetron in the prevention of nausea and emesis associated with cyclophosphamide–doxorubicin chemotherapy. J. Clin. Oncol. 9:1268–1274, 1991.

Gralla, R.J.: Antiemetic drugs for chemotherapeutic support: Current treatment and rationale for development of newer agents. Cancer 15(Suppl. 4):1003–1006, 1992.

Hockenberry-Eaton, M., and Benner, A.: Patterns of nausea and vomiting in children: Nursing assessment and intervention. Oncol. Nurs. Forum 17:575–584, 1990.

Hogan, C.A.: Advances in the management of nausea and vomiting. Nurs. Clin. North Am. 25:475–497, 1991.

Jones, A.L., et al.: Comparison of dexamethasone and ondansetron in the prophylaxis of emesis induced by moderately emetogenic chemotherapy. Lancet 338(8675):483–487, 1991.

Jurgens, H., and McQuade, B.: Ondansetron as prophylaxis for chemotherapy and radiation-induced emesis in children. Oncology 49:279–285, 1992.

Kris, M.G., et al.: Controlling delayed nausea and vomiting: Double-blind, randomized trial comparing placebo, dexamethasone alone and metoclopramide plus dexamethasone in patients receiving cisplatin. J. Clin. Oncol. 7:108–114, 1989.

Kris, M.G., et al.: Oral ondansetron for the control of delayed emesis after cisplatin: Report of a Phase II study and review of completed trials to manage delayed emesis. Cancer 70:1012–1016, 1992.

Laszlo, J., and Cotanch, P.H.: Nausea and vomiting of chemotherapy. In Holland, J.L., et al. (eds.): Cancer Medicine, 3rd ed. (pp. 2261–2267). Philadelphia, Lea and Febiger, 1993.

Lucarelli, C.D., and Grant, M.: Nausea and vomiting: Problems experienced in cancer treatment. In Nursing Management of Common Problems (pp. 16–24). Atlanta, American Cancer Society, 1988.

Marshall, G., et al.: Antiemetic therapy for chemotherapy-induced nausea and vomiting: Metoclopramide, benztropine, dexamethasone and lorazepam regimen compared with lorazepam alone. J. Pediatr. 115:156–160, 1989.

Mitchell, E.P., and Schein, P.S.: Gastrointestinal toxicity of chemotherapeutic agents. In Perry, M.C. (ed.): The Chemotherapy Source Book (pp. 620–634). Baltimore, Williams & Wilkins, 1992.

Morrow, G.R.: Anticipatory nausea and vomiting in cancer patients undergoing chemotherapy treatment. Clin. Psych. Rev. 8:517–556, 1988.

Nelson, K., and Walsh, D.: Management of the anorexia cachexia syndrome. Cancer Bull. 43:403–406, 1991.

Plezia, P.M., et al.: Randomized crossover comparison of high-dose intravenous metoclopramide versus a five-day antiemetic regimen. J. Pain Symptom Management 5(2):101–108, 1990.

Plosker, G.L., and Goa, K.L.: Granisetron: A review of its pharmacological properties and therapeutic use as an antiemetic. Drugs 42(5):805–824, 1991.

Portenoy, R.K.: Constipation in the cancer patient: Causes and management. Med. Clin. North Am. 71:303–311, 1987.

Ramstack, J.L., and Rosenberg, E.: Nutrition for the Chemotherapy Patient. Palo Alto, CA, Bull Publishing, 1990.

Redd, W.H., et al.: Nausea induced by mental images of chemotherapy. Cancer 72(2):629–636, 1993.

Rhodes, V.A., et al.: Patterns of nausea, vomiting, and distress in patients receiving antineoplastic drug protocols. Oncol. Nurs. Forum 14:435–447, 1987.

Richardson, A.: Theories of self-care: Their relevance to chemotherapy-induced nausea and vomiting. J. Adv. Nurs. 16:671–676, 1991.

Rosenberg, S.A.: Interleukin 2: Clinical applications. In DeVita, V.T., Jr., Hellman, S., and Rosenberg, S.A. (eds.): Biologic Therapy of Cancer (pp. 159–177). Philadelphia, J.B. Lippincott, 1991.

Ross Laboratories: Enteral Nutrition—Ready Reference (chart). Columbus, OH, Ross Laboratories, 1993.

Schmitt, R.M.: Controlling nausea and vomiting in outpatients. Oncol. Nurs. Forum 17:277, 1990.

Shike, M., and Brennan, M.F.: Supportive care of the cancer patient. In DeVita, V.T., Jr., Hellman, S., and Rosenberg, S.A. (eds.): Cancer, Principles and Practice of Oncology, 3rd ed. (pp. 2029–2044). Philadelphia, J.B. Lippincott, 1989.

Skipper, A., Szeluga, D.J., and Groenwald, S.L.: Nutritional disturbances. In Groenwald, S.L., et al. (eds.): Cancer Nursing: Principles and Practice, 3rd ed. (pp. 620–643). Boston, Jones and Bartlett, 1993.

Smith, D.B., et al.: Comparison of ondansetron and ondansetron plus dexamethasone as antiemetic prophylaxis during cisplatin-containing chemotherapy. Lancet 338(8675):487–490, 1991.

Stefanek, M.E., Sheilder, V.R., and Fetting, J.H.: Anticipatory nausea and vomiting: Does it remain a significant clinical problem? Cancer 62:2654–2657, 1988.

Warr, D., Willian, A., Fine, S., et al.: Superiority of granisetron to dexamethasone plus prochlorperazine in the prevention of chemotherapy-induced emesis. J. Natl. Cancer Inst. 83(16):1169–1173, 1991.

Wujick, D.: Current research in side effects of high-dose chemotherapy. Semin. Oncol. Nurs. 8:102–112, 1992.

Chapter 9

Effects on Reproduction/ Sexual Function

Marianne Glasel, R.N., M.S., M.A.

Antineoplastic agents have mild to profound effects on reproduction and sexual function. These may include alterations in self-concept, body image, sexual identity, sex role, relationships, gonadal function, fertility, and sexual functioning.

The effects of therapy on gonadal function, fertility, and sexual functioning vary depending on the agent(s), total dose, duration of treatment, gender and age of client, and time from completion of therapy. Some losses in fertility may be temporary, although lasting for years; others may be permanent. In some cases, the effects of antineoplastic drugs are not known. Many agents or combinations of agents have not been studied for their alterations of fertility and sexuality; for drugs still in the investigational phase, little or nothing is known about their overall effects. Of the agents that have been investigated, the alkylating agents and those used in combination chemotherapy have been shown to have the greatest adverse effects on gonadal function and fertility. As the importance of these alterations in gonadal and sexual function becomes more evident, we can anticipate further research into their effects. Until then, we must rely on the information that has been gathered to date.

Many patients receive chemotherapy prior to or during their reproductive years. It is a nursing responsibility to discuss donor egg program or sperm-banking with these patients and, when indicated, a parent or significant other.

The antineoplastic agents that have effects on gonadal function, fertility, and sexual function can be found in Table 9–1. A plan of care for the client experiencing alterations in sexuality can be found in Table 9–2.

Table 9–1   Effects of Antineoplastic Agents on Reproductive/Gonadal Function and Sexual Function

AGENT	EFFECT
Aminopterin	Teratogenic
Androgens (e.g., Halotestin, Methosorb, Teslac)	*Female:* Hirsutism, decreased breast size, deepening of voice, increased libido, enlarged clitoris, hot flashes, undetermined effects on fertility
Busulfan	Decreased gonadal function and fertility, gynecomastia; possibly teratogenic
Carmustine	Decreased testicular function and fertility
Chlorambucil	Affects testicular function and fertility (azoospermia may be permanent); possibly teratogenic
Cisplatin (Platinol, DDP, CIS)	*Male:* Oligospermia and low sperm motility, decreased libido; teratogenic *Female:* Irregular menses
Corticosteroids	*Male:* Oligospermia and low sperm motility *Female:* Irregular menses
Cyclophosphamide (Cytoxan, Endoxan, Neosar, Procytox, CTX)	Severely decreased gonadal function and fertility, with possible permanent sterility; teratogenic
Cytosine arabinoside (Arabinosyl, Cytosar-U, Tarabine, ARA-C)	Decreased testicular function and fertility; may cause vaginitis; teratogenic
Dactinomycin (Cosmegen, Actinomycin-D, ACT-D)	Decreased gonadal function and fertility
Daunorubicin	Teratogenic and embryotoxic
Diethylstilbestrol (and all estrogens)	*Male:* Decreased libido, gynecomastia, breast tenderness, decreased testicular size, possible ejaculatory disorder, decreased semen volume, erectile dysfunction
Doxorubicin	Decreased gonadal function and fertility; may cause irritation of vagina; teratogenic

Table 9–1 Effects of Antineoplastic Agents on Reproductive/
Gonadal Function and Sexual Function (Continued)

AGENT	EFFECT
Estramustine phosphate	Gynecomastia, breast tenderness
Etoposide (VePesid)	May affect ovarian function.
Floxuridine (FUDR)	Teratogenic
5-Fluorouracil	Rarely affects gonadal function and fertility; may cause vaginitis; teratogenic
Fludarabine (Fludara)	May decrease testicular function; possibly teratogenic
Fluoxymesterone	*Female:* Virilization, menstrual irregularities, enlarged clitoris, hot flashes, increased libido *Male:* Gynecomastia
Flutamide (in combination with LHRH analogue/agonist)	*Male:* Hot flashes, gynecomastia, decreased libido, erectile dysfunction
Goserelin acetate	*Male:* Hot flashes, erectile dysfunction, decreased libido, azoospermia, gynecomastia, breast tenderness
Hydroxyurea	Decreased gonadal function and fertility
Interferon alfa	*Male:* Transient erectile dysfunction, decreased libido
Leuprolide acetate	*Male:* Hot flashes, testicular atrophy, erectile dysfunction, decreased libido, azoospermia, gynecomastia, breast tenderness
Levamisole (Ergamisol)	Possibly embryotoxic, especially in combination with 5-fluorouracil
Lomustine	Decreased testicular function and fertility
Mechlorethamine hydrochloride (Nitrogen mustard)	Decreased gonadal function and fertility; teratogenic
Medroxyprogesterone acetate	Decreased ovarian function and fertility, breast tenderness, galactorrhea, libido changes
Megestrol acetate (Megace)	Decreased ovarian function and fertility, breast tenderness
Melphalan	Decreased gonadal function and fertility
Mercaptopurine	Decreased gonadal function and fertility; teratogenic. May cause vaginitis
Methotrexate	Rarely affects gonadal function and fertility; may cause vaginitis; teratogenic
Methylprednisolone sodium succinate	Menstrual abnormalities

(Continued)

Table 9–1 Effects of Antineoplastic Agents on Reproductive/ Gonadal Function and Sexual Function (Continued)

AGENT	EFFECT
Mitotane (Lysodren)	Gynecomastia
Mitoxantrone (Novantrone)	May be teratogenic
Plicamycin (Mithracin)	May cause azoospermia
Procarbazine (Matulane, Natulan)	Erectile dysfunction, severely decreases gonadal function and fertility; may be teratogenic and embryotoxic
Progestins (e.g., Amen, Depo-Provera)	*Female:* Libido changes, may cause breast tenderness and menstrual abnormalities, decreased ovarian function and fertility
Tamoxifen citrate (Nolvadex)	*Premenopausal female:* Highly teratogenic; menopausal symptoms *Postmenopausal female:* Exacerbation of menopausal symptoms
Thioguanine	Decreases gonadal function and fertility; may cause vaginitis; may be teratogenic
Thiotepa	Decreases gonadal function and fertility; teratogenic
Vinblastine (Velban)	May decrease gonadal function and fertility; teratogenic, embryotoxic
Vincristine (Oncovin)	Decreases gonadal function and fertility, possible erectile dysfunction and/or retrograde ejaculation

Combination Therapy†

ABVD—doxorubicin, bleomycin, vinblastine, and dacarbazine	Less gonadal toxicity than MOPP or COPP; if ovarian failure occurs, recovery of function is rare
CMF—cyclophosphamide, methotrexate, and 5-fluorouracil	Affects ovarian function and fertility
COPP—cyclophosphamide, vincristine, procarbazine, and prednisone	Severely affects gonadal function and fertility, with greater effects for males
CVB—cisplatin, vinblastine, and bleomycin, with or without doxorubicin	Affects testicular function and fertility
CVP—cyclophosphamide, vincristine, and prednisone	Affects gonadal function and fertility
MOPP—mechlorethamine, vinblastine, procarbazine, and prednisone	Affects gonadal function and fertility; irreversible azoospermia

Table 9–1   Effects of Antineoplastic Agents on Reproductive/
Gonadal Function and Sexual Function   (Continued)

AGENT	EFFECT
MVPP—mechlorethamine, vinblastine, procarbazine, and prednisolone	Affects gonadal function and fertility, with high incidence of permanent infertility; may cause persistent decrease in libido in males.
POMB/ACE—cisplatin, vincristine, methotrexate, bleomycin, actinomycin D, cyclophosphamide, and etoposide	Affects testicular function and fertility, usually with recovery of spermatogenesis
PVB±-A—cisplatin, vinblastine, and bleomycin, + or − doxorubicin	Produces azoospermia, with recovery of spermatogenesis in majority of males
VAB-6—cyclophosphamide, vinblastine, bleomycin, cisplatin, and actinomycin D	Affects testicular function and fertility

*Effects are dependent on total dose, duration of treatment, age of patient, and time from completion of therapy. Some fertility losses are permanent.

†Effects on fertility are greater and more prolonged than with single agents and are related to total dose, time off treatment, and age of patient.

NOTE: (1) The effect of chemotherapeutic agents on the prepubertal testis appears to be less than on the adult testis; however, high doses of alkylating agents and some combination therapy regimens may cause damage. (2) The effect of chemotherapeutic agents on prepubertal ovaries appears to be less than on adult ovaries. (3) The effects of chemotherapy on fertility will increase with the addition of radiation therapy.

Table 9–2 Plan of Care for the Patient with Alterations in Sexuality

PATIENT PROBLEM	EXPECTED OUTCOMES	STANDARD OF PRACTICE
Knowledge deficit related to potential alterations in sexuality related to chemotherapy/biotherapy • sexual dysfunction • infertility • altered sexuality patterns • altered body image	The patient/significant other will: State potential alterations that may affect sexuality and/or fertility. Describe measures that may be used to facilitate sexual functioning or continue sexual relations using alternate means when necessary. Verbalize feelings regarding body image and identify specific measures to improve self-concept. Describe available community resources. Discuss reproductive alternatives.	1. Assess level of knowledge. 2. Instruct patient/significant other about potential effects of treatment on sexuality and fertility. 3. Provide information about measures that may be taken to facilitate sexual functioning. 4. Counsel for effective use of birth control measures, if applicable. 5. Discuss groups and resources that may assist the person experiencing alterations in sexuality (e.g., sexual encounter groups, reproductive or genetic counselor, sperm banks). 6. Encourage patient/significant other to discuss feelings regarding body image and, when indicated, provide information about measures that can improve self-concept and appearance. 7. Provide written and/or visual learning aids to reinforce teaching. 8. Provide time and climate to allow for questions, discussion, and feedback as needed. 9. Assist patient/significant other in coping process by providing emotional support.

	The patient/significant other will:	Male and female:
Potential for sexual dysfunction related to effects of chemotherapy/biotherapy	Identify potential or actual alterations in sexual function. Recognize that fatigue associated with the disease process and/or therapy may play a role in altered sexual patterns. State measures that can be taken to facilitate sexual activity. Attain a satisfying level of sexual activity compatible with functional capacity. Identify alternative methods for expressing sexuality.	1. Inform patient that this may be a temporary or permanent condition. 2. Encourage the patient to explore alternative means of sexual gratification. *Female:* 1. Advise use of artificial lubricants (e.g., K-Y jelly, Ortho Personal Lubricant) if dyspareunia is present. 2. Discuss use of vaginal dilator if indicated. *Male:* 1. Advise patient of potential for erectile dysfunction. 2. Assure patient that sexual pleasure is still possible even if ejaculation is altered. 3. Discuss surgical interventions (e.g., penile implants) for the patient with permanent erectile dysfunction.

Disturbance in body image and/or self-concept related to effects of chemotherapy/biotherapy	The patient will:
	List clinical signs and symptoms of alterations associated with specific cytotoxic agents (e.g., gynecomastia, alopecia, impaired integrity of vaginal membranes).
	State measures to prevent or manage alterations.
	Communicate feelings about altered body image resulting from chemotherapy.
		1. Encourage patient/significant other to discuss feelings regarding body image.
		2. When indicated, inform patient that this may be a temporary, reversible condition (e.g., alopecia).
		3. Discuss measures that can be taken to improve self-concept and appearance.
		  a. Psychological (e.g., counselling, self-help groups).
		  b. Cosmetic (e.g., "Look Good, Feel Better" Program, assist with grooming).
		  c. Medical/surgical (e.g., radiation therapy to reduce gynecomastia).

(Continued)

279

Table 9–2 Plan of Care for the Patient with Alterations in Sexuality (Continued)

PATIENT PROBLEM	EXPECTED OUTCOMES	STANDARD OF PRACTICE
Alteration in sex role performance related to sexual alterations	The patient and significant other will: Continue to maintain a satisfying sexual relationship, using alternative means as necessary. Recognize that the cause of the sexual dysfunction is a common side effect of the chemo/biotherapy agent(s) administered. Identifies and/or demonstrates measures that can be taken to promote acceptance of self as a sexual being. Verbalized satisfaction with sexual expression.	1. Discuss expected alterations in sexual function that frequently occur with antineoplastic agents. 2. Assess sexual response cycle and functioning, and utilize information in developing an individualized plan of care for the patient and significant other. 3. Encourage patient and significant other to: a. Express feelings about alterations in sexual role performance. b. Explore alternative means of sexual gratification. 4. Inform significant other of the importance of his (her) support throughout the period of altered sexual role performance.

Grieving related to potential or actual infertility related to effects of chemotherapy/biotherapy, or grieving related to altered sexuality and fertility related to effects of chemotherapy/biotherapy

The patient will demonstrate adaptation to and/or a healthy way of coping with alterations as evidenced by:
Describing some possible strategies for coping with alterations.
Participation in self-care activities within physical capabilities.
Statement of realistic goals for readjustment in lifestyle and sexual relationship.

1. Encourage patient and significant other to express feelings, fears, and concerns.
2. Inform patient that stages of grieving are expected and normal responses to any loss.
3. Teach patient about coping strategies.
4. Encourage patient to identify and utilize coping strategies that were successful in the past in accommodating current alterations.
5. Show empathy for and be supportive of patient and significant other.
6. Observe for signs of grieving (e.g., anger, denial, insomnia).
7. If alteration is temporary, provide this information to client.
8. Enlist support of family, friends, clergy, when indicated.
9. Facilitate contact with persons who have successfully adapted to the sexual alterations associated with chemotherapy.
10. Evaluate need for referral for psychological and/or sexual counselling, when indicated.

(Continued)

Table 9–2 Plan of Care for the Patient with Alterations in Sexuality (Continued)

PATIENT PROBLEM	EXPECTED OUTCOMES	STANDARD OF PRACTICE
Decreased libido related to fatigue or ovarian or testicular function	The patient will: Maintain a healthy sexual relationship with significant other. Verbalize a plan of adaptation to accommodate alterations.	1. Encourage patient to verbalize concerns about sexual activity alterations with significant other. 2. Establish a pattern of rest and activity that will allow for fulfillment of maximal physical and sexual activity, based on patient's expressed needs and desires. 3. Include partner in planning and elicit his (her) support. 4. Instruct patient to get adequate rest before and after sexual activity.

Potential for gonadal dysfunction related to the effects of antineoplastic agents	The patient/significant other will:
	List signs and symptoms and potential consequences of gonadal dysfunction associated with specific antineoplastic agents.
	State measures to manage alterations in gonadal dysfunction.
	Describe available interventions and resources (e.g., reproductive alternatives).
		Male and female:
		1. Inform patient that this may be a temporary or permanent condition.
		2. Encourage patient to discuss feelings regarding gonadal dysfunction.
		
		Female:
		1. Assess menstrual history, presence of menopausal symptoms, reproductive/fertility history, and presence of pregnancy.
		2. Discuss potential alterations in sexuality related to gonadal dysfunction that may occur with antineoplastic agents:
		  a. Irregular or absent menses.
		  b. Menopausal symptoms (e.g., hot flashes, night sweats, irritability, decreased libido, decreased vaginal lubrication).
		  c. Temporary infertility or sterility.
		  d. Premature osteoporosis.

3. Identify available interventions and resources to prevent or manage alterations in sexuality related to gonadal dysfunction (e.g., donor egg programs, hormone replacement therapy, artificial vaginal lubricants)

4. Encourage patient to discuss feelings regarding gonadal dysfunction.

Male:

1. Assess reproductive/fertility history and genitourinary function.

2. Discuss potential alterations in sexuality related to gonadal dysfunction (e.g., testosterone production, spermatogenesis) that may occur with specific antineoplastic agents:
   a. Decreased libido.
   b. Retrograde ejaculation.
   c. Erectile dysfunction.
   d. Temporary infertility or sterility.
   e. Gynecomastia and breast tenderness (with chemical castration).

3. Identify available interventions and resources to manage alterations in sexuality related to gonadal dysfunction (e.g., sperm banking, sexual dysfunction clinics, medications to reverse retrograde ejaculation, support groups such as US TOO).

References

American Cancer Society: *Proceedings of the Workshop on Psychosexual and Reproductive Issues Affecting Patients with Cancer—1987.* New York, American Cancer Society, 1987.

Aubier, F., et al.: Male gonadal function after chemotherapy for solid tumors in childhood. J. Clin. Oncol. *7*:304–309, 1989.

Auchincloss, S.S.: Sexual dysfunction in cancer patients: Issues in evaluation and treatment. In Holland, J.C., and Rowland, J.H. (eds.): *Handbook of Psychooncology* (pp. 383–413). New York, Oxford University Press, 1989.

Averette, H.E., Boike, G.M., and Jarrell, MA.: Effects of cancer chemotherapy on gonadal function and reproductive capacity. Cancer *40*:199–209, 1990.

Barton, C., and Waxman, J.: Effects of chemotherapy on fertility. Blood Rev. *4*:187–195, 1990.

Byrne, J.S.: Fertility and pregnancy after malignancy. Semin. Perinatol. *14*:423–429, 1990.

Byrne, J., et al.: Effects of treatment on fertility in long-term survivors of childhood or adolescent cancer. N. Engl. J. Med. *317*:1315–1321, 1987.

Chamorro, T.: Gonadal and reproductive sequelae of cancer therapy. Curr. Issues Cancer Nurs. Pract. 1–14, November, 1990.

Charak, B.S., et al.: Testicular dysfunction after cyclophosphamide-vincristine-procarbazine-prednisolone chemotherapy for advanced Hodgkin's disease. A long-term follow-up study. Cancer *65*:1903–1906, 1990.

DeCensi, A.U., et al.: Evidence for testicular impairment after long-term treatment with a luteinizing hormone-releasing hormone agonist in elderly men. J. Urol. *142*:1235–1238, 1989.

Deirio, G., et al.: Hypothalamic-pituitary-ovarian axis in women with operable breast treated with adjuvant CMF and tamoxifen. Tumor *72*:53–61, 1986.

Dowsett, M., and Richner, J.: Effects of cytotoxic chemotherapy on ovarian and adrenal steroidogenesis in premenopausal breast cancer patients. Oncology *48*:21–220, 1991.

Dudas, S.: Altered body image and sexuality. In Groenwald, S.L., et al. (eds.): *Cancer Nursing: Principles and Practice*, 2nd ed. (pp. 581–593). Boston, Jones and Bartlett, 1990.

Feldman, J.E.: Ovarian failure and cancer treatment: Incidence and interventions for the premenopausal woman. Oncol. Nurs. Forum *16*(19):651–657, 1989.

Gershenson, D.M.: Menstrual and reproductive function after treatment with combination chemotherapy for malignant ovarian germ cell tumors. J. Clin. Oncol. *6*:270–275, 1988.

Gradishar, W.J., and Schilsky, R.L.: Ovarian function following radiation and chemotherapy for cancer. Semin. Oncology *16*:425–436, 1989.

Guy, J.L.: Medical oncology—the agents. In Baird, S.B., McCorkle, R., and Grant, M. (eds.): *Cancer Nursing: A Comprehensive Textbook* (pp. 266–290). Philadelphia, W.B. Saunders, 1991.

Hansen, S.W., Berthelsen, J.G., and von der Maase, H.: Long-term fertility and Leydig cell function in patients treated for germ cell cancer with cisplatin, vinblastine, and bleomycin versus surveillance. J. Clin. Oncol. *8*:1695–1698, 1990.

Heiney, S.P.: Adolescents with cancer: Sexual and reproductive issues. Cancer Nurs. *12*:95–101, 1989.

Hobbie, W.L., and Schwartz, C.L.: Endocrine late effects among survivors of cancer. Semin. Oncol. Nurs. *5*:14–21, 1989.

Kantoff, P.W., and Barnick, M.B.: Late toxicities, long-term follow-up, less intensive treatment: Leading issues in the therapy of testis cancer. J. Clin. Oncol. *6*:1216–1219, 1988.

Kinsella, T.J.: Effects of radiation therapy and chemotherapy on testicular function. Prog. Clin. Biol. Res. *302*:171–177, 1989.

Kirshon, B., et al.: Teratogenic effects of first-trimester cyclophosphamide therapy. Obstet. Gynecol. *72*(3, Pt. 2):462–464, 1988.

Krebs, L.U.: Sexual and reproductive dysfunction. In Groenwald, S.L., et al. (eds.): *Cancer Nursing: Principles and Practice,* 2nd ed. (pp. 563–580). Boston, Jones and Bartlett, 1990.

Kreuser, E.D., et al.: Reproductive and endocrine gonadal capacity in patients treated with COPP chemotherapy for Hodgkin's disease. J. Cancer Res. Clin. Oncol. *113:*260–266, 1987.

Kreuser, E.D., et al.: Gonadal toxicity following cancer therapy in adults: Significance, diagnosis, prevention and treatment. Cancer Treat. Rev. *17:*169–175, 1990.

Lamb, M.A.: Psychosexual issues: The woman with cancer. Semin. Oncol. Nurs. *6:*237–243, 1990.

Levy, M.J., and Stillman, R.J.: Reproductive potential in survivors of childhood malignancy. Pediatrician *18:*61–70, 1991.

Loescher, L.J., et al.: Surviving adult cancers, Part 1: Physiologic effects. Ann. Intern. Med. *111:*411–432, 1989.

Russo, A., et al.: Histologic and hormonal evaluation of the ovarian function in leukemic girls after successful treatment. Pediatr. Hematol. Oncol. *7(19):*301–306, 1990.

Rustin, G.J., et al.: Fertility after chemotherapy for male and female germ cell tumors. Int. J. Androl. *10:*389–392, 1987.

Sanger, W.G., Olson, J.H., and Sherman, J.K.: Semen cryobanking for men with cancer: Criteria change. Fertil. Steril. *58:*1024–1027, 1992.

Schain, W.S.: The sexual and intimate consequences of breast cancer treatment. In *Psychosocial Issues and Cancer* (pp. 26–33). Atlanta, American Cancer Society, 1988.

Schover, L.R., Schain, W.S., and Montague, D.K.: Sexual problems of patients with cancer. In DeVita, V.T., Jr., Hellman, S., and Rosenberg, S.A. (eds.): *Cancer: Principles and Practice of Oncology,* 3rd ed. (pp. 2206–2224). Philadelphia, J.B. Lippincott, 1989.

Shalev, O., Rahav, G., and Milwidsky, A.: Reversible busulfan-induced ovarian failure. Eur. J. Obstet. Gynecol. Reprod. Biol. *26:*239–242, 1987.

Sherins, R.J., and Mulvihill, J.J.: Gonadal dysfunction. In DeVita, V.T., Jr., Hellman, S., and Rosenberg, S.A. (eds.): *Cancer: Principles and Practice of Oncology,* 3rd ed. (pp. 170–180). Philadelphia, J.B. Lippincott, 1989.

Shilsky, R.L.: Male fertility following cancer chemotherapy. J. Clin. Oncol. *7:*295–297, 1989.

Shilsky, R.L., et al.: Gonadal and sexual function in male patients with hairy cell leukemia: Lack of adverse effects of recombinant alpha 2-interferon treatment. Cancer Treat. Rep. *71:*179–181, 1987.

Smith, D.B., and Babaian, S.: The effects of treatment for cancer on male fertility and sexuality. Cancer Nurs. *15:*271–275, 1992.

Steele, D.: Drugs causing sexual dysfunction and their alternatives: A reference tool. Urol. Nurs. *9:*10–12, 1989.

Wang, D.Y., Moore, J.W., and Rubens, R.D.: Ovarian function and adjuvant chemotherapy for early breast cancer. Eur. J. Cancer Clin. Oncol. *23:*745–748, 1987.

Chapter 10

Alterations in the Integumentary System

Linda Tenenbaum, R.N., M.S.N., O.C.N.
Debi Leshin, R.N., B.S.N., O.C.N.

The integumentary system includes the skin, hair, nails, and the mucous membranes that line the oral, gastrointestinal, and female reproductive cavities. Problems affecting this system include alterations in skin and nails, alopecia, and alterations in mucous membranes.

Although alterations in the integumentary system usually are not life-threatening, they may be overwhelming and may have a devastating effect on the comfort, body image, and emotional well-being of the patient. To some patients, changes that occur in the skin, hair, and nails may be more traumatic than the actual diagnosis of cancer. Therefore, the emotional support of the patient with integumentary alterations should be of paramount consideration when developing a standard of practice for the care of these patients.

Alopecia

Alopecia, or loss of hair, is the result of interference with synthesis in basal hair cells, and weakened hair shafts, which break off at the scalp with minimal force (Yarbro, 1992). This usually occurs within 2 to 3 weeks after a course of chemotherapy. Alopecia is noted predominately in the scalp hair, which is actively growing. There may be thinning of the hair or partial or complete loss of scalp hair. Body hair, including eyebrows, eyelashes, axillary hair, and pubic hair, is less frequently lost.

The cytotoxic agents most commonly associated with alopecia are antitumor antibiotics and alkylating agents. Alopecia occurs to a lesser extent with antimetabolites, *Vinca* alkaloids, and interferons.

Hair regrowth usually occurs after termination of treatments. The new hair frequently has a different texture or color than the hair that was lost. This change is usually temporary, and the hair returns to its original type within 1 year (Goodman et al., 1993, p. 761).

Alopecia is not physiologically threatening, but may have devastating effects on body image, self-esteem, social interactions, and sexuality. Males and females and young and old alike share the fear of an altered body image; thus, alopecia is a primary consideration of the patient deciding whether to receive a course of chemotherapy.

The scalp tourniquet and scalp hypothermia have been used in the past to prevent alopecia; however, there are dangers involved with these devices including micrometastases to the scalp and cancer recurrence (Keller and Blausey, 1988). Commercial distribution of these devices was halted by the Food and Drug Administration (Seipp, 1993, p. 2395). The nurse should discuss the safety factors of such devices with the patient. The current focus is on psychological and emotional preparation and support of the patient anticipating or experiencing alopecia, rather than prevention of hair loss. Support systems such as an *I Can Cope* group and programs such as the American Cancer Society/National Cosmetology Association's *Look Good, Feel Better* are described in more detail in Appendix C. The nurse should discuss the use of appropriate headcoverings, such as a wig, turban, scarf, or cap, and should help the patient select the one that is most appropriate.

Alterations in Oral Mucosa

The integrity of oral mucous membranes may be affected by many chemotherapeutic and biologic agents, most commonly antimetabolites, *Vinca* alkaloids, antitumor antibiotics, interleukin-2 (IL-2), and lymphokine activated killer (LAK) cells. Oral complications will occur in approximately 40% of all patients who receive chemotherapy, and are seen more frequently in patients with leukemias and lymphomas than those with solid tumors (Sonis, 1993). Other factors which may increase the risk for developing oral complications include radiation therapy to the head and neck region, malnutrition, dehydration, smoking, alcohol consumption, advanced age, preexisting dental or periodontal disease, and bone marrow transplantation.

Common alterations in the oral mucosa may include inflammation; desquamation and ulceration; mucositis (stomatitis, dryness, and/or burning); discomfort or pain, especially when eating hot or spicy foods; bleeding; taste alterations (dysgeusia); and the potential for oral infection and/or bleeding. These may be the result of the disease process or may be direct or indirect effects of therapy.

Direct stomatoxicity represents interference with the process of cell renewal caused by chemotherapeutic or biotherapy agents or radiation therapy to the head and neck region. **Indirect stomatoxicity** is secondary to myelosuppression, and can be expected to occur around the time of the drug's nadir (Sonis, 1993, p. 2387). This includes oral infections due to granulocytopenia, and bleeding due to thrombocytopenia. See Chapter 7 for further information on myelosuppression.

Xerostomia, or dryness of the oral mucosa, is the result of decreased production of saliva. This may cause alterations in taste, difficulty in chewing or swallowing, and poor fit of dentures. Xerostomia may also be responsible for ill-fitting dentures and added difficulty with solid food intake. Xerostomia may be exacerbated by concomitant radiation therapy to the head and neck region.

Mucositis is inflammation of epithelial cells in response to cancer therapies. This may affect mucous membranes that line the oral, gastrointestinal, and/or female reproductive cavities.

Stomatitis is an inflammatory response affecting the oral cavity (lips, gums, gingiva, tongue, palate, floor of the mouth) and/or throat. Stomatitis can be manifested by inflammation, desquamation, ulceration, dryness, burning, discomfort, and/or pain. In the early stages, stomatitis may not be visually detectable on oral assessment; thus, it is imperative that the patient who is receiving antineoplastic agents be taught to report any sensations of tingling, numbness, burning, or pain in the oral cavity. Mucositis and stomatitis may cause pain and discomfort that can be more pronounced when eating, thus causing a potential nutritional deficit. There is increased risk for localized infection when the integrity of the oral mucosa is compromised. This risk is compounded when neutropenia is also present (see Chapter 7).

Nursing Interventions

Nursing care of the patient receiving agents that may dry or irritate the oral mucosa includes prevention and early detection of alterations, assessment, maintenance of comfort and nutritional intake, and patient education. The severity of alterations varies with each individual's status. The oral assessment can be recorded using descriptive terms or a standardized reference or form. The World Health Organization (WHO) numeric guide (Table 10–1) is a more simplified grading scale. The Oral Cavity Assessment Form (Table 10–2) is a more specific and comprehensive grading scale.

Good oral hygiene and comfort measures must be an integral part of the nursing care given to the patient with potential or actual alterations of the oral mucosa. Management of xerostomia includes oral rinses before meals, avoidance of dry, spicy, and acidic foods, and use of sauces and gravies. Lubricating agents, such as artificial saliva, or antibacterial moisturizing gels (Table 10–3) can be used as well. Nonmedicinal measures that the patient may employ to moisten the oral cavity and stimulate saliva include maintaining adequate fluid intake, or sucking on ice chips or salivary-stimulants such as hard candies or sugar-free lemon drops.

Periodic re-evaluation of the condition of the oral cavity is essential to determine if mucosal alterations are progressing or returning to a normal state. A plan of care for the client with alterations in oral mucosa can be found in Table 10–4.

Skin Alterations

The skin is constantly growing new layers from beneath and shedding old cells. Chemotherapeutic agents interfere with the metabolism of these rapidly growing cells. Alterations that may affect the skin include erythema, urticaria, photosensitivity, radiation recall, acnelike reactions, hyperkeratosis, or hyperpigmentation.

Erythema and Urticaria

Both of these disorders may occur with aldesleukin, aminoglutethimide, altretamine, bleomycin, cylcophosphamide, cytarabine, dacarbazine, dactinomycin, epirubicin, erythropoietin alfa, fludarabine, 5-fluorouracil (topical), hydroxyurea, idarubicin, interleukin-2, leukeran, melphalan, methotrexate, mitotane, mitoxantrone, monoclonal antibodies, paclitaxel, procarbazine, sargramostim, thiotepa, or vindesine. Urticaria may also be part of an anaphylactic or hypersensitivity reaction (HSR), a rare occurrence that may be seen with some antineoplastic agents. For further information on HSRs, see Chapter 13.

Photosensitivity

This condition may occur with chemotherapeutic agents that possess radiosensitizing properties. These include bleomycin, dacarbazine, daunorubicin, doxorubicin, floxuridine, 5-fluorouracil, idarubicin, and methotrexate.

With photosensitivity, an acute burn may occur upon minimal exposure to the sun's rays. This is particularly prominent within the first 48 hours after the drug is administered. The client receiving photosensitizing medications must be taught to avoid direct exposure to the sun's rays.

1. Stay out of the sun's direct path at all times, especially during periods of peak emission of ultraviolet rays. This usually is between 10:00 A.M. and 2 P.M., but varies depending on geographic location and time of year.
2. Wear clothing to cover areas of exposed skin (usually the arms, face, shoulders, and back). Clothing should include long sleeves, preferably of cotton, and a wide-brimmed hat.
3. Apply a high-efficiency sunscreen (#25 or higher).

Radiation Recall

Radiation recall may occur when certain medications are administered simultaneously with or following a course of radiation therapy. These agents include bleomycin, cyclophosphamide, dactinomycin, daunorubicin, doxorubicin, 5-fluorouracil, hydroxyurea, idarubicin, ifosfamide, and methotrexate.

Radiation recall may occur weeks or months after radiation therapy has been administered. It initially presents as an erythematous rash in the area that was irradiated. This may be followed by a period of dry desquamation. Severe reactions can result in vesicle formation, wet desquamation, and permanent discoloration and/or hyperpigmentation of the skin in the affected region.

Hyperpigmentation

Hyperpigmentation may involve the skin, tongue, mucous membranes, and/or nails. It is seen more commonly in dark-skinned persons and those receiving alkylating agents or antitumor antibiotics (Goodman et al., 1993, p. 744). 5-Fluorouracil and bleomycin administered intravenously may cause hyperpigmentation along the veins of the extremity in which the medication was infused. Hyperpigmentation occurs within a few weeks after chemotherapy administration and is usually a temporary alteration. The nurse should inform the client that it will disappear within 2 to 3 months after termination of chemotherapeutic agents.

Alterations in Nails

Nails may be altered in persons receiving bleomycin, cyclophosphamide, doxorubicin, floxuridine, 5-fluorouracil, idarubicin, and ifosfamide. Changes include hyperpigmentation, thickening, brittleness, and horizontal or linear "banding." Changes usually occur 5 to 10 weeks after administration of the chemotherapeutic agent. Most nails will resume normal growth after therapy has been completed. A plan of care for the client with alterations in integrity of skin or nail can be found in Table 10–4.

Table 10–1 World Health Organization Toxicity Grading—Oral Membranes

0	1	2	3	4
Normal	Soreness/ erythema	Erythema, ulceration; can eat solids	Ulceration; requires liquid diet only	Alimentation not possible

Reprinted with permission from Miller, A.B., Hoogstraten, B., Staquet, M., and Winkler, A.: Reporting results of cancer treatment. Cancer 47:207–214, 1981.

Table 10–2 A Guide to Physical Assessment of the Oral Cavity: Numeric and Descriptive Ratings

CATEGORY	RATING	1	2	3	4
Lips	1 2 3 4	Smooth, pink, moist, and intact	Slightly wrinkled and dry; one or more isolated reddened areas	Dry and somewhat swollen; may have one or two isolated blisters; inflammatory line of demarcation	Very dry and edematous; entire lip inflamed; generalized blisters or ulceration
Gingiva and oral mucosa	1 2 3 4	Smooth, pink, moist, and intact	Pale and slightly dry, one or two isolated lesions, blisters, or reddened areas	Dry and somewhat swollen; generalized redness; more than two isolated lesions, blisters, or reddened areas	Very dry and edematous; entire mucosa very red and inflamed; multiple confluent ulcers
Tongue	1 2 3 4	Smooth, pink, moist, and intact	Slightly dry; one or two isolated reddened areas; papillae prominent particularly at base	Dry and somewhat swollen; generalized redness but tip and papillae are redder; one or two isolated lesions or blisters	Very dry and edematous; thick and engorged; entire tongue very inflamed, tip very red and demarcated with coating; multiple blisters or ulcers
Teeth	1 2 3 4	Clean, no debris	Minimal debris, mostly between teeth	Moderate debris, clinging to ½ of visible enamel	Teeth covered with debris
Saliva	1 2 3 4	Thin, watery, plentiful	Increase in amount	Saliva scanty and may be somewhat thicker than normal	Saliva thick and ropy, viscid or mucid

Oral dysfunction score: TOTAL _____	No dysfunction 5	Mild dysfunction 6–10	Moderate dysfunction 11–15	Severe dysfunction 16–20

From Beck, S.L., and Yasko, J.M.: *Guidelines for Oral Care* (p. 28). Crystal Lake, IL, Sage Products, 1993. Reprinted with permission.

Table 10–3 Specific Features of Mouthcare Products

PRODUCT	FEATURES
Biotene antibacterial dental chewing gum	Replenishes reduced lactoperoxidase system found in xerostomia.
Biotene antibacterial toothpaste with fluoride	Contains the bacteriocidal lactoperoxidase enzyme system similar to that found in saliva.
Lip balm, K-Y jelly, petroleum jelly	Moistens lips, prevents cracking and bleeding.
Soft toothbrush	Removes debris, gentler than regular bristle toothbrush. Use with platelet count < 50,000/mm^3.
Toothettes	Removes debris, gentler than soft toothbrush. Use with platelet count <50,000/mm^3, or with mucositis, stomatitis.
Normal saline solution	Removes debris, moistens oral mucosa.
Oral lubricants or artificial saliva (Moi-Stir, Mouthkote, Oral Balance Oralube, Salivart, Xerolube)	Moistens, lubricates, protects oral mucosa; assists with moistening mouth when eating. Use with xerostomia.
Orabase, Hurricane, Oratec-gel, Zilactin	Coating agents in gel or spray forms, contain topical anesthetic. (NOTE: Mild, transient stinging may be present upon application of Oratec gel, Zilactin.)
Xylocaine viscous, dyclonine HCl, Ulcerease	Oral rinses for relief of pain. Xylocaine—swish and swallow; others—swish and spit.
"Stomatitis cocktail" (Xylocaine + Benadryl + Maalox); MouthKote P/R	Relief of oral pain due to mucositis/stomatitis. Swish and swallow, or swish and spit. NOTE: Benadryl may exacerbate xerostomia.
Cetacaine spray, Mouthkote P/R spray or gel, viscous xylocaine	Short-acting topical anesthetics. Mouthkote P/R—anesthetic/moisturizer combination.
Biotene, Peridex rinse	Decreases bacterial load in mouth.
Sodium bicarbonate	Neutralizes oral pH, dissolves mucin, loosens debris.
Mylanta, Maalox	Alkalinizes oral pH.
Nystatin, Ketaconazole	Prevents/treats fungal infection. Swish and swallow.
Mycelex Troches	Anticandida/antifungal lozenge.
Avoid the Following:	
Commercial mouthwash containing alcohol	Irritates and dries oral mucosa.
Glycerine or lemon-glycerine swabs	Dries oral mucosa.

Adapted from Galbraith, 1991, p. 236, and Goodman et al., 1993, pp. 776–778.

Table 10-4 Plan of Care for the Patient with Potential Alterations in Integumentary Status

PATIENT PROBLEM	EXPECTED OUTCOMES	STANDARD OF PRACTICE

Knowledge deficit related to potential alterations of the integumentary system related to chemotherapy/biotherapy:
• skin alterations
  • erythema, urticaria
  • photosensitivity
  • radiation recall
  • hyperpigmentation
• alteration in nails
• alopecia
• alterations in oral mucosa
  • xerostomia
  • mucositis/stomatitis
	The patient/significant other will:
	State clinical signs of integumentary changes caused by specific antineoplastic agents.
	Discuss measures utilized to ameliorate integumentary effects of antineoplastic agents.
	Explain the potential for infection associated with integumentary alterations and the measures that may be utilized to prevent or control infection.
	State resources available that assist in coping with effects of integumentary alterations.
		1. Assess level of knowledge.
		2. Instruct patient/significant other about potential integumentary alterations of specific antineoplastic agents that he/she will receive (see the tables in Section 2 and information about specific medications in Chapters 3 and 4).
		3. Instruct patient/significant other about methods for management of integumentary effects of antineoplastic agents.
		4. Provide information regarding resources available to assist in coping with integumentary changes.
		5. Provide written learning aids to reinforce teaching.
		6. Provide time and climate to allow for questions, discussion, and feedback as needed.
		7. Assist patient/significant other in coping process by providing emotional support.

(Continued)

295

Table 10-4 Plan of Care for the Patient with Potential Alterations in Integumentary Status (Continued)

PATIENT PROBLEM	EXPECTED OUTCOMES	STANDARD OF PRACTICE

Alteration in skin and/or nail integrity resulting from potential:
• erythema, urticaria
• photosensitivity
• radiation recall
• hyperpigmentation
• alteration in nails
Potential altered body image secondary to skin and/or nail changes
	The patient will:
	List clinical signs and symptoms of skin or nail alterations associated with specific cytotoxic agents.
	State measures to prevent or manage skin irritation or infection.
	Demonstrate appropriate hygienic measures to maintain skin integrity.
	Communicate feelings about altered body image resulting from integumentary changes.
		For all potential alterations:
		1. Assess skin daily and report onset, location, and description of cutaneous reactions.
		2. Teach and administer hygienic and preventive measures:
		  a. Use mild soap (e.g., Basis, Dove, Ivory) and tepid water.
		  b. Avoid abrasive cleansing action and gently pat area when bathing or washing.
		  c. Avoid tight-fitting clothing or irritating fabrics (e.g., linen, wool).
		  d. Avoid exposing skin to extreme heat or cold (e.g., heating pad, ice bag, sun lamp).
		  e. Avoid chemical irritants such as scented sprays, deodorants.
		  f. Instruct patient to avoid scratching any irritated areas.
		3. Apply topical medication as ordered for pain and/or irritation.
		4. Encourage patient to ventilate feelings regarding altered body image and offer support.
		5. Refer patient to support groups for additional aid in coping with body image changes.
		6. Perform nursing measures indicated specific to the following alterations:

A. **For photosensitivity:**

1. Instruct patient to avoid exposure to sunlight and other forms of ultraviolet light by:

   a. Wearing protective clothing over face, arms, and other exposed areas (e.g., cotton fabric, long sleeves, wide-brim hat).

   b. Using a sunscreen with SPF of 15 or higher on skin areas exposed to sunlight.

B. **For radiation recall:**

1. Inform patient who has had or is receiving radiation therapy and an anthracycline antibiotic or high-dose methotrexate of possible occurrence.

2. Inform client that this is an expected side effect that will gradually disappear when therapy is discontinued.

3. Instruct patient to report signs and symptoms of radiation recall (erythema, vesicle formation).

C. **For hyperpigmentation:**

1. Inform patient that this is an expected side effect that will gradually disappear when therapy is discontinued.

D. **For nail alterations:**

1. Teach patient about anticipated alterations in nails (e.g., brittleness, banding, hyperpigmentation) and inform that alterations are temporary and will subside gradually upon completion of therapy.

(Continued)

Table 10–4 Plan of Care for the Patient with Potential Alterations in Integumentary Status (Continued)

PATIENT PROBLEM	EXPECTED OUTCOMES	STANDARD OF PRACTICE
Potential altered self-concept or body image secondary to alopecia	The patient/significant other will: State specific cytotoxic agents they will receive that cause partial or complete alopecia. Describe hair care measures that should be taken when partial alopecia is present. Describe measures that can be taken to help adapt to physical changes caused by alopecia. Address feelings about potential hair loss and alteration in body image and self-concept. Describe resources available to the person anticipating or experiencing alopecia.	1. Prior to hair loss, instruct patient/significant other about specific cytotoxic agents that cause partial or complete alopecia. 2. Encourage patient to select a wig, turban, or other head cover prior to hair loss. 3. Instruct patient about use of gentle hair care practices to minimize hair loss whenever possible. 　a. Brush hair gently. 　b. Wash hair with mild shampoo. 　c. Refrain from use of permanent wave or hair dyes. 　d. Avoid use of curling irons, etc. 　e. Use blow dryer on cool, gentle setting. 4. Encourage patient/significant other to verbalize feelings regarding hair loss and body image alteration, and effects on intimacy (see Chapter 9). 5. Provide information about resources (e.g., American Cancer Society wig loan policy), insurance coverage for hairpiece, or other head covering. 6. Discuss support systems available in the community (e.g., local support group; *I Can Cope; Look Good, Feel Better*) (see Appendix D). 7. Answer questions and provide emotional support.

Alteration in comfort:
Pain related to alterations in oral mucosa
- xerostomia
- mucositis
- stomatitis

The patient will:
List specific cytotoxic agents that may cause mucosal alterations.
List clinical signs and symptoms of xerostomia, mucositis/stomatitis.
State measures to prevent or manage xerostomia, mucositis, and/or stomatitis.
Demonstrate appropriate oral assessment and hygiene measures.
Demonstrate oral comfort by maintaining adequate food and fluid intake.

1. Obtain dental history.
2. Assess oral mucosa with and without dental appliances in place, and instruct patient how to do daily self-assessment of the oral cavity.
3. Instruct patient in performance of daily oral hygiene measures.
   a. Gently brush teeth after meals and before bedtime.
   b. Gently floss daily with unwaxed floss, unless contraindicated by thrombocytopenia.
   c. If applicable, remove dentures and replace at mealtime.
4. Instruct patient to utilize preventive measures (e.g., saline rinse, baking soda, soft toothbrush or Toothettes, avoid alcohol-containing mouthwash). See sample products in Table 10–3.
5. Encourage adequate intake of P.O. fluids unless contraindicated.
6. Encourage high-protein, soft, bland diet and avoidance of hot, spicy, acidic foods or other irritating foods.
7. Discourage use of tobacco and alcohol.
8. Instruct patient to avoid elective dental procedures.
9. Recommend use of lip balm or artificial saliva if xerostomia is present.
10. Encourage patient to report pain, tingling, dryness, numbness, or burning of oral cavity.
11. Reinforce and administer oral hygiene protocol as ordered.
12. Administer local and/or systemic pain medication as ordered.

References

Beck, S.L., and Yasko, J.M.: *Guidelines for Oral Care*. Crystal Lake, IL, Sage Products, 1993.

Goodman, M., Ladd, L.A., and Purl, S.: Integumentary and mucous membrane alterations. In Groenwald, S.L., et al. (eds.): *Cancer Nursing: Principles and Practice*, 3rd ed. (pp. 734–799). Boston, Jones and Bartlett, 1993.

Keller, J.F., and Blausey, L.A.: Nursing issues and management in chemotherapy-induced alopecia. Oncol. Nurs. Forum 15(5):603–607, 1988.

Miller, A.B., Hoogstraten, B., Staquet, M., and Winkler, A.: Reporting results of cancer treatment. Cancer 47:207–214, 1981.

Seipp, C.A.: Hair loss. In DeVita, V.T., Jr., Hellman, S., and Rosenberg, S.A. (eds.): *Cancer: Principles and Practices of Oncology*, 4th ed. (pp. 2394–2395). Philadelphia, J.B. Lippincott, 1993.

Sonis, S.T.: Oral complications of cancer therapy. In DeVita, V.T., Jr., Hellman, S., and Rosenberg, S.A. (eds.): *Cancer: Principles and Practices of Oncology*, 4th ed. (pp. 2385–2394). Philadelphia, J.B. Lippincott, 1993.

Yarbro, C.H.: Nursing implications in the administration of cancer chemotherapy. In Perry, M.C. (ed.): *The Chemotherapy Source Book* (pp. 873–883). Baltimore, Williams & Wilkins, 1992.

Recommended Readings

General Information

Goodman, M.: Managing the side effects of chemotherapy. Semin. Oncol. Nurs. 5(2, Suppl.): 29–52, 1989.

Alopecia

Camp-Sorrell, D.: Scalp hypothermia devices: Current status. ONS News 6(8):1,5, 1991.

Perez, J.E., Macchiavelli, M., and Leone, B.A.: High dose alpha-tocopherol as a preventative of doxorubicin-induced alopecia. Cancer Treat. Rep. 70:1213–1214, 1986.

Schlesselman, S.M.: Helping your patient cope with alopecia. Nursing 18(12):43–45, 1988.

Stomatitis/Mucositis

Amigoni, N.A., Johnson, G.K., and Kalwarf, K.L.: The use of sodium bicarbonate and hydrogen peroxide in periodontal therapy: A review. J. Am. Dent. Assoc. 114:217–221, 1981.

Barrett, P.: Clinical characteristics and mechanisms involved in chemotherapy-induced oral ulceration. Oral Surg. Oral Med. Oral Pathol. 63:424–428, 1987.

Beck, S.L.: Prevention and management of oral complications in the cancer patient. In Hubbard, S.M., Greene, P.E., and Knobf, M.T. (eds.): *Current Issues in Cancer Nursing Practice Updates* (pp. 1–11). Philadelphia, J.B. Lippincott, 1990.

Betcher, D., and Burnham, N.: Chlorehexidine. J. Pediatr. Oncol. Nurs. 7(2):82–83, 1990.

Childers, N.K., et al.: Oral complications in children with cancer. Oral Surg. Oral Med. Oral Pathol. 55:40–47, 1993.

Daeffler, R.J.: Impaired mucous membranes. In Daeffler, R.J., and Petrosino, B.M.: *Manual of Oncology Nursing Practice* (pp. 98–108). Rockville, MD, Aspen Publishers, 1990.

Daeffler, R.J., and Landrum, B.: Impaired skin and/or tissue integrity. In Daeffler, R.J., and Petrosino, B.M.: *Manual of Oncology Nursing Practice* (pp. 109–115). Rockville, MD, Aspen Publishers, 1990.

Eilers, J.G.: Oral cavity problems experienced in cancer treatment. In *Nursing Management of Common Problems* (pp. 9–16). Atlanta, American Cancer Society, 1989.

Eilers, J., Berger, A.M., and Petersen, M.C.: Developmental testing of the oral assessment guide. Oncol. Nurs. Forum *15*:325–330, 1988.

Fattore, L., Larson, R.A., and Mostofi, R.: Dental management of cancer patients receiving chemotherapy. Illinois Med. J. *169*:223–226, 1986.

Ferretti, G.G., et al.: Effect of chlorhexidine mouthrinse on mucositis in patients receiving intensive chemotherapy. J. Dent. Res. *99*:342–356, 1987.

Galbraith, L.K., et al.: Treatment for alteration in mucosa related to chemotherapy. Pediatr. Nurs. *17*(3):233–236, 1991.

Goodman, M., and Stoner, C.: Mucous membrane integrity, impairment of, related to stomatitis. In McNally, J.C., et al. (eds.): *Guidelines for Oncology Nursing Practice*, 2nd ed. (pp. 241–251). Philadelphia, W.B. Saunders, 1991.

Griefzu, S., Radjeski, D., and Winnick, B.: Oral care is part of cancer care. RN *53*(6):43–46, 1990.

Hubbard, S.M., et al.: Prevention and management of oral complications in the cancer patient. Curr. Issues Cancer Nurs. Pract. Updates *1*(6):1–12, 1992.

Hyland, S.: Selecting a tool for measuring stomatitis. Oncol. Nurs. Forum *13*(2):119–120, 1986.

Janmohamed, R., et al.: Herpes simplex in oral ulcers in neutropenic patients. Br. J. Cancer *61*:469–470, 1990.

Kenny, S.A.: Effect of two oral care protocols on the incidence of stomatitis in hematology patients. Cancer Nurs. *13*:345–353, 1990.

Kremery, V., Jr., et al.: Fluconazole in the treatment of mycotic oropharyngeal stomatitis and esophagitis in neutropenic cancer patients. Chemotherapy *37*:343–345, 1991.

Kusler, D.L., and Rambur, B.A.: Treatment for radiation-induced xerostomia: An innovative remedy. Cancer Nurs. *15*:191–195, 1992.

LeVeue, F.G., et al.: Clinical evaluation of MGI 209, an anesthetic, film-forming agent for relief from painful oral ulcers associated with chemotherapy. J. Clin. Oncol. *10*:1963–1968, 1992.

Mahood, D.J., et al.: Inhibition of fluorouracil-induced stomatitis by oral cryotherapy. J. Clin. Oncol. *9*:449–452, 1991.

National Institutes of Health Consensus Development Conference: Oral complications of cancer therapies: Diagnosis, prevention and treatment: The National Institutes of Health Consensus Development Conference Statement. Oncology *5*(7):64–83, 1991.

Nieweg, R., Poelhuis, E.K., and Abraham-Inpijn, L.: Nursing care for oral complications associated with chemotherapy. Cancer Nurs. *15*:313–321, 1992.

Peterson, D.E., and Schubert, M.M.: Oral toxicity. In Perry, M.C. (ed.): *The Chemotherapy Source Book* (pp. 508–530). Baltimore, Williams & Wilkins, 1992.

Poland, J.: Prevention and treatment of oral complications in the cancer patient. Oncology *5*(7):45–50, 1991.

Sonis, S., and Clark, J.: Prevention and management of oral mucositis induced by antineoplastic therapy. Oncology *5*:11–21, 1992.

Toth, B.B., and Fleming, T.J.: Oral care for the patient with cancer. Highlights Antineoplastic Drugs *8*:27–35, 1990.

Toth, B.B., Martin, J., and Fleming, T.J.: Oral and dental care associated with cancer therapy. Cancer Bull. *43*:397–402, 1991.

Western Consortium for Cancer Nursing Research: Development of a staging system for chemotherapy-induced stomatitis. Cancer Nurs. *14*:6–12, 1991.

Zerbe, M.B., et al.: Relationships between oral mucositis and treatment variables in bone marrow transplant patients. Cancer Nurs. *15*:196–205, 1992.

Cutaneous Alterations

Bork, K.: *Cutaneous Side Effects of Drugs.* Philadelphia, W.B. Saunders, 1988.

Hood, A.F.: Cutaneous side effects of cancer chemotherapy. Med. Clin. North Am. *70:* 187–209, 1986.

Kerker, B.J., and Hood, A.F.: Chemotherapy-induced cutaneous reactions. Semin. Dermatol. *8:*173–181, 1989.

Richards, C., and Wujick, D.: Cutaneous toxicity associated with high-dose cytosine arabinoside. Oncol. Nurs. Forum *19:*1191–1195, 1992.

Wood, H.A., and Ellerhorst-Ryan, J.M.: Delayed adverse skin reactions associated with mitomycin-C administration. Oncol. Nurs. Forum *11*(4):14–18, 1984.

Chapter 11

Alterations in Behavior

Cheryl A. Bean, D.S.N., R.N., C.S.,
O.C.N.

Introduction

During the course of treatment with antineoplastic agents, hormones, or biological response modifiers (BRMs), clients may manifest subtle or dramatic changes in their cognitive, emotional, or behavioral functioning. While there is relative consensus in the literature regarding many of the neuropsychiatric side effects of cancer chemotherapy, their overall incidence and subsequent impact on functional capacity, psychological distress, and quality of life remains unknown. Moreover, psychological depression, a common neuropsychiatric side effect of cancer chemotherapy, may influence immunologic and hormonal functioning, thereby further impacting morbidity or mortality (Zonderman, Costa, and McCrae, 1989). This chapter discusses the neuropsychiatric side effects of antineoplastic agents, hormonal agents, and BRMs. The reader is referred to Chapter 13 for further discussion of chemotherapy-associated neurotoxicities.

Intrapersonal and interpersonal behaviors or response patterns for every individual diagnosed with cancer are unique, highly personal, complex, dynamic, nonlinear, and nonhierarchial. Numerous, inter-related factors such as past experiences with cancer or its treatment, the goal(s) of cancer therapy, beliefs, values, personality, resources, cultural biases, developmental level, psychological preparation, problem-solving and coping abilities, and actual or perceived disease- or treatment-related threats or demands influence these behavioral disturbances and neuropsychiatric symptoms (Clark, 1992).

Because appropriate management depends on accurate assessment and diagnosis of patient problems, clinicians and researchers are directing increasing attention to possible pathophysiologic mechanisms of psychologic sequelae with current therapies for cancer treatment (Holland and Lesko, 1989). Although frequently included under the general heading of acute and chronic central nervous system (CNS) toxicity, more systematic information through well-controlled studies is needed on the neuropsychiatric side effects of cancer chemotherapy on psychological and psychiatric functioning (Holland and Lesko, 1989; Peterson and Popkin, 1980).

Several factors, however, confound accurate assessment of the neuropsychiatric side effects of chemotherapeutic agents for cancer. These include but are not limited to (1) direct and indirect CNS alterations attributed to the malignancy itself; (2) the additive or synergistic neurotoxic effects of multiagent chemotherapeutic regimens; (3) multimodality therapy combining chemotherapy with radiation therapy or biotherapy, e.g., methotrexate and cranial radiotherapy; and (4) the addition of a corticosteroid, most commonly prednisone in doses greater than 60 mg/d for 5 to 14 days every 3 to 4 weeks, in many multiagent treatment protocols. An additional factor that must be considered is disease- or therapy-induced metabolic alterations that may occur with the enzyme L-asparaginase, which may cause the pancreas to produce less insulin, resulting in psychomotor retardation with mental depression as the blood sugar level increases. Another example is the gonadotropin-releasing hormone analog aminoglutethimide, which may alter the hormone system, resulting in hypothyroidism with subsequent lethargy, somnolence, and depression (MacDonald, 1992; Peterson and Popkin, 1980; Post-White, 1986).

Antineoplastic Agents

Table 11–1 outlines specific neuropsychiatric toxicities associated with many commonly used antineoplastic agents, hormonal agents, and BRMs. For most of these medications, the incidence and severity of neuropsychiatric toxicity are dose- and schedule-dependent. Although long-term or permanent deficits have been reported, reversal or resolution of neuropsychiatric side effects commonly occurs quickly with discontinuation of the drug, reduction of the dosage, or adjustment of the schedule (Furlong, 1993; Peterson and Popkin, 1980).

(Text continued on page 310)

Table 11–1 Neuropsychiatric Effects of Chemotherapeutic Agents

AGENT	TOXICITY	INCIDENCE	REMARKS
Alkylating Agents			
Chlorambucil (Leukeran)	Cerebral dysfunction Delirium	Rare	See 5-fluorouracil below Drug overdose
Cisplatin (Platinol)	Encephalopathy Confusion		May be due to electrolyte imbalance
Ifosfamide (Ifex)	CNS toxicity Confusion Somnolence Hallucinations Psychosis	Variable	Alkylator-like agent Dose limiting CNS symptoms documented at all ages & range from mild to severe HD 3–5 gm/m^2 Usually resolve within 24–48 h following withdrawal Co-causative & predisposing factors: brain edema with hyperhydration, decreased renal function, concomitant drugs affecting the CNS, & metabolic acidosis
Nitrogen mustard (Mustargen)	Cerebral dysfunction Delirium Hallucinations Lethargy		See 5-fluorouracil below With HD for BMT
Nitrosoureas			
Carmustine (BCNU)	Encephalopathy Confusion/ disorientation		Reversible
Antimetabolites			
HD Cytosine arabinoside (Cytosar-U, Tarabine, Ara-C)	Cerebellar dysfunction Somnolence	0–25%	Cumulative dose >36 gm/ m^2
	Cerebral dysfunction Confusion/ disorientation Memory loss Cognitive dysfunction Encephalopathy	0–25%	Liver dysfunction Renal insufficiency Prior neurologic disorder Prior CNS therapy Cerebral dysfunction usually concomitant with cerebellar dysfunction Generally reversible, but can be permanent or incomplete

(Continued)

Table 11–1 Neuropsychiatric Effects of Chemotherapeutic Agents
(Continued)

AGENT	TOXICITY	INCIDENCE	REMARKS
5-Fluoroura-cil (Adrucil)	Cerebral dysfunction Delirium		Onset sudden, can pro-gress rapidly Clinical manifestations in the domains of cognition, orientation, attention, wakefulness, psychomo-tor behavior, & mood Caused by altered cere-bral metabolism, im-pairing neuronal func-tioning
Methotrexate IT (Folex, Mexate, Uro-mitexan)	Acute Lethargy	5–40%	Attributed to meningeal ir-ritation/arachnoiditis
	Delayed Confusion Somnolence Irritability Delirium Dementia	<1%	Attributed to leuko-encephalopathy (LEC) See 5-fluorouracil above
HD	Acute Somnolence Confusion Disorientation Irritability Dementia	10% 2–22% 2–22%	Meningeal irritation/arachnoiditis
IT & CNS irradiation	Subacute Lethargy Irritability	>50%	"Somnolence syndrome"
	Delayed Learning deficits Neuropsychologi-cal deficits Confusion Dementia	>50% 5% 5%	LEC LEC
HD & CNS irradiation	Delayed Confusion Somnolence Irritability Dementia	15%	LEC
IT & HD	Delayed Same as HD & CNS irradiation	2%	LEC
IT, HD, & CNS irradi-ation	Delayed Same as HD & CNS irradiation Neuropsychologic deficits	45–55% Common	LEC

Table 11–1   Neuropsychiatric Effects of Chemotherapeutic Agents
(Continued)

AGENT	TOXICITY	INCIDENCE	REMARKS
Mitotic inhibitors			
Etoposide (VePesid, VP-16)	CNS toxicity Confusion Somnolence	Rare	HD therapy Reversible
Vincristine (Oncovin, Vincasar), Vinblastine (Velbe, Velsar), Vindesine (Eldisine)	CNS toxicity Confusion Depression Insomnia Hallucinations	Rare	Reversible
Antitumor antibiotics			
Pliamycin (Mithracin)	CNS toxicity Agitation Irritability	86%	Reversible
Miscellaneous Agents			
Altretamine (oral) (Hexalen)	CNS toxicity Depression Hallucinations Somnolence Confusion Agitation Suicide thoughts or plans	13–25%	Incidence 28–50% with HD therapy (>225 mg/m^2/d) In combination with vincristine (inconclusive) In combination with dacarbazine Daily therapy >3 mo Reversible
Enzymes			
L-asparaginase (Elspar, Kidrolase)	Encephalopathy/ cerebral dysfunction Lethargy Drowsiness/ somnolence Confusion Depression Hallucinations Stupor Delirium	21–60% Rare Rare	Reversible Liver dysfunction See 5-fluorouracil above
Mitotane (Lysodren)	Encephalopathy Lethargy Somnolence Depression	Common	Mild

(Continued)

Table 11–1 Neuropsychiatric Effects of Chemotherapeutic Agents
(Continued)

AGENT	TOXICITY	INCIDENCE	REMARKS
Procarbazine (oral) (Matulane, Natulan)	CNS depression Drowsiness/stupor Confusion Agitation Hallucinations Delirium Psychosis	8–30%	Reversible See 5-fluorouracil above
Hormonal agents			

Corticosteroids (various brand names)	Psychiatric symptoms
	Depression
	Mania
	Delirium
	Cognitive impairment
	Psychosis
	  Emotional lability
	  Anxiety
	  Pressured speech
	  Sensory flooding
	  Agitation
	  Hallucinations
	  Body image alterations
	  Delusions
	Panic disorder
	Obsession-compulsion
	Catatonia
		6–62%
		40%
		28%
		10%
		
		14%
		
		Rare
		Rare
		Rare
			5%—severe
			Dosage >40 mg/d (prednisone)
			See 5-fluorouracil above
			Memory, attention, concentration, mental speed

	Neuropsychiatric symptoms Hyperkinesia Tremor Nervousness Sleep disturbances Euphoria/dysphoria Agitation	Common	Dosage >40 mg/d (prednisone) Reversible
Antiestrogens			
Tamoxifen (Nolvadex, Tamofen)	Encephalopathy Confusion Lethargy	Uncommon	
Investigational agents			
Acivicin (AT-125)	Encephalopathy Confusion Delirium Hallucinations		Reversible See 5-fluorouracil above

Table 11–1 Neuropsychiatric Effects of Chemotherapeutic Agents
(Continued)

AGENT	TOXICITY	INCIDENCE	REMARKS
PALA	Encephalopathy Confusion Lethargy Delirium Hallucinations		See 5-fluorouracil above
Spiromustine	Encephalopathy Confusion Lethargy Hallucinations		
Thymidine	Encephalopathy Confusion Hallucinations		Toxicity increased with concomitant 5-fluorouracil
Biological response modifiers			

Interferon (alpha, beta, & gamma)	Neurobehavioral symptoms
	Behavioral changes
	  Lethargy
	  Hypersomnia
	Affective disorders
	  Depression
	Cognitive changes
	  Confusion
	  Impaired memory
	  Deficits in verbal abstraction & visuographic skills
	  Impaired concentration
	  Hallucinations
	Delirium
		
		Unusual
		
		Rare
		
		Unusual
		
		Rare
		Rare
			Systemic interferon-alpha primarily
			Usually prompt resolution following cessation (several days to 2 wks), but may persist
			
			See 5-fluorouracil

HD recombinant IL-2	CNS symptoms Confusion Restlessness Hallucinations Delirium Psychoses	 Common Common Unusual Unusual Rare	Extension of infusion time & decrease in total dose under investigation to reduce CNS symptoms CNS symptoms vary with concomitant IL-2/LAK cell therapy

IT = intrathecal; HD = high dose; IA = intra-arterial.
Adapted from Cameron, J.C.: Ifosfamide neurotoxicity. Cancer Nurs. 16:40–46, 1993; Furlong, T.G.: Neurologic complications of immunosuppressive cancer therapy. Oncol. Nurs. Forum 20:1337–1354, 1993; MacDonald, D.R. In Perry, M.C. (ed.): The Chemotherapy Source Book (pp. 666–679). Baltimore: Williams & Wilkins, 1992; Myers, C.A., Scheibel, R.S., and Forman, A.D.: Persistent neurotoxicity of systematically administered interferon-alpha. Neurology 41:672–676, 1991; Peterson, L.G., and Popkin, M.K.: Neuropsychiatric effects of chemotherapeutic agents for cancer. Psychosomatics 21:141–153, 1980; Post-White, J.: Glucocorticosteroid-induced depression in the patient with leukemia or lymphoma. Cancer Nurs. 9:15–22, 1986; Strauman, J.J.: The nurse's role in the biotherapy of cancer: Nursing research of side effects. Oncol. Nurs. Forum 15(6)(Suppl):35–39, 1988; Zimberg, M., and Berenson, S.: Delirium in patients with cancer: Nursing assessment and intervention. Oncol. Nurs. Forum 17:529–538, 1990.

Alkylating Agents

The neuropsychiatric effects of ifosfamide, an aklylator-like agent, are variable and dose-limiting, occurring more frequently with high-dose therapy (3 to 5 gm/m^2). Clinical manifestations include confusion, somnolence, hallucinations, and even psychosis and usually resolve within 48 hours following discontinuation of therapy (Cameron, 1993).

Neuropsychiatric disturbances with mechlorethamine (nitrogen mustard, Mustargen) most often occur with high-dose therapy for bone marrow transplantation. Delirium and hallucinations are symptoms that have been reported with mechlorethamine (Peterson and Popkin, 1980).

Cisplatin (Platinol) in doses greater than 60 mg/kg may cause encephalopathy with confusion; however, this side effect may be due to drug-induced fluid and electrolyte imbalances (MacDonald, 1992; Peterson and Popkin, 1980).

Nitrosoureas

Carmustine (BiCNU, BCNU) produces little or no neuropsychiatric side effects at usual intravenous doses (200 or 80 mg/m^2/d × 3 days); however, an encephalopathy with confusion and seizures may result from high-dose, intravenous therapy (600 to 800 mg/m^2 or more) with autologous bone marrow transplantation.

Antimetabolites

Methotrexate (Mexate, Folex) principally acts as a competitive inhibitor of the enzyme dihydrofolate reductase, thereby inhibiting DNA, RNA, and protein synthesis by limiting available reduced folates. While little or no neuropsychiatric side effects have been reported with oral or intravenous methotrexate in usual doses, an acute encephalopathy characterized by seizures, confusion, hemiparesis, and coma occasionally follows high-dose (>1 gm/m^2) intravenous use. The encephalopathy typically occurs after several treatments with high-dose methotrexate; however, it may not recur with subsequent infusions and usually is transient and reversible (MacDonald, 1992).

A progressive leukoencephalopathy (LEC) may follow high-dose intravenous methotrexate and cranial irradiation. A severe delayed neurotoxicity that resembles multiple sclerosis, progressive LEC most often is seen in children with acute lymphoblastic leukemia (ALL). This may be due to the lowering of cerebrospinal fluid (CSF) folate, as intravenous folate may reverse the syndrome. Progressive LEC often begins insidiously during the first year after treatment and resembles a fulminant dementing process, with features including irritability, insomnia, confusion, tremor, ataxia, and personality and intellectual decline (Furlong, 1993; MacDonald, 1992; Peterson and Popkin, 1980).

The type, dosage, and combination of treatment modalities, as well as the cumulative dose of methotrexate, the radiation dose with intravenous methotrexate, and the cumulative intrathecal dose of methotrexate after cranial irradiation, appear to influence the development of progressive LEC. A higher risk is associated with multimodality therapy; single-modality therapy has demonstrated only a 1 to 2% incidence of progressive LEC (Furlong, 1993).

Meningeal irritation, or arachnoiditis, most commonly occurs with intrathecal methotrexate. Numerous factors appear to influence its development, including drug diluent and formulation, dosage, administration schedule, drug pharmacokinetics, presence of meningeal disease, and concomitant therapies. A subacute toxicity with intrathecal methotrexate and CNS irradiation (1,800 to 2,400 cGy) is the somnolence syndrome, clinically characterized by lethargy, irritability, fever, nausea and vomiting, and diarrhea (Furlong, 1993).

Delirium, an irreversible pathophysiological disorder, is caused by altered cerebral metabolism that impairs neuronal functioning. Characterized by impaired cognitive functioning and perceptual, emotional, and behavioral alterations, delirium may occur with intrathecal methotrexate as well as with 5-fluorouracil, L-asparaginase, nitrogen mustard, procarbazine, chlorambucil, steroids, recombinant interleukin-2 (IL-2), lymphokine activated killer (LAK) cells, and interferon. Moreover, other medications such as narcotic analgesics, anticholinergics-antihistamines, antifungal agents (e.g., amphotericin B), and antiviral agents (e.g., acyclovir) increase the risk for delirium (Zimberg and Berenson, 1990).

In its early (mild) stages, delirium frequently is mistaken for anxiety or depression. This may delay diagnosis, supportive and protective interventions, and appropriate pharmacological management with oral neuroleptics until severe symptoms are present (Zimberg and Berenson, 1990). Early behavioral symptoms of delirium include a change in sleep patterns with restlessness and transient disorientation; increased irritability, anger, and temper outbursts; withdrawal from family, friends, and caregivers; and forgetfulness (a behavior not previously manifested by the patient). Severe behavioral changes include refusal to cooperate with reasonable requests; swearing, shouting, or abusive language; and illusions, delusions, and hallucinations (Fleishman & Lesko, 1989).

Cytosine arabinoside (Cytosar-U, Ara-C) can be administered by two routes. The intravenous route is common when treating adult-onset acute myelogenous leukemia (AML). Intrathecal administration, used in treating CNS leukemia, allows the medication to cross the blood-brain barrier. There is little or no neurotoxicity associated with usual intravenous doses; dose-related cerebellar and cerebral toxicity may occur with high-dose treatment (2 to 3 gm/m^2 every 12 hours for 8 to 12 doses). Manifestations of these toxicities are usually reversible, with symptom improvement in 4 to 7 days after onset. Administration of the drug over 2 to 3 hours may decrease the incidence of cerebellar toxicity. Other predisposing factors in the development of cerebellar toxicity with high-dose treatment include (1) age greater than 50 years (it is recommended that the dose be decreased to 1.5 to 2 gm/m^2, with 24 gm/m^2 total to prevent excessive and irreversible effects); (2) preexisting and progressive hepatic dysfunction; (3) previous neurologic dysfunction; (4) renal insufficiency; and (5) previous CNS therapy (Furlong, 1993).

Vinca Alkaloids

Neurotoxic side effects are greatest with vincristine (Oncovin, Vincasar), followed by vindesine (Eldisine) and then vinblastine (Velban, Velbe, Velsar). The CNS effects of vincristine most often appear late and range from irritability and depression to seizure and coma with high dosages. While the overall incidence is less than 5%, patients receiving 75 μg/kg may experience hallucinations. With vinblastine therapy, a variety of temporary mood and behavioral alterations, including mental depression or anxiety, have been noted in up to 80% of patients.

Antitumor Antibiotics

At certain dosage levels, all antitumor antibiotics have the potential to produce CNS side effects, as demonstrated experimentally in animal models; however, the development of severe bone marrow toxicity has limited their use in humans at these levels (Peterson and Popkin, 1980).

At clinical doses, plicamycin (Mithracin), principally used in the treatment of embryonal cell carcinoma and for palliation for certain types of hypercalcemia, is associated with a high incidence of irritability and anxiety. CNS side effects are not significant with doxorubicin (Adriamycin) and daunorubicin (Cerubidine) (Peterson and Popkin, 1980).

Miscellaneous Antineoplastic Agents

The incidence of encephalopathy/cerebral dysfunction with L-asparaginase (Elspar, Kidrolase, L-ASP), especially in the presence of liver dysfunction, ranges from 21 to 60%, with clinical manifestations including lethargy, drowsiness/somnolence, confusion, depression, hallucinations, stupor, and delirium. These neuropsychiatric side effects are reversible with discontinuation of therapy (Furlong, 1993; MacDonald, 1992).

Three miscellaneous agents that warrant discussion because of their neuropsychiatric side effects are altretamine, mitotane, and procarbazine. Altretamine (Hexalen, Hexastat, hexamethylmelamine, HMM), an ethylenimine derivative, has been reported to cause confusion, depression, hallucinations, and possibly suicidal tendencies. The neuropsychiatric effects do not appear to be dose- or schedule-related. These behavioral symptoms appear several days to several weeks after initiation of therapy, with full recovery within days to weeks following discontinuation of the drug (MacDonald, 1992; Peterson and Popkin, 1980).

Mental depression, which is dose-related and reversible, is a common side effect with mitotane (Lysodren), a derivative of the insecticide DDT. Procarbazine (Matulane, Natulan), a hydrazine, crosses the blood-brain barrier and may produce CNS depression, as evidenced by a pattern of diffuse slow waves on EEG. Symptoms begin shortly after initiation of therapy and usually are reversible with drug discontinuation. Clinical manifestations include drowsiness/stupor, confusion, agitation, hallucinations, delirium, and psychosis. Moreover, procarbazine is synergistic with alcohol, barbiturates, and phenothiazines, thereby potentiating their CNS side effects (MacDonald, 1992; Peterson and Popkin, 1980).

Corticosteroids

While initial side effects to steroids, such as an increased sense of well-being and an increased appetite, can be clinically useful, it is well-known that prednisone can produce a broad spectrum of untoward psychiatric reactions (termed organic affective syndromes), e.g., major mood changes, depression, and, although infrequent (approximately a 5% incidence), psychosis. In addition to prednisone, methylprednisolone and dexamethasone may produce similar neuropsychiatric symptoms. While uncommon, other clinically significant steroid-induced disturbances include panic disorder, obsessive-compulsive behavior, and catatonia (Furlong, 1993; Post-White, 1986).

Behavioral responses to corticosteroids are independent of dosage; however, a linear relationship between corticosteroid dosage and untoward psychiatric sequelae has been reported, i.e., more severe drug-induced mental aberrations with higher doses (>40 mg/d). The neuropsychiatric side effects of prednisone are reversible with discontinuation of therapy (Fleishman and Lesko, 1989; Furlong, 1993; Peterson and Popkin, 1980).

Table 11–2 lists the risk factors and clinical manifestations of depression. Hepatic dysfunction increases susceptibility to all neurotoxicities and may mandate dose reduction, up to as much as 50%, or discontinu-

Table 11–2   Depression: Risk Factors and Clinical Manifestations

Risk factors

Personal	History of depression (patient or family)
	Prior psychiatric illness
	Depression or manic episodes
	Alcoholism and/or drug abuse
	Suicide attempt or family history of suicide
Illness and treatment	Advanced stage disease
	Uncontrolled pain
	Pharmacologic
	Corticosteroids (prednisone, dexamethasone)
	Chemotherapeutic agents
	Vincristine/vinblastine/vindesine
	Hexamethylmelamine (oral)
	L-asparaginase
	Mitotane
	Interferon
	Other medications
	Estrogens
	Cimetidine
	Diazepam
	Phenobarbital
	Propranolol
	Rauwolfia alkaloids
	Indomethacin
	Levodopa
	Methyldopa
	Pentazocine
	Phenmetrazine
	Other medical conditions
	Metabolic
	Nutritional
	Endocrine
	Neurological

Clinical manifestations	***Psychological***
	Dysphoric mood, e.g., sad, depressed, anxious, crying; diurnal mood changes
	Pessimistic thoughts
	Feelings of hopelessness, helplessness, powerlessness
	Loss of interest and pleasure
	Withdrawal from social interactions
	Lowered self-esteem
	Inappropriate & excessive guilt
	Burden on others
	Feelings of worthlessness/inadequacy
	Impaired concentration
	Disorientation in elderly ("pseudodementia")
	Mood with prognosis
	Suicidal ideation
	Delusional thoughts
	Somatic
	Insomnia
	Anorexia with weight loss
	Fatigue
	Psychomotor impairment or agitation
	Constipation
	Decreased sexual interest

Adapted from Gorman, L.M., Sultan, D., and Luna-Raines, M.: *Psychosocial Nursing Handbook for the Nonpsychiatric Nurse.* Baltimore: Williams and Wilkins, 1989; Massie, M.J.: Depression. In Holland, J.C., and Rowland, J.H. (eds.): *Handbook of Psychooncology: Psychological Care of the Patient with Cancer* (pp. 283–290). New York: Oxford University Press, 1989.

ation of therapy in patients with bilirubin levels of 30 mg/dl or more. Moreover, the additive or synergistic effect of combining vinca alkaloids with other potentially neurotoxic drugs, such as etoposide (VP-16) or teniposide (VM-26), potentiates development of neurotoxicities (Furlong, 1933; Peterson and Popkin, 1980).

Biological Response Modifiers (BRMs)

The neuropsychiatric side effects associated with interferon, and primarily with systemic interferon-alpha, include behavioral changes, e.g., lethargy and hypersomnia; affective disorders, e.g., depression; and cognitive changes, e.g., confusion, hallucinations, and impaired memory. Interferon also may cause delirium. EEG abnormalities, e.g., diffuse slowing of background activity and intermittent frontally dominant delta activity, often accompany the neurobehavioral symptoms. While these neurobehavioral symptoms may persist, there usually is prompt resolution following cessation of therapy (Irwin, 1987; Meyers, Scheibel, and Forman, 1991; Zimberg and Berenson, 1990).

CNS toxicity is common with high-dose recombinant IL-2, particularly with concomitant administration of LAK cells. Common neuropsychiatric side effects include confusion and restlessness. Extending the infusion time and/or decreasing the total dose delivered may reduce CNS symptoms. Continuous infusion over 5 days usually is tolerated better than a single bolus injection. While their incidence is uncommon, hallucinations, delirium, and even psychosis may occur (Fleishman and Lesko, 1989; Strauman, 1988).

Nursing Management

All of the neuropsychiatric toxicities associated with antineoplastic drugs, hormones, and BRMs can have a devastating impact on the patient, family, and caregivers and can severely limit continued treatment, functional capacity, and quality of life while increasing psychological distress. Most of the toxicities are dose- or schedule-related and reversible within hours or days of adjustment or discontinuation of therapy. The goals of treatment, e.g., cure versus palliation, are a critical element in all management decisions.

An individualized and comprehensive assessment of symptoms, mental status, and physical status that is repeated at frequent intervals during therapy is the key to prompt diagnosis of neuropsychiatric side effects, supportive and protective interventions, and appropriate pharmacologic, psychologic, or psychiatric management as needed. The use of a standardized neurobehavioral assessment tool, e.g., the Neurobehavioral Rating Scale (assesses behavior, cognition, and memory) or the Mini-Mental State Examination (assesses cognition and memory), can provide helpful confirmatory evidence of alterations and facilitate assessment and communication of changes in memory and cognitive and behavioral function (Fleishman and Lesko, 1989; Furlong, 1993).

Patient and family education is critical to prompt diagnosis and appropriate management, since it may be necessary to monitor the patient's mental status daily or several times daily if it is changing rapidly. This is especially important when titrating medication dosage according to the patient's behavior.

Communications that utilize active, nonjudgmental listening will reduce anxiety, increase security, and facilitate development of a trusting nurse-patient/family relationship and therapeutic environment for early recognition and management of actual and potential neuropsychiatric side effects.

Because physiological variables (e.g., fluid and electrolyte imbalances, liver dysfunction, or renal insufficiency) and pre-existing or concurrent illnesses (e.g., patient or family history of affective disorder or history of alcohol or drug abuse) and concurrent life stresses may contribute to the development or severity of neuropsychiatric side effects with cancer chemotherapy, their ongoing assessment is essential to timely and accurate diagnosis and effective management of cognitive, emotional, or behavioral alterations. Many metabolic, nutritional, endocrine, and neurological disorders produce clinical manifestations that can be mistaken for depression, anxiety, or other neuropsychiatric toxicities and require assessment and appropriate treatment in the cancer patient showing symptoms.

References

Cameron, J.C.: Ifosfamide neurotoxicity: A challenge for nurses, a potential nightmare for patients. Cancer Nurs. 16:40–46, 1993.

Clark, J.: Psychosocial dimensions: The patient. In Groenwald, S.L., Frogge, M.H., Goodman, M., and Yarbro, C.H. (eds.): Cancer Nursing: Principles and Practice, 2nd ed. (pp. 346–364). Boston, Jones and Bartlett, 1992.

DeVita, V.T., Hellman, S., and Rosenberg, S.A. (eds.): Biologic Therapy of Cancer. Philadelphia: J.B. Lippincott, 1991.

Fleishman, S., and Lesko, L.: Delirium and dementia. In Holland, J.C., and Rowland, J.H. (eds.): Handbook of Psychooncology: Psychological Care of the Patient with Cancer (pp. 342–355). New York: Oxford University Press, 1989.

Furlong, T.G.: Neurologic complications of immunosuppressive cancer therapy. Oncol. Nurs. Forum 20:1337–1354, 1993.

Gabrilove, J.L.: Colony-stimulating factors: Clinical status. In DeVita, V.T., Jr., et al.: Important Advances in Oncology, 1991 (pp. 215–237). Philadelphia: J.B. Lippincott, 1991.

Gorman, L.M., Sultan, D., and Luna-Raines, M.: *Psychosocial Nursing Handbook for the Nonpsychiatric Nurse*. Baltimore: Williams and Wilkins, 1989.

Holland, J.C., and Lesko, L.M.: Chemotherapy, endocrine therapy, and immunotherapy. In Holland, J.C., and Rowland, J.H. (eds.): *Handbook of Psychooncology: Psychological Care of the Patient with Cancer* (pp. 146–162). New York, Oxford University Press, 1989.

Irwin, M.M.: Patients receiving biological response modifiers: Overview of nursing care. Oncol. Nurs. Forum 14(6)(Suppl.):32–37, 1987.

MacDonald, D.R.: Neurotoxicity of chemotherapeutic agents. In Perry, M.C. (ed.): *The Chemotherapy Source Book* (pp. 666–679). Baltimore: Williams & Wilkins, 1992.

Massie, M.J.: Depression. In Holland, J.C., and Rowland, J.H. (eds.): *Handbook of Psychooncology: Psychological Care of the Patient with Cancer* (pp. 283–290). New York: Oxford University Press, 1989.

Meyers, C.A., Scheibel, R.S., and Forman, A.D.: Persistent neurotoxicity of systemically administered interferon-alpha. Neurology 41:672–676, 1991.

Peterson, L.G., and Popkin, M.K.: Neuropsychiatric effects of chemotherapeutic agents for cancer. Psychosomatics 21:141–153, 1980.

Post-White, J.: Glucocorticosteroid-induced depression in the patient with leukemia or lymphoma. Cancer Nurs. 9:15–22, 1986.

Strauman, J.J.: The nurse's role in the biotherapy of cancer: Nursing research of side effects. Oncol. Nurs. Forum 15(6)(Suppl.):35–39, 1988.

Zimberg, M., and Berenson, S.: Delirium in patients with cancer: Nursing assessment and intervention. Oncol. Nurs. Forum 17:529–538, 1990.

Zonderman, A.B., Costa, P.T., and McCrae, R.R.: Depression as a risk for cancer morbidity and mortality in a nationally representative sample. JAMA 262:1191–1195, 1989.

Chapter 12

Chemotherapy-Induced Second Malignancies

Catherine A. Hydzik, R.N., M.S., O.C.N.
Christine Miaskowski, R.N., Ph.D.,
F.A.A.N.

A second malignancy, also known as a treatment-related malignancy, is defined as the development of a new cancer in a patient following treatment for a primary malignancy. This chapter will focus on the development of second malignancies following treatment with chemotherapy. Chemotherapy-induced second malignancies are one of the most serious long-term effects of chemotherapy treatment because they are usually associated with a poor prognosis.

This chapter is organized into several sections. The first section reviews the common epidemiological approaches used to determine the prevalence rates and risk factors associated with the development of second malignancies. The major risk factors associated with the development of second malignancies that are common to all types of primary cancer treatment are summarized in section two. The third section of the chapter provides a comprehensive review of the major studies that have determined prevalence rates, relative risk ratios, and specific risk factors for the following primary malignancies: pediatric cancers, Hodgkin's disease, breast cancer, ovarian cancer, lung cancer, multiple myeloma, gastrointestinal cancer, testicular cancer, and non-Hodgkin's lymphoma. The chapter concludes with a discussion of the nursing implications of caring for patients who are at potential risk for developing a chemotherapy-induced second malignancy.

Approaches to Studying Second Malignancies

Two epidemiologic methods are utilized to determine risk factors and identify the relative risk for second malignancies. One method, the cohort study, identifies patients with a specific tumor type who had received treatment and observes them over time to determine the incidence of second malignancies. Participants are recruited from tumor registries, multicenter trials, or hospitals. These patients have the same primary diagnosis but may not have received the same treatment.

Cohort studies are used to analyze actuarial or life table risks. The first step is to assess whether there is an increased risk or probability of developing a second malignancy based on treatment for the primary cancer. The risk probability or relative risk of developing a second malignancy is calculated by taking the actual number of second malignancies observed in the study population and dividing by the expected number from data on the general population. The cumulative risk is the probability of developing a second malignancy over a period of time.

The case control method is the second approach used to analyze the relationship between cancer treatment and the development of a second malignancy. Individuals who developed a second malignancy are compared to a control group of individuals who have not developed cancer. In the case control method, data collection is smaller, more easily managed, less time consuming, and cost efficient. However, the potential for bias is much greater. The bias in selecting the control group can skew the results or lead to inaccurate associations or conclusions. The control group must be representative of the entire group.

Risk Factors Associated with Chemotherapy-Induced Second Malignancies

Because cancer survival rates have increased, it is now possible to study the development of second malignancies. Both children and adults receiving chemotherapy for a primary cancer are at risk for the development of a treatment-related malignancy. The specific patient risk factors, as well as the exact relationship between chemotherapy administration and the development of a second malignancy are extremely complex. Epidemiological approaches as described previously, are used to determine the prevalence rates, as well as the relationship between chemotherapy regimens, patient characteristics, tumor types, and the development of second malignancies. Systematic investigations have identified several risk factors that are summarized in Table 12–1.

Chemotherapy-Specific Risk Factors

The first group of risk factors associated with the development of a second malignancy are related to the chemotherapy regimen itself. The chemotherapy-specific risk factors that have been identified include the specific chemotherapeutic drug, total cumulative dose administered, and administration schedule.

As outlined in Table 12–2, the chemotherapeutic agents have been classified into three categories: group 1 agents are carcinogenic to humans; group 2a agents are probably carcinogenic to humans; group 2b agents are possibly carcinogenic to humans; and group 3 agents are not carcinogenic. Many of the agents in groups 1, 2a, and 2b are part of chemotherapy regimens used to treat human cancers. The two largest groups of chemotherapy agents that are implicated in the development of second malignancies are the alkylating agents and the nitrosoureas. In addition, there are data to suggest that etoposide (VePesid, VP-16) and teniposide (VM-26) may produce secondary leukemias.

Besides the specific chemotherapy agent administered, the risk for a second malignancy may depend on the total cumulative dose of the drug administered. Recent data suggest that the risk of a secondary leukemia increases proportionally with the total cumulative dose of chemotherapy administered.

Another risk factor associated with the development of a second malignancy is the administration schedule of an agent. For example, the risk of epipodophyllotoxin-induced acute myeloid leukemia appears to depend on the drug administration schedule. Prolonged treatment with

Table 12–1 Potential Risk Factors Associated with the Development of a Second Malignancy

Treatment-related risk factors
  Chemotherapy
    Specific agent
    Total cumulative dose
    Administration schedule
    Time period after treatment
  Radiation therapy
  Multimodality therapy
Genetic/familial predisposition
Age
Immune status
Environmental factors
Splenectomy in Hodgkin's disease

Table 12–2 Carcinogenicity Classification
of Chemotherapeutic Agents

Group 1

Carcinogenic to humans

Busulfan (Myleran)
Chlorambucil (Leukeran)
Cyclophosphamide (Cytoxan)
Melphalan (Alkeran)
MOPP (Mechlorethamine [Nitrogen Mustard], Oncovin [Vincristine], Procarbazine
hydrochloride [Matulane], Prednisone)
Semustine (Methyl-CCNU)
Tresulfan

Group 2a

Probably carcinogenic to humans

Carmustine (BCNU)
Cisplatin (Cis-Diamminedichloroplatinum, Platino)
Doxorubicin (Adriamycin)
Lomustine (CCNU)
Mechlorethamine (Nitrogen Mustard)
N-methyl-N-nitrosourea
Procarbazine hydrochloride (Matulane, Natulan)
Thiotepa (triethylenethiophosphoramide)

Group 2b

Possibly carcinogenic to humans

Bleomycin (Blenoxane)
Dacarbazine (DTIC)
Daunomycin (Daunorubicin)
Medroxyprogesterone acetate (Depo-Provera)
Mitomycin C (Mitomycin)
Streptozotocin (Zanosar)
Uracil mustard (Uracil)

Group 3

Noncarcinogenic to humans

Actinomycin D (Dactinomycin)
5-Azacytidine
5-Fluorouracil (5-Fu)
Methotrexate (Folex, Mexate)
Prednisone

From the International Agency for Research on Cancer (IARC), 1987, 1990. Reprinted with
permission.

weekly or twice weekly doses of an epipodophyllotoxin resulted in an increased risk for the development of leukemia compared to other schedules of drug administration.

The time period after chemotherapy treatment needs to be considered when analyzing risk factors related to the chemotherapy regimen. The risk of developing a secondary leukemia appears to be greatest within the first few years following treatment. Typically, leukemia will occur between the second and tenth years after therapy, with the peak incidence at around five years. In contrast, the time period after treatment for the development of solid tumors is usually greater than ten years.

Another risk factor associated with the development of second malignancies is multimodal therapy. The exact relationship between the development of a second malignancy and multimodal therapy (i.e., chemotherapy, and/or surgery, and/or radiation therapy) is unclear. Several studies have found that the combination of alkylating agents and radiation therapy does not appear to increase the risk of leukemia. However, several studies have documented an increased risk of leukemia in Hodgkin's patients treated with multimodal therapy. The relationship between multimodal therapy and the development of second malignancies in the form of solid tumors is currently unknown.

Additional Risk Factors

Besides the treatment itself, additional risk factors associated with the development of a second malignancy include genetic predisposition, age, immune status, environmental factors, and splenectomy in patients with Hodgkin's disease. Some studies have suggested a relationship between a genetic predisposition and the development of a second malignancy. However, the data on the relationship between age and the development of a second malignancy are inconclusive. Several studies found a correlation between increasing age (i.e., >40 years of age at the time of treatment) and increased incidence of secondary leukemias. However, these data are confounded by the fact that in the general population, the overall incidence of leukemia increases with age.

An additional risk factor associated with the development of second malignancies is the immune status of the host. Prolonged immunosuppression may increase the incidence of second malignancies.

Finally, the environment may pose an additional risk. Some data suggest that exposure to chemicals or petroleum products may increase the risk of secondary leukemias. In addition, personal habits (i.e., smoking, alcohol consumption) may add to an individual's risk. The problem with establishing the exact causal relationship between environmental factors and personal habits and the relative risk of second malignancies is that these risk factors are extremely difficult to isolate and quantify.

Types of Second Malignancies

Second malignancies can be subdivided into two types. The most common type of second malignancy is leukemia, with acute non-lymphocytic leukemia (ANLL) being the most common subtype. A solid tumor in any one of the major organs is the other type of second malignancy. This chapter provides a review of the literature on chemotherapy-induced second malignancies in pediatric patients as well as in patients with the following primary tumors: Hodgkin's disease, breast cancer, ovarian cancer, lung cancer, multiple myeloma, gastrointestinal cancer, testicular cancer, and non-Hodgkin's lymphoma. In addition, malignancies occurring in patients with nonmalignant diseases treated with chemotherapeutic agents will be discussed.

The remainder of this chapter is organized by patient population or primary tumor type. For each patient population or tumor type, a synthesis of the literature on second malignancies is provided with the major risk factors highlighted. In addition, a table summarizing the studies done to date on second malignancies is included. This table provides, at a glance, information on the types of second malignancies that occur in a given patient population, the associated risk factors, and the relative and cumulative risk for developing a second malignancy. Nurses can use this resource when screening patients who have the potential to develop a second malignancy.

Pediatric Malignancies

Survival rates for childhood cancers have increased dramatically. Therefore, a population of patients in which one can study the late effects of chemotherapy is now available. Evidence suggests that if a child develops one malignancy, he or she is at a 10 times greater risk to develop a second malignancy compared with an age-matched individual. Recent estimates suggest that 3% to 12% of childhood cancer survivors will develop a second malignancy within 20 years after their diagnosis.

The results of studies of pediatric cancer survivors who developed a second malignancy during the period from 1985 to 1993 are summarized in Table 12–3. The most common primary cancers were retinoblastoma, followed by Hodgkin's disease, soft tissue sarcomas, Wilm's tumor, and brain cancers. Approximately 68% of the second malignancies observed in childhood cancer survivors were associated with radiation therapy. The most frequently documented radiation-associated second malignancies were bone sarcomas, followed by soft tissue sarcomas, leukemias/

lymphomas, and thyroid cancers. However, the most common second malignancies associated with chemotherapy were leukemias/lymphomas, and brain tumors.

Chemotherapy, particularly the alkylating agents, administered with or without radiation therapy markedly increased the risk for secondary leukemias in the pediatric population. Recently, etoposide has been linked to the increased risk of leukemia in this population. In addition, in pediatric patients, genetic and familial factors (i.e., retinoblastoma) may predispose an individual to develop a second malignancy. Pediatric nurses must evaluate cancer survivors well into adolescence and adulthood because the latency period to developing these secondary neoplasms may be longer than 10 years.

Hodgkin's Disease

The development of second malignancies in patients with Hodgkin's disease is well documented. The studies on second malignancies associated with Hodgkin's disease conducted from 1982 to 1991 are summarized in Table 12–4.

The majority of Hodgkin's disease patients who develop a secondary leukemia were treated with chemotherapy or combined multimodal therapy. Yet, several unanswered questions and some controversial issues exist around the identified risk factors for secondary malignancies following chemotherapy treatment for Hodgkin's disease.

While the administration of alkylating agents is associated with the development of secondary leukemia, one question that remains to be answered is whether combined multimodal therapy, as compared to single agent therapy, increases the risk of leukemia. The person's age at the time of treatment is another factor that influences the development of leukemia. Recent data suggest that as age increases so does the relative risk of secondary leukemia. In addition, researchers are attempting to determine if splenectomy contributes to an increased risk of leukemia. The spleen may play a potential role in tumor immunosurveillance. If this is the case, splenectomy may decrease the patient's immunosurveillance capacity to "filter-out" leukemic cells and may increase the patient's risk for a secondary chemotherapy-induced leukemia.

The risk of developing a secondary cancer, following treatment for Hodgkin's disease, seems to increase over time. Finally, patients who smoke may be at increased risk of developing a secondary solid tumor following chemotherapy for Hodgkin's disease.

In conclusion, the risk of secondary malignancies following treatment for Hodgkin's disease seems to be closely related to the type and intensity of therapy. MOPP therapy (i.e., mechlororethamine, vincristine, procarbazine, and prednisone) containing alkylating agents is the most common regimen that has been linked to second malignancies. However, it was also one of the most common regimens used to treat Hodgkin's disease. Other risk factors that have been associated with the potential for developing a second malignancy following treatment for Hodgkin's disease include age (i.e., over 40 years), multimodal therapy, stage of disease (i.e., increased stage), and/or a splenectomy.

Nurses caring for Hodgkin's disease patients must be able to identify the high-risk patient and perform ongoing surveillance evaluations.

Breast Cancer

The potential for a leukemogenic effect from adjuvant chemotherapy for breast cancer, despite its benefits, has raised some concern. Cases of leukemia have been documented in patients who have received adjuvant chemotherapy. However, the subjects were so heterogenous, that it was impossible to determine the exact incidence and draw definitive conclusions. The studies on secondary malignancies following chemotherapy treatment for breast cancer conducted from 1985 to 1990 are summarized in Table 12–5.

The administration of alkylating agents, particularly melphalan, is associated with an increased risk for a secondary leukemia. The total dose of the agent administered seems to correlate with the risk for second malignancy. Andersson and colleagues (1990) suggested that an increased risk of leukemia was associated with prednimustine alone and that, in addition, a synergetic effect may exist between prednimustine and the other agents. Lavey and colleagues (1990) indicated that the overall risk of second malignancy in breast cancer patients treated with radiation or chemotherapy did not increase during the first 10 years following treatment. Interestingly, some research suggests that chemotherapy, with or without radiation, may decrease a woman's risk of contralateral breast cancer.

Nurses need to continue to evaluate the effectiveness of treatment and the late effects of chemotherapy in breast cancer survivors. The risks appear to be much lower in the breast cancer population compared to the Hodgkin's disease population. However, breast cancer is a more common tumor and while the relative risk for developing a secondary malignancy is lower, more patients may actually go on to develop a treatment-related malignancy.

Ovarian Cancer

Ovarian cancer is primarily treated with surgery and chemotherapy. An increased risk of leukemia following chemotherapy treatment for ovarian cancer has been documented. The studies of second malignancies in ovarian cancer conducted from 1977 to 1990 are summarized in Table 12–6.

These studies clearly document the increased risk of leukemia in ovarian cancer patients treated with alkylating agents. Data from these studies suggest that there is a positive correlation between drug dosage and increased risk for leukemia. Recent reports suggest that administration of cisplatin may be linked to the development of a secondary leukemia. Greene (1992) identified 45 cases from the literature of patients who developed a cisplatin-associated second malignancy. However, none of these reported studies proved that cisplatin was the cause of the subsequent malignancy. In addition, cisplatin was used in conjunction with one or more chemotherapeutic agents, thus making it difficult to determine a definitive linkage between cisplatin administration and the development of a secondary cancer. Only one case was cited in which cisplatin was the only agent administered to the patient. Epidemiologic studies are required to determine whether cisplatin is a human carcinogen. Ideally, patients should be exposed to cisplatin as a single agent, not as part of a combination regimen, to determine the exact causal relationship.

Because ovarian cancer patients are living longer, the relationship between primary treatment and treatment-related malignancies will begin to be more clearly delineated.

Lung Cancer

The studies on second malignancies associated with lung cancer, conducted from 1984 to 1989, are summarized in Table 12–7. The specific chemotherapeutic agents administered to treat the primary lung cancer appear to be the greatest risk factor associated with the development of a secondary leukemia. Several studies documented that an association exists between the dose of etoposide administered and the risk of developing leukemia. Also, a shorter latency period for leukemia was observed in the patients treated with etoposide compared to the patients treated with alkylating agents.

Because lung cancer patients are living longer, the exact relationships between treatment of the primary disease and development of a second malignancy will be further defined in the next several years.

Multiple Myeloma

Multiple myeloma was the first oncologic diagnosis associated with an increased risk of secondary acute leukemia. In 1970, four cases of acute myelomonocytic leukemia were reported in multiple myeloma patients who were treated with melphalan for 30 to 57 months. This number of cases could not be explained by chance and prompted a systematic investigation. The available data suggest that melphalan is the etiological agent in the development of secondary leukemia.

Two studies on second malignancies associated with multiple myeloma are reviewed and summarized in Table 12–8. It has been suggested that chemotherapy may be associated with the development of acute leukemia. It also has been hypothesized that patients diagnosed with myeloma may have a predisposition to develop acute leukemia because patients who are not treated develop leukemia. Such an occurrence may be part of the natural history of this disease. There is a need for well-documented studies to explore this relationship.

Gastrointestinal Cancer

The one study on second malignancies associated with chemotherapy treatment for gastrointestinal cancer is summarized in Table 12–9. Semustine (methyl-CCNU) was the chemotherapeutic agent implicated in the development of a secondary leukemia. The data suggest that receiving larger doses of semustine increased the risk of developing secondary malignancies.

Testicular Cancer

The literature suggests that some patients who have been successfully treated for testicular germ cell tumors may have an increased risk of developing a second malignancy. The studies done in this area, from 1984 to 1991, are summarized in Table 12–10.

The increased risk of developing a second malignancy following treatment for testicular cancer may be associated, only in part, with treatment given for the primary cancer. Incidence rates suggest that some patients with testis cancer may be at an increased risk of developing a second primary testicular germ cell tumor independent of treatment, although the exact reason is unknown.

Survivors of testicular cancer appear to have an increased risk of developing the following second malignancies: contralateral testis cancer, leukemia, renal carcinoma, bladder cancer, pancreatic cancer, melanoma, non-Hodgkin's lymphoma, and prostate cancer.

Several reports have documented the occurrence of acute nonlymphocytic leukemia following chemotherapy for germ cell tumors. A majority of these patients were treated with chemotherapy or combined multimodal therapy. The risk of second malignancy may be attributed to treatment with alkylating agents or high-dose etoposide. The risk factors associated with the development of acute nonlymphocytic leukemia remain to be elucidated in this patient population.

Non-Hodgkin's Lymphoma

The studies on second malignancies in non-Hodgkin's lymphoma, conducted from 1988 to 1991, are summarized in Table 12–11. The literature suggests that non-Hodgkin's lymphoma patients may be at increased risk for developing a secondary leukemia or bladder cancer. Patients treated with combined multimodal therapy (i.e., chemotherapy and radiation therapy) may be at increased risk of developing a secondary leukemia. The risk of a secondary bladder cancer seems to be attributed to chemotherapy. The specific agent correlated with the increased risk is cyclophosphamide. Also, there seems to be an association with the total cumulative dose of the drug administered. Nurses must identify patients at high risk of developing a secondary cancer and monitor all non-Hodgkin's lymphoma survivors for the late effects of chemotherapy.

Nonmalignant Diseases Treated with Chemotherapeutic Agents

Lupus nephritis, polyarteritis nodosa, polycythemia vera, primary systemic amyloidosis, rheumatoid arthritis, and Wegener's granulomatosis are nonmalignant diseases that may be treated with chemotherapeutic agents and that have been associated with the development of malignancies. The chemotherapeutic agents that may be used are cyclophosphamide, melphalan, methotrexate, and uracil mustard. Health care professionals caring for patients with nonmalignant diseases who are receiving one of these agents should be aware of the potential risk effects. It is important for the patient to be aware of the risks and benefits from the chemotherapy treatment and to make an informed decision. In addition, the patient should be carefully monitored to assess for expected and unexpected effects of the treatment.

Nursing Implications

Nurses play a crucial role in caring for patients at risk of developing a second malignancy. The nursing implications are outlined in Table 12–12. First, the nurse must be knowledgeable about the relative risk for developing second malignancies associated with each primary tumor type and must be able to identify patients at risk. Once high-risk patients are identified, an accurate assessment is critical to ensure early diagnosis. Patients at risk for second malignancies should be educated about the late effects of therapy and the importance of ongoing follow-up and health-promoting behaviors. The ongoing assessment and care of these patients must be documented.

Fergusson and colleagues (1987) analyzed the time required to conduct a late effects evaluation compared to a routine follow-up evaluation. A late effects evaluation, conducted as part of a routine follow-up visit, required approximately an additional 15 minutes of the provider's time. However, while this study focused on the time required to conduct a late effects physical evaluation, additional studies are needed to document the additional time required to counsel and educate patients and families about the late effects of treatment.

An essential role of nursing is to teach the patient about the significance of ongoing evaluation, the need for lifelong follow-up care, and the need for ongoing communication with the oncology team. The oncology team can provide multidisciplinary care and support to the patient and his or her family. Follow-up care must be individualized based on the patient's primary cancer diagnosis and health history.

Ongoing surveillance of the cancer survivor should consist of periodic physical examinations and specific laboratory tests. The patient's status and surveillance evaluation must be documented. Meticulous documentation is needed because these charts may be used in subsequent epidemiologic studies. Accurate records will make it easier to abstract vital information to determine prevalence rates and risk factors. Nurses are responsible for maintaining accurate records and documenting any counseling or educating they do with these patients.

Patients who develop a second malignancy often are a challenge to health care providers. These patients have a poor prognosis and require physical care as well as intense psychosocial support. They may express or exhibit a myriad of feelings, emotions, and concerns including sadness, disbelief, despair, anger, or blame. In addition, the patient's family may also express a myriad of feelings, emotions, and concerns.

Similarly, the health care professional may experience an emotional response, especially if the patient is a cancer survivor with whom there is a shared relationship. Nurses must examine their own feelings about second malignancies and must deal appropriately with these emotions.

Often the patient and family need time to deal with the new diagnosis and may require extra support to handle the crisis. When the patient and family are ready, they will need information that will foster a partnership in planning care. Nursing care must include an assessment of the patient's and family's coping strategies and abilities to problem solve. Nurses can provide education and emotional support as well as physical care throughout the patient's illness. These interventions may assist the patient and family to cope more effectively with the disease and treatment.

Summary

This chapter provided an overview of chemotherapy-induced second malignancies and highlighted the risk factors associated with the development of second malignancies. The development of second malignancies following chemotherapy treatment for pediatric tumors, Hodgkin's disease, ovarian cancer, breast cancer, lung cancer, multiple myeloma, gastrointestinal cancer, testicular cancer, non-Hodgkin's lymphoma, and nonmalignant diseases was reviewed.

A significant number of patients are surviving longer as a result of chemotherapy. As nurses caring for the cancer survivor, we must be knowledgeable about cancer chemotherapeutic agents and the potential or actual impact of this treatment on the cancer patient's life. Health care professionals have a responsibility to keep abreast of the late effects of treatment and an obligation to minimize the potential side effects. We must be creative in our approach to addressing the needs of the survivor and studying the long-term effects of various cancer treatments on the survivor. Research is warranted to determine the incidence and degree of long-term effects of chemotherapy and to develop strategies to limit them. In addition, research would allow us to offer patients the best treatment options and the information regarding risks and benefits of treatment.

Table 12–3 Second Malignancies Associated with the Treatment
of Pediatric Malignancies

REFERENCE	PRIMARY DIAGNOSIS/ SAMPLE SIZE		SECOND MALIGNANCY		RISK FACTOR(S) AND ASSOCIATED FINDING(S)	RELATIVE RISK	CUMULATIVE RISK
	TYPE	NO.	TYPE	NO.			
Meadows and Silber, 1985	Total = 292		Total = 308		• Genetic predisposition seen with retinoblastoma and Wilm's tumor.	Not reported	Not reported
	Primary cancers in which second malignancies developed:		Bone sarcoma	67			
	Retinoblastoma	52	Soft tissue sarcomas	59			
	Hodgkin's disease	40			• Treatment with chemotherapy (alkylating agents).		
	Soft tissue sarcomas	40	Leukemia/lymphoma	59			
	Wilm's tumor	36	(acute nonlymphocytic				
	Brain tumor	31	leukemia was the most		• MOPP regimen.		
	Neuroblastoma	28	common type)		• Median latency period was 5.5 years.		
	Leukemia	13					
	Non-Hodgkin's lymphoma	12					
	Other	22					

332

	Other cancers: Skin cancer Brain tumors Thyroid cancers Other neoplasms	31 29 13 24		• Median latency period was 9.5 years. • Overall median latency period to develop a second malignancy was 10 years for patients whose second malignancy developed in the radiation therapy field and 5 years for those not associated with radiation therapy (range, 1 month to 34 years).
Tucker et al, 1987	Total = 9,170 Primary cancers in which second malignancies developed: Hodgkin's disease 12 Wilm's tumor 4 Ewing's sarcoma 2 Medulloblastoma 1 Neuroblastoma 1 Rhabdomyosarcoma 1 Glioblastoma 1	Total = 22 Acute nonlymphocytic leukemia 20 Acute lymphoblastic leukemia 1 Chronic myeloid leukemia 1	14	• Treatment with chemotherapy. • Higher total dose with an alkylating agent. • Administration of doxorubicin. • Median latency period was 3.5 years (range, 2.6 to 12 years).
			Not reported	

(Continued)

Table 12–3 Second Malignancies Associated with the Treatment of Pediatric Malignancies (Continued)

REFERENCE	PRIMARY DIAGNOSIS/ SAMPLE SIZE		SECOND MALIGNANCY		RISK FACTOR(S) AND ASSOCIATED FINDING(S)	RELATIVE RISK	CUMULATIVE RISK
	TYPE	NO.	TYPE	NO.			
Tucker et al, 1987	Total = 9,170 Childhood cancers	9,170	Total = 64 Bone cancer (most common second malignancy for retinoblastoma survivors)	64	• Treatment with chemotherapy. • Cyclophosphamide was the most frequently administered agent. • Higher cumulative doses. • Combined multimodal therapy (i.e., chemotherapy and radiation therapy). • Median latency period was 10 years (range, 3 to 25 years).	133	2.8 ± 0.7% at 20 years.

Study			Second malignancy		Risk factors	Relative risk	Notes
De Vathaire et al, 1989	Total = 634		Total = 32		• Treatment with chemotherapy. • Dactinomycin. • Combined multimodal therapy (i.e., chemotherapy and radiation therapy).	2.7	Not reported
	Primary cancers in which second malignancy developed:		Thyroid cancer	6			
	Neuroblastoma	6	Bone cancer	6			
	Non-Hodgkin's lymphoma	2	Breast cancer	2			
	Rhabdomyosarcoma	5	Skin cancer	5			
	Ewing's sarcoma	3	Brain cancer	3			
	Retinoblastoma	1	Stomach cancer	1			
			Soft tissue cancer	5			
Meadows et al, 1989	Total = 979		Total = 38		• Treatment with radiation therapy. • Median latency period was 12 years (range, 0.8 to 21 years).	9	Any second malignancy: 2% at 5 years, 5% at 10 years, 9% at 15 years.
	Childhood Hodgkin's disease	979	Solid tumors	18			
			Nonlymphocytic leukemia	17	• Treatment with radiation therapy. • Most common regimen was MOPP. • Higher cumulative doses with an alkylating agent. • Therapy of 6 months or more with at least two alkylating agents.		

(Continued)

Table 12–3 Second Malignancies Associated with the Treatment
of Pediatric Malignancies (Continued)

REFERENCE	PRIMARY DIAGNOSIS/ SAMPLE SIZE		SECOND MALIGNANCY		RISK FACTOR(S) AND ASSOCIATED FINDING(S)	RELATIVE RISK	CUMULATIVE RISK
	TYPE	NO.	TYPE	NO.			
			Non-Hodgkin's lymphoma	3	• Splenectomy. • Median latency period was 4.5 years (range, 2 to 10 years). • Treatment with chemotherapy. • Splenectomy. • Median latency period was 5 years (range, 0.8 to 9.5 years).		
Neglia et al, 1991	Total = 9,720 Acute lymphoblastic leukemia	9,720	Total = 43 Neoplasms of the central nervous system New leukemia/lymphoma Other neoplasms	24 10 9	• Age < 5 years. • Treatment with radiation therapy, especially for tumors arising in the central nervous system.	Not reported	2.5% at 15 years.

Pui et al, 1991	Total = 731		Not reported	3.8% within 6 years.
	Acute lymphoblastic leukemia	731		
	Total = 21			
	Acute myeloid leukemia	21	• Major risk factors: prolonged treatment with epipodophyllotoxins (etoposide and teniposide) on a weekly or twice weekly schedule. • Patient characteristics: a. T-cell immunophenotype. b. Mediastinal mass. c. Initial central nervous system involvement. • Higher total cumulative doses. • Combined multimodal therapy (i.e., chemotherapy and radiation therapy). • Median latency period was 40 months (range, 15 to 100 months).		

(Continued)

Table 12–3 Second Malignancies Associated with the Treatment of Pediatric Malignancies (Continued)

REFERENCE	PRIMARY DIAGNOSIS/ SAMPLE SIZE TYPE	NO.	SECOND MALIGNANCY TYPE	NO.	RISK FACTOR(S) AND ASSOCIATED FINDING(S)	RELATIVE RISK	CUMULATIVE RISK
Whitlock et al, 1991	Case report of patient with yolk sac tumor and lung metastases	1	Total = 1 Acute nonlymphocytic leukemia	1	• Treatment with chemotherapy (etoposide and cisplatin). • Actual latency period was 17 months. • Authors found 36 cases of leukemia in the literature: a. Treatment included the use of etoposide-containing chemotherapeutic regimens. b. Shorter latency period. c. Higher cumulative doses of etoposide. d. Translocation involving 11q 23 (chromosomal abnormality).	Not reported	Not reported

Jeha et al, 1992	142	Total = 142 Osteosarcoma				
		Total = 2 Acute nonlymphocytic leukemia	2	• Treatment with chemotherapy: Cisplatin, methotrexate, and Adriamycin. • Actual latency period was 3 and 4 years.	Not reported	Not reported
Kaplinsky et al, 1992	1	Case report of rhabdomyosarcoma				
		Total = 1 T-cell acute lymphoblastic leukemia	1	• Combined multimodal therapy. • Treatment with D-VACA chemotherapy (vincristine, Actinomycin D, cyclophosphamide, Adriamycin, and DTIC) for 6 cycles and radiation therapy to the involved field. • Actual latency period was 41 months.	Not reported	Not reported

(Continued)

Table 12–3 Second Malignancies Associated with the Treatment of Pediatric Malignancies (Continued)

REFERENCE	PRIMARY DIAGNOSIS/ SAMPLE SIZE TYPE	NO.	SECOND MALIGNANCY TYPE	NO.	RISK FACTOR(S) AND ASSOCIATED FINDING(S)	RELATIVE RISK	CUMULATIVE RISK
Verdeguer et al, 1992	Total = 62 Acute lymphoblastic leukemia	62	Total = 3 Acute nonlymphoblastic leukemia	3	• Treatment with chemotherapy (teniposide and ARA-C). • Mean latency period was 20 months (range, 13 to 29 months).	Not reported	Not reported
Haupt et al, 1993	Case report of Langerhans' cell histiocytosis of bone	1	Total = 1 Acute myeloid leukemia	1	• Treatment with chemotherapy. • Specific agent was etoposide (VP-16). • Total cumulative dose was 8,400 mg/m^2. • Actual latency period was 18 months.	Not reported	Not reported

Winick et al, 1993	Total = 203					
	Acute lymphoblastic leukemia	203				
	Total = 10					
	Acute myeloid leukemia	10	• Treatment with chemotherapy.	Not reported	5.9 ± 3.2% at 4 years.	
			• Specific agent was etoposide (VP-16).			
			• Median total dose was 7.9 g/m^2 (range, 5.1 to 9.9 g/m^2).			
			• Therapy was administered twice weekly every 9 weeks.			
			• Overall latency period ranged from 23 to 68 months.			

Table 12–4 Second Malignancies Associated with the Treatment of Hodgkin's Disease

REFERENCE	SAMPLE SIZE	SECOND MALIGNANCY		RISK FACTOR(S) AND ASSOCIATED FINDING(S)	RELATIVE RISK	CUMULATIVE RISK
		TYPE	NO.			
Grunwald and Rosner, 1982		Total = 216			Not reported	Not reported
		Acute myeloid leukemia	216	• Combined multimodal therapy (i.e., chemotherapy and radiation therapy). • Most common regimen was MOPP. • Pancytopenia prior to onset of leukemia. • Median latency period was 73.4 months (range, 9 to 222 months).		
Pedersen-Bjergaard and Larsen, 1982	Total = 391	Total = 17		• Treatment with chemotherapy. • Combined multimodal therapy. • Age > 40 years.	Not reported	3.9 ± 1.3% at 5 years. 9.9 ± 2.9% at 9 years.
		Final secondary malignancy	17			
		Preleukemia	4			
		Acute myeloproliferation	3			
		Acute nonlymphocytic leukemia	10			

Study	No. of patients	Second malignancies		Risk factors		
Aisenberg, 1983	Total = 408	Total = 9			Not reported	4.9% at 12 years. 9.1% for patients treated with MOPP.
		Acute nonlymphocytic leukemia	8	• Treatment with MOPP chemotherapy.		
		Non-Hodgkin's lymphoma	1	• Age > 40 years.		
				• Stage IV disease.		
				• Relapse after MOPP chemotherapy.		
Tester et al. 1984	Total = 473	Total = 34			Not reported	Not reported
		Acute nonlymphocytic leukemia	8	• Age > 40 years for solid tumors.		
		Chronic myeloid leukemia	1	• Incidence of solid tumors increases over time.		
		Non-Hodgkin's disease	3			
		Sarcomas	3			
		Other tumors	19			
Koletsky et al, 1986	Total = 183	Total = 14			Not reported	5.9 ± 2.8% at 10 years.
		Acute nonlymphocytic leukemia	5	• Treatment with chemotherapy (alkylating agents and procarbazine).		
		Non-Hodgkin's lymphoma	3			
		Lung cancer	3			
		Thyroid cancer	1			
		Vulvar cancer	1			
		Gastric cancer	1			

(Continued)

343

Table 12–4 Second Malignancies Associated with the Treatment of Hodgkin's Disease (Continued)

REFERENCE	SAMPLE SIZE	SECOND MALIGNANCY TYPE	NO.	RISK FACTOR(S) AND ASSOCIATED FINDING(S)	RELATIVE RISK	CUMULATIVE RISK
Valagussa et al, 1986	Total = 1,329	Total = 68			Not reported	Not reported
		Acute nonlymphocytic leukemia	19	• Treatment with chemotherapy.		
		Non-Hodgkin's lymphoma	6	• Treatment with combined multimodal therapy.		
		Solid tumors	43	• Age > 40 years. • Latency period for solid tumors was within 12 years for a majority of patients. • There were 25 cases which occurred in previously irradiated areas.		
Blayney et al, 1987	Total = 192	Total = 12			95.7	0.03 ± 0.015% at 5 years. 0.10 ± 0.03% at 10 years.
		Acute nonlymphocytic leukemia	5	• Treatment with MOPP chemotherapy.		
		Myelodysplastic syndrome	5	• Treatment with combined multimodal therapy.		
		Erythroleukemia	1	• Latency period ranged from 3 to 9 years.		
		Chronic myelogenous leukemia	1			

Study	Total	Type	No.	Comments	Value	Results
Boivin and O'Brien, 1988	Total = 6,513	Solid tumors	154	• Shorter duration of follow-up for the chemotherapy patients. • Latency period ranged from 10 to 15 years.	2.1 By treatment groups: radiation—2.2, Chemotherapy alone—1.1	Not reported
Tucker et al, 1988	Total = 1,507	Leukemia Lymphoma	28 9	• Treatment with adjuvant chemotherapy or chemotherapy alone. • Splenectomy. • Latency period ranged from a few years to the first 10 years.	5.2	All second cancers: 17.6 ± 3.1% at 15 years. Leukemia—3.3 ± 0.6% after 10 years.
		Solid tumors	46	• Treatment with adjuvant chemotherapy. • Latency period has increased over time.		Solid tumors: 13.2 ± 3.1% at 15 years.

(Continued)

Table 12–4 Second Malignancies Associated with the Treatment of Hodgkin's Disease (Continued)

REFERENCE	SAMPLE SIZE	SECOND MALIGNANCY		RISK FACTOR(S) AND ASSOCIATED FINDING(S)	RELATIVE RISK	CUMULATIVE RISK
		TYPE	NO.			
Van Leeuwen et al, 1989	Total = 744	Total = 45				Overall risk: 20.6 ± 2.9% at 15 years.
		Lung cancer	14	• Treatment with radiation therapy. • Increase with time since diagnosis.	4.9	6.2 ± 1.9% at 15 years.
		Non-Hodgkin's lymphoma	9	• Treatment with combined modality therapy. • Latency period of 10 years or more.	31	5.9 ± 2.1% at 15 years.
		Leukemia	16	• Treatment with chemotherapy. • Splenectomy. • Age > 40 years. • Latency period ranged from 5 to 10 years.	45.7	6.3 ± 1.7% at 15 years.
		Myelodysplastic syndrome	6			
Zulian and Mirimanoff, 1989	Total = 69 Nodular sclerosis Hodgkin's 69	Total = 6		• Treatment with MOPP and extensive radiation therapy.	Not reported	Not reported
		Acute non-lymphoblastic leukemia	3			
		Preleukemia	2			
		Non-Hodgkin's lymphoma	1			

Andrieu et al, 1990	Total = 441	Acute nonlymphocytic leukemia	10	• Treatment with MOPP and radiation therapy. • Increased risk of combined multimodal therapy.	Not reported	3.5 ± 2.7% at 15 years.
Kaldor et al, 1990	Total = 163	Leukemia	163	• Treatment with MOPP chemotherapy. • Increased risk when treated with 6 or more cycles (dose-related). • Splenectomy. • Advanced stages of Hodgkin's disease. • Latency period ranged from 5 to 9 years.	Chemotherapy alone: 9	Not reported
Cimino et al, 1991	Total = 947	Leukemia Non-Hodgkin's lymphoma Solid tumors	23 5 28	• Treatment with multimodal therapy.	Not reported	2 ± 0.6% at 10 years. 13 ± 3.8% at 19 years.

Table 12–5 Second Malignancies Associated with the Treatment of Breast Cancer

REFERENCE	SAMPLE SIZE	SECOND MALIGNANCY		RISK FACTOR(S) AND ASSOCIATED FINDING(S)	RELATIVE RISK	CUMULATIVE RISK
		TYPE	NO.			
Fischer et al, 1985	Total = 8,483 Primary breast cancer Total = 5,299 Patients treated adjuvant chemotherapy	Total = 34 Leukemia Myeloproliferative syndrome	27 7	• Treatment with adjuvant chemotherapy regimens containing L-phenylalanine mustard (L-PAM).	Not reported	1.68 ± 0.33% at 10 years.
Valagussa et al, 1987	Total = 845 Resectable breast cancer N = 666 Received adjuvant chemotherapy with CMF (cyclophosphamide, methotrexate, fluorouracil)	Total = 21 Solid tumors	21	• No increased risk of second malignancies following CMF as administered in this study.	Not reported	4.2 ± 1.03% following adjuvant chemotherapy.

Study					
Geller et al, 1989	Case report Total = 2	Acute leukemia Total = 2	2	• Treatment with CMF chemotherapy. • Pancytopenia 3 years after treatment. • Postmenopausal.	Not reported	Not reported
Andersson et al, 1990	Total = 71 Advanced breast cancer	Acute non-lymphocytic leukemia Total = 5	5	• Treatment with combination chemotherapy (prednimustine, methotrexate, 5-fluorouracil, mitoxantrone, and tamoxifen). • Prednimustine was suspected to have a high leukemogenic effect. • Advanced age (mean, 61 years). • Developed refractory cytopenia. • Latency period ranged from 9 to 37 months.	339	25.4 ± 10.3% at 37 months after treatment.
Curtis et al, 1990	Total = 13,734	Acute non-lymphocytic leukemia Total = 24	24	• Treatment with chemotherapy (alkylating agents). • Duration of alkylating agent therapy. • Melphalan was the major overall risk factor.	11.5 following chemotherapy.	0.7 ± 0.2% at 10 years.

Table 12–6 Second Malignancies Associated with the Treatment of Ovarian Cancer

REFERENCE	SAMPLE SIZE	SECOND MALIGNANCY		RISK FACTOR(S) AND ASSOCIATED FINDING(S)	RELATIVE RISK	CUMULATIVE RISK
		TYPE	NO.			
Reimer et al, 1977	Total = 5,455	Total = 13 Acute nonlymphocytic leukemia	13	• Treatment with chemo-therapy (alkylating agents). • Median latency period was 41.5 months (range, 30 to 90 months).	21 Treatment with che-mother-apy: 36.1.	Not reported
Greene et al, 1982	Total = 1,399 Of the 1,399 women, 998 had been treated with alkylating agents.	Of these 998 women, 12 developed acute nonlymphocytic leukemia		• Treatment with chemo-therapy (alkylating agents). • Two specific agents were melphalan and chlorambucil. • Higher cumulative doses of alkylating agents. • Duration of treatment. • Median latency period was 47 months (range, 2 to 7 years).	110	9.6 ± 3.3% at 7 years.

Greene et al, 1986	Total = 3,363	Total = 35			23.5	After chemotherapy—8.4 ± 1.6% at 10 years.
		Acute nonlymphocytic leukemia	28	• Treatment with chemotherapy. • Alkylating agents. • Two specific agents were melphalan and chlorambucil. • Melphalan therapy was two to three times more likely to cause leukemia disorders than cyclophosphamide therapy. • Higher cumulative dose of alkylating agents. • Highest risk was 5 to 6 years after the first treatment and appears to decrease.		
		Preleukemia	7			
Chambers et al, 1989	Case report Total = 2	Total = 2			Not reported	Not reported
		Acute nonlymphocytic leukemia	1	• Treatment with chemotherapy. • Two specific agents were cisplatin and doxorubicin *without* alkylating agents or radiation therapy.		
		Preleukemia	1			

(Continued)

Table 12–6 Second Malignancies Associated with the Treatment of Ovarian Cancer (Continued)

REFERENCE	SAMPLE SIZE	SECOND MALIGNANCY		RISK FACTOR(S) AND ASSOCIATED FINDING(S)	RELATIVE RISK	CUMULATIVE RISK
		TYPE	NO.			
Kaldor et al, 1990	Total = 99,113	Total = 114				
		Leukemia (most common type: acute)	114	• Treatment with chemotherapy. • Alkylating agents. • Specific agents were melphalan, chlorambucil, thiotepa, and treosulfan. • Melphalan was the most leukemogenic. • Higher cumulative doses. • Increasing age. • Two patients were treated with doxorubicin and cisplatin.	Chemotherapy alone: 12.	Not reported
Reed and Evans, 1990	Case report Total = 1	Total = 1				
		Acute nonlymphocytic leukemia	1	• Combined multimodal therapy with cyclophosphamide and altretamine irradiation to pelvis and abdomen, and cisplatin.	Not reported	Not reported

Table 12–7 Second Malignancies Associated with the Treatment of Lung Cancer

REFERENCE	SAMPLE SIZE		SECOND MALIGNANCY		RISK FACTOR(S) AND ASSOCIATED FINDING(S)	RELATIVE RISK	CUMULATIVE RISK
	TYPE	NO.	TYPE	NO.			
Chak et al, 1984	Total = 158		Total = 3				
	Small cell carcinoma of the lung	158	Acute nonlymphocytic leukemia	3	• Treatment with chemotherapy. • Specific regimens: POCC (procarbazine, vincristine, cyclophosphamide, and CCNU) and VAM (etoposide, doxorubicin, and methotrexate). • Most likely to be attributed to the development of leukemia were procarbazine, cyclophosphamide, and CCNU. • Higher cumulative doses. • Combined multimodal therapy (i.e., chemotherapy and radiation therapy). • Actual latency period was 2.3, 2.7, and 3 years.	316	25 ± 13% at 3.1 years.

(Continued)

Table 12-7 Second Malignancies Associated with the Treatment of Lung Cancer (Continued)

REFERENCE	SAMPLE SIZE		SECOND MALIGNANCY		RISK FACTOR(S) AND ASSOCIATED FINDING(S)	RELATIVE RISK	CUMULATIVE RISK
	TYPE	NO.	TYPE	NO.			
Johnson et al, 1986	Total = 377		Total = 2				
	Small cell lung cancer	377	Acute nonlymphocytic leukemia	2	• Treatment with chemotherapy. • Specific regimen: CAV (cyclophosphamide, doxorubicin, and vincristine) with or without methotrexate, etoposide, and hexamethylmelamine. • Combined multimodal therapy (i.e., chemotherapy and radiation therapy) was given to 93% of the study sample. • Actual latency period was 22 and 81 months.	154	1.9 ± 1.4% at 7 years.

| Yu et al, 1986 | Case report of a man with small cell carcinoma of the lung

Total = 1 | Total = 1

Metastatic liver disease after 10 cycles of MEPH (mitomycin, etoposide, cisplatinum [platinol], and hexamethylmelamine [altretamine]). | • Treatment with chemotherapy.
• Combined multimodal therapy (i.e., chemotherapy and radiation therapy).
• Specific regimens: MACC (methotrexate, doxorubicin, cyclophosphamide, and lomustine) and MEPH.
• Authors found 15 cases of leukemia in the literature:
  a. All patients received combination chemotherapy.
  b. Most were treated with combined multimodal therapy (i.e., chemotherapy and radiation therapy).
  c. Alkylating agents or nitrosoureas.
  d. Etoposide was administered in ⅔ of the patients.
  e. Mean latency period was 32 months (range, 10 to 58 months). | Not reported | Not reported |

(Continued)

355

Table 12–7 Second Malignancies Associated with the Treatment of Lung Cancer (Continued)

REFERENCE	SAMPLE SIZE TYPE	NO.	SECOND MALIGNANCY TYPE	NO.	RISK FACTOR(S) AND ASSOCIATED FINDING(S)	RELATIVE RISK	CUMULATIVE RISK
Ratain et al, 1987	Total = 119		Total = 4			Not reported	44 ± 24% at 2.5 years.
	Advanced non-small cell carcinoma of the lung	119	Acute nonlymphocytic leukemia	4	• Treatment with etoposide and cisplatin with or without vindesine. • Higher cumulative doses. • Median etoposide dose was 6,795 mg/m^2 in the four leukemia patients. • Combined multimodal therapy (i.e., chemotherapy and radiation therapy). • Smoking. • Actual latency period: 13, 18, 19, and 35 months.		
Brenez et al, 1990	Case report of a man with non-small cell carcinoma of the lung Total = 1		Total = 1 Acute nonlymphocytic leukemia	1	• Treatment with chemotherapy (etoposide and cisplatin). • Actual latency period was 2 years.	Not reported	Not reported

Table 12-8 Second Malignancies Associated with the Treatment of Multiple Myeloma

REFERENCE	SAMPLE SIZE	SECOND MALIGNANCY		RISK FACTOR(S) AND ASSOCIATED FINDING(S)	RELATIVE RISK	CUMULATIVE RISK
		TYPE	NO.			
Gonzales et al, 1977	Total = 476	Total = 11		• Treatment with chemotherapy. • Melphalan with prednisone for a median of 3 years. • First clue: unexplained panctopenia.	100	Not reported
		Acute leukemia	6			
		Cideroblastic anemia	5			
Bergsagel et al, 1979	Total = 364	Total = 14		• Treatment with chemotherapy. • All patients received the alkylating agent melphalan.	214	17.4% at 50 months.
		Acute leukemia	14			

357

Table 12–9 Second Malignancies Associated with the Treatment of Gastrointestinal Cancer

REFERENCE	SAMPLE SIZE	SECOND MALIGNANCY		RISK FACTOR(S) AND ASSOCIATED FINDING(S)	RELATIVE RISK	CUMULATIVE RISK
		TYPE	NO.			
Boice et al, 1983	Total = 3,633	Total = 14		• Treatment with semustine (methyl-CCNU). • Dose-response relationship. • Increases over time.	12.4 after semustine.	4.0 ± 2.2% at 6 years after semustine.
		Acute nonlymphocytic leukemia	7			
		Myelodyplastic syndromes	2			
		Preleukemia	5			

Table 12–10 Second Malignancies Associated with the Treatment of Testicular Cancer

REFERENCE	SAMPLE SIZE		SECOND MALIGNANCY		RISK FACTOR(S) AND ASSOCIATED FINDING(S)	RELATIVE RISK	CUMULATIVE RISK
	TYPE	NO.	TYPE	NO.			
Hoekman et al, 1984	Total = 99		Total = 3				
	Inoperable germ cell tumors	99	Acute leukemia	3	• Treatment with combined multimodal therapy (i.e., chemotherapy and radiation therapy). • One patient received chemotherapy alone. • Actual latency period was 4, 17, and 61 months.	Not reported	Not reported
Redman et al, 1984	Total = 722		Total = 5				
	Germ cell tumors	722	Acute nonlymphocytic leukemia	4	• Treatment with chemotherapy (alkylating agents). • Median latency period was 44 months.	13.7 for total population to 50.1 in the group treated with chemotherapy alone.	Not reported
			Chronic myelomonocytic leukemia	1			
			Acute leukemia reviewed from the literature	14			

(Continued)

Table 12–10 Second Malignancies Associated with the Treatment of Testicular Cancer (Continued)

| REFERENCE | SAMPLE SIZE | | SECOND MALIGNANCY | | RISK FACTOR(S) AND ASSOCIATED FINDING(S) | RELATIVE RISK | CUMULATIVE RISK |
	TYPE	NO.	TYPE	NO.			
Van Imhoff et al, 1986	Case report Disseminated testicular cancer	1	Total = 1 Acute lymphocytic leukemia	1	• Treatment with PVB (cisplatin, vinblastine, and bleomycin) chemotherapy. • Latency period was 5 years.	Not reported	Not reported
De Vore et al, 1989	Case report Seminoma	1	Total = 1	1	• Treatment with chemotherapy (cisplatin, etoposide, and bleomycin). • Actual latency period was 33 months.	Not reported	Not reported

Study		Second malignancy		Comments		
Fossa et al, 1990	Total = 876 Testicular cancer 876	Total = 65 Malignant melanoma 7 Leukemia 3 Lung cancer 12 Stomach cancer 6 Colon cancer 5 Bladder cancer 5 Other 27		• Combined multimodal therapy (i.e., chemotherapy and radiation therapy). • Most common used drugs: Adriamycin and cyclophosphamide. • Genetic predisposition.	1.58	Not reported
Roth et al, 1988	Total = 229 Disseminated germ cell tumors 229	Total = 3 Oropharyngeal squamous cell carcinoma 1 Multiple intra-abdominal angiosarcoma 1 Metastatic gastric adenocarcinoma 1		• Short course, intensive PVB does *not* predispose to the development of a second malignancy.	Not reported	Not reported
Pedersen-Bjergaard et al, 1991	Total = 212 Germ cell tumors 212	Total = 5 Acute myeloid leukemia 4 Myelodysplasia 1		• Treatment with chemotherapy. • High-dose etoposide (> 2,000 mg/m^2).	336	4.7 ± 2.3% at 5 to 7 years.

Table 12–11 Second Malignancies Associated with the Treatment of Non-Hodgkin's Lymphoma

REFERENCE	SAMPLE SIZE	SECOND MALIGNANCY		RISK FACTOR(S) AND ASSOCIATED FINDING(S)	RELATIVE RISK	CUMULATIVE RISK
		TYPE	NO.			
Gomez et al, 1982	Total = 117	Total = 5 Acute nonlymphocytic leukemia Myeloproliferative syndrome	4 1	• Treatment with radiation therapy or combined multimodal therapy. • Treatment with chemotherapy including BCNU, mechlorethamine, cyclophosphamide, vincristine, and prednisone. • Increasing cumulative dose.	Not reported	Not reported
Greene et al, 1983	Total = 517	Total = 9 Acute nonlymphocytic leukemia	9	• Treatment with combined multimodal therapy (i.e., chemotherapy and radiation therapy). • Advancing age. • Mean latency period was 68 months.	Risk for leukemia: 105	7.9 ± 3.2% at 10 years.

Pedersen-Bjergaard et al, 1991	Total = 471	Total = 7 Bladder cancer	7	• Treatment with chemotherapy (cyclophosphamide). • Higher cumulative doses. • Median latency period was 93 months (range, 65 to 141 months).	6.8	3.5 ± 1.8% at 8 years. 10.7 ± 4.9 at 12 years.
Travis et al, 1989	Total = 17,261	Total = 42 Bladder cancer	42	• Treatment with chemotherapy. • No specific drug used. • Most widely accepted drug was cyclophosphamide.	Not reported	Not reported
Sigal et al, 1991	Case report Total = 1	Total = 1 Leiomyosarcoma and an invasive transitional cell carcinoma	1	• Treatment with chemotherapy. • Cyclophosphamide (240 g) over 6½ years.	Not reported	Not reported

Table 12–12 Nursing Implications for Patients at Risk for a Second Malignancy

Case Finding

Identify high-risk population.

Patient and Family Education

Patient and family education at time of primary diagnosis should include:
The potential side effects and relative risks.
The importance of ongoing follow-up.
Health promotion behaviors (i.e., no smoking).

Patient Assessment

Assess patients for the late effects of treatment on an ongoing basis.

Interventions If a Second Malignancy Develops

Assess patient and family ability to cope.
Allow patient and family to verbalize.
Offer emotional support to patient and family.
Assist patient and family to problem solve.
Provide physical care.

Documentation

Perform a comprehensive history and physical examination (review of systems).
Chart accurately and precisely.
Flow sheet/form to systematically collect data.
Charts often are used in epidemiologic studies.

Research

Participate in research studies.
Keep abreast of the results of studies.

References

Aisenberg, A.: Acute nonlymphocytic leukemia after treatment for Hodgkin's disease. Am. J. Med. 75:449–454, 1983.

Andersson, M., Preben, P., and Pedersen-Bjergaard, J.: High risk of therapy-related leukemia and preleukemia after therapy with prednimustine, methotrexate, 5-fluorouracil, mitoxantrone, and tamoxifen for advanced breast cancer. Cancer 65:2460–2464, 1990.

Andrieu, J.M., et al.: Increased risk of secondary acute nonlymphocytic leukemia after extended-field radiation therapy combined with MOPP chemotherapy for Hodgkin's disease. J. Clin. Oncol. 8:1148–1154, 1990.

Bergsagel, D.E., et al.: The chemotherapy of plasma-cell myeloma and the incidence of acute leukemia. N. Engl. J. Med. 301:743–748, 1979.

Blayney, D.W., et al.: Decreasing risk of leukemia with prolonged follow-up after chemotherapy and radiotherapy for Hodgkin's disease. N. Engl. J. Med. 316:710–714, 1987.

Boice, J.D., et al.: Leukemia and preleukemia after adjuvant treatment of gastrointestinal cancer with semustine (methyl-CCNU). N. Engl. J. Med. *309:*1079–1084, 1983.

Boice, J.D., et al.: Leukemia after adjuvant chemotherapy with semustine (methyl-CCNU): Evidence of a dose-response effect. N. Engl. J. Med. *314:*119–120, 1986.

Boivin, J.F., and O'Brien, K.: Solid cancer risk after treatment of Hodgkin's disease. Cancer *61:*2541–2546, 1988.

Brenez, D., et al.: Acute nonlymphocytic leukemia following chemotherapy with cisplatin and etoposide for non-small-cell carcinoma of the lung: Case report. Cancer Chemother. Pharmacol. *26:*235–236, 1990.

Chak, L.Y., et al.: Increased incidence of acute nonlymphocytic leukemia following therapy in patients with small cell carcinoma of the lung. J. Clin. Oncol. *2:*385–390, 1984.

Chambers, S.K., et al.: Development of leukemia after doxorubicin and cisplatin treatment for ovarian cancer. Cancer *64:*2459–2461, 1989.

Cimino, G., et al.: Second primary cancer following Hodgkin's disease: Updated results of an Italian multicentric study. J. Clin. Oncol. *9:*432–437, 1991.

Coleman, M.P., Bell, C.M.J., and Fraser, P.: Second primary malignancy after Hodgkin's disease, ovarian cancer and cancer of the testis: A population-based cohort study. Br. J. Cancer *56:*349–355, 1987.

Curtis, R.E., et al.: Leukemia following chemotherapy for breast cancer. Cancer Res. *50:*2741–2746, 1990.

De Vathaire, F., et al.: Role of radiotherapy and chemotherapy in the risk of second malignant neoplasms after cancer in childhood. Br. J. Cancer *59:*792–796, 1989.

De Vore, R., et al.: Therapy-related acute nonlymphocytic leukemia with monocytic features and rearrangement of chromosome 11q. Ann. Intern. Med. *110:*740–742, 1989.

Fergusson, J., et al.: Time required to assess children for the late effects of treatment: A report from the Children's Cancer Study Group. Cancer Nurs. *10:*300–310, 1987.

Fischer, B., et al.: Leukemia in breast cancer patients following adjuvant chemotherapy or postoperative radiation: The NSABP experience. J. Clin. Oncol. *15:*1640–1658, 1985.

Fossa, S.D., et al.: Second non-germ malignancies after radiotherapy of testicular cancer with or without chemotherapy. Br. J. Cancer *61:*639–643, 1990.

Geller, R.B., et al.: Secondary acute myelocytic leukemia after adjuvant therapy for early-stage breast carcinoma. Cancer *64:*629–634, 1989.

Gomez, G.A., Aggarwal, K.K., and Han, T.: Post-therapeutic acute malignant myeloproliferative syndrome and acute nonlymphocytic leukemia in non-Hodgkin's lymphoma. Cancer *50:*2285–2288, 1982.

Gonzales, F., Trujillo, J.M.S., and Alexanian, R.: Acute leukemia in multiple myeloma. Ann. Intern. Med. *86:*440–443, 1977.

Greene, M.H.: Is cisplatin a human carcinogen? J. Natl Cancer Inst. *84:*306–312, 1992.

Greene, M.H., et al.: Acute nonlymphocytic leukemia after therapy with alkylating agents for ovarian cancer. N. Engl. J. Med. *307:*1416–1421, 1982.

Greene, M.H., et al.: Evidence of a treatment dose response in acute nonlymphocytic leukemias which occur after therapy of non-Hodgkin's lymphoma. Cancer Res. *43:*1891–1898, 1983.

Greene, M.H., et al.: Melphalan may be a more potent leukemogen than cyclophosphamide. Ann. Intern. Med. *10:*360–367, 1986.

Grunwald, H.W., and Rosner, F.: Acute myeloid leukemia following treatment of Hodgkin's disease: A review. Cancer *50:*676–683, 1982.

Haupt, R., et al.: Acute myeloid leukemia after single-agent treatment with etoposide for Langerhan's cell histiocytosis of bone. Am. J. Pediatr. Hematol./Oncol. *15:*255–257, 1993.

Hoekmann, K., et al.: Acute leukemia following therapy for teratoma. Eur. J. Cancer Clin. Oncol. *20:*501–502, 1984.

International Agency for Research on Cancer: Overall evaluation of carcinogenicity: An update of IARC monographs 1–42. IARC Monogr. Eval. Carcinog. Risk Chem. Hum. 47(Suppl. 7):37–74, 1987.

International Agency for Research on Cancer: IARC monographs programme of the evaluation of carcinogenic risks to humans. IARC Monogr. Eval. Carcinog. Risk Chem. Hum. 50:11–31, 1990.

Jeha, S., Jaffe, N., and Robertson, R.: Secondary acute nonlymphoblastic leukemia in two children following treatment with a cis-diamminedichloroplatinum-II-based regimen for osteosarcoma. Med. Pediatr. Oncol. 20:71–74, 1992.

Johnson, D.H., et al.: Acute nonlymphocytic leukemia after treatment of small cell lung cancer. Am. J. Med. 81:962–968, 1986.

Kaldor, J.M., et al.: Leukemia following Hodgkin's disease. N. Engl. J. Med. 322:7–13, 1990.

Kaldor, J.M., et al.: Leukemia following chemotherapy for ovarian cancer. N. Engl. J. Med. 322:1–6, 1990.

Kaplinsky, C., et al.: T-cell acute lymphoblastic leukemia following therapy of rhabdomyosarcoma. Med. Pediatr. Oncol. 20:229–231, 1992.

Koletsky, A.J., et al.: Second neoplasms in patients with Hodgkin's disease following combined modality therapy: The Yale experience. J. Clin. Oncol. 4:311–317, 1986.

Kyle, R.A., Pierre, R.V., and Bayrd, E.D.: Multiple myeloma and acute myelomonocytic leukemia. N. Engl. J. Med. 283:1121–1125, 1970.

Lavey, R.S., Eby, N.L., and Prosnitz, L.R.: Impact of radiation therapy and/or chemotherapy on the risk for a second malignancy after breast cancer. Cancer 66:874–881, 1990.

Meadows, A.T., et al.: Second malignant neoplasms in children: An update from the late effects study group. J. Clin. Oncol. 3:532–538, 1985.

Meadows, A.T., Obringer, A.C., and Marredo, O.: Second malignant neoplasms following childhood Hodgkin's disease: Treatment and splenectomy as risk factors. Med. Pediatr. Oncol. 17:477–484, 1989.

Meadows, A.T., and Silber, J.: Delayed consequences of therapy for childhood cancer. CA: A Cancer Journal for Clinicians 35:271–286, 1985.

Neglia, J.P., et al.: Second neoplasms after acute lymphoblastic leukemia in childhood. N. Engl. J. Med. 325:1330–1336, 1991.

O'Keane, J.C.: Carcinoma of the urinary bladder after treatment with cyclophosphamide. N. Engl. J. Med. 319:871, 1988.

Pedersen-Bjergaard, J., et al.: Increased risk of myelodysplasia and leukemia after etoposide, cisplatin and bleomycin for germ cell tumors. Lancet 338:359–363, 1991.

Pedersen-Bjergaard, J., Ersboll, J., and Hansen, V.L.: Carcinoma of the urinary bladder after treatment with cyclophosphamide for non-Hodgkin's lymphoma. N. Engl. J. Med. 318:1028–1032, 1988.

Pedersen-Bjergaard, J., and Larsen, S.O.: Incidence of ANLL, preleukemia and acute myeloproliferative syndrome up to 10 years after treatment of Hodgkin's disease. N. Engl. J. Med. 307:965–971, 1982.

Pui, C.H., et al.: Acute myeloid leukemia in children treated with epipodophyllotoxins for acute lymphoblastic leukemia. N. Engl. J. Med. 325:1682–1687, 1991.

Ratain, M.J., et al.: Acute nonlymphocytic leukemia following etoposide and cisplatin combination chemotherapy for advanced non-small-cell carcinoma of the lung. Blood 70:1412–1417, 1987.

Redman, J.R., et al.: Leukemia following treatment of germ cell tumors in men. J. Clin. Oncol. 2:1080–1087, 1984.

Reed, E., and Evans, M.K.: Acute leukemia following cisplatin-based chemotherapy in a patient with ovarian cancer. J. Natl Cancer Inst. 82:431–432, 1990.

Reimer, R.R., et al.: Acute leukemia after alkylating agent therapy of ovarian cancer. N. Engl. J. Med. 297:177–181, 1977.

Rosner, F., and Grunwald, H.: Multiple myeloma terminating in acute leukemia: Report of 12 cases and review of the literature. Am. J. Med. 57:927–939, 1974.

Rosner, F., and Grunwald, H.W.: Simultaneous occurrence of multiple myeloma. Ann. Intern. Med. 86:440–443, 1977.

Roth, B.J., et al.: Cisplatin-based combination chemotherapy for disseminated germ cell tumors: Long-term follow-up. J. Clin. Oncol. 6:1239–1247, 1988.

Sigal, S.H., et al.: Carcinosarcoma of bladder following long-term cyclophosphamide therapy. Arch. Pathol. Lab. Med. 115:1049–1051, 1991.

Tester, W.J., et al.: Second malignant neoplasms complicating Hodgkin's disease: The National Cancer Institute experience. J. Clin. Oncol. 2:762–769, 1984.

Travis, L.B., et al.: Bladder cancer after chemotherapy for non-Hodgkin's lymphoma. N. Engl. J. Med. 321:544–545, 1989.

Tucker, M.A., et al.: Bone sarcomas linked to radiotherapy and chemotherapy in children. N. Engl. J. Med. 317:588–593, 1987.

Tucker, M.A., et al.: Leukemia after therapy with alkylating agents for childhood cancer. J. Natl Cancer Inst. 78:459–464, 1987.

Tucker, M.A., et al.: Risks of second cancers after treatment for Hodgkin's disease. N. Engl. J. Med. 318:76–81, 1988.

Valagussa, P., et al.: Second acute leukemia and other malignancies following treatment for Hodgkin's disease. J. Clin. Oncol. 4:830–837, 1986.

Valagussa, P., et al.: Second malignancies after CMF for resectable breast cancer. J. Clin. Oncol. 5:1138–1142, 1987.

Van Imhoff, G.W., et al.: Acute nonlymphocytic leukemia 5 years after treatment with cisplatin, vinblastine and bleomycin for disseminated testicular cancer. Cancer 57:984–987, 1986.

van Leeuwen, F.E., et al.: Increased risk of lung cancer, non-Hodgkin's lymphoma and leukemia following Hodgkin's disease. J. Clin. Oncol. 7:1046–1058, 1989.

Verdeguer, A., et al.: Acute nonlymphoblastic leukemia in children treated for acute lymphoblastic leukemia with an intensive regimen including teniposide. Med. Pediatr. Oncol. 20:48–52, 1992.

Whitlock, J.A., Greer, J.P., and Lukens, J.N.: Epipodophyllotoxin-related leukemia. Cancer 68:600–604, 1991.

Winick, N., et al.: Secondary acute myeloid leukemia in children with acute lymphoblastic leukemia treated with etoposide. J. Clin. Oncol. 11:209–217, 1993.

Yu, P.P., et al.: Acute myelogenous leukemia following complete remission of small cell carcinoma of the lung. Med. Pediatr. Oncol. 14(2):100–103, 1986.

Zulian, G.B., and Mirimanoff, R.O.: Ten-year nodular sclerosis Hodgkin's disease and second malignancies. Eur. J. Cancer Clin. Oncol. 25:659–665, 1989.

Recommended Readings

Anderson, N., and Lokich, J.: Bilateral breast cancer after cured Hodgkin's disease. Cancer 65:221–223, 1990.

Bajorin, D.F., et al.: Acute nonlymphocytic leukemia in germ cell tumor patients treated with etoposide-containing chemotherapy. J. Natl Cancer Inst. 85:60–62, 1993.

Baker, G.L., et al.: Malignancy following treatment of rheumatoid arthritis with cyclophosphamide. Am. J. Med. 83:1–9, 1987.

Ballen, K.K., and Antin, J.H.: Treatment of therapy-related acute myelogenous leukemia and myelodysplastic syndromes. Hematol. Oncol. Clin. North Am. 7:477–493, 1993.

Boivin, J.F.: Second cancer and other late side effects of cancer treatment: A review. Cancer 65:770–775, 1990.

Boyer, M., and Raghavan, D.: Toxicity of treatment of germ cell tumors. Semin. Oncol. 19:128–142, 1992.

DeGramont, A., et al.: Erythrocyte mean corpuscular volume during cytotoxic therapy is a predictive parameter of secondary leukemia in Hodgkin's disease. Cancer 59:301–304, 1987.

DeLaat, C.A., and Lampkin, B.C.: Long-term survivors of childhood cancer: Evaluation and identification of sequelae of treatment. CA: A Cancer Journal for Clinicians 42:263–282, 1992.

Duffner, P.K., and Cohen, M.E.: The long-term effects of central nervous system therapy on children with brain tumors. Neurol. Clin. North Am. 9:479–495, 1991.

Ellman, M.H., et al.: Lymphoma developing in a patient with rheumatoid arthritis taking low dose weekly methotrexate. J. Rheumatol. 18:1741–1743, 1991.

Erban, S.B., and Sokas, R.K.: Kaposi's sarcoma in an elderly man with Wegener's granulomatosis treated with cyclophosphamide and corticosteroids. Arch. Intern. Med. 148:1201–1203, 1988.

Escolante, A., Kaufman, R.L., and Beardmore, T.D.: Acute myelocytic leukemia after the use of cyclophosphamide in the treatment of polyarteritis nodosa. J. Rheumatol. 16:1147–1149, 1989.

Ettinger, L.J., et al.: Adjuvant adriamycin and cisdiamminedichloroplatinum in primary osteosarcoma. Cancer 47:248–254, 1981.

Fraser, M.C., and Tucker, M.A.: Late effects of cancer therapy: Chemotherapy-related malignancies. Oncol. Nurs. Forum 15(1):67–77, 1988.

Fraser, M.C., and Tucker, M.A.: Second malignancies following cancer therapy. Semin. Oncol. Nurs. 5(1):43–55, 1989.

Gertz, M.A., and Kyle, R.A.: Acute leukemia and cytogenetic abnormalities complicating melphalan treatment of primary systemic amyloidosis. Arch. Intern. Med. 150:629–633, 1990.

Gibbons, R.B., and Westerman, E.: Acute nonlymphocytic leukemia following short-term intermittent intravenous cyclophosphamide treatment of lupus nephritis. Arthritis Rheum. 31:1552–1554, 1988.

Glicksman, A.S., et al.: Second malignant neoplasms in patients successfully treated for Hodgkin's disease: A Cancer Leukemia Group B study. Cancer Treat. Rep. 66:1035–1044, 1982.

Hawkins, M.M., Draper, G.J., and Kingston, J.E.: Incidence of second primary tumours among childhood cancer survivors. Br. J. Cancer 56:339–347, 1987.

Hydzik, C.A.: Late effects of chemotherapy: Implications for patient management and rehabilitation. Nurs. Clin. North Am. 25:423–446, 1990.

Klastersky, J., and Leleux, A.: Secondary neoplasms following cancer treatment with a special emphasis on lung tumors. Neoplasma 38:253–256, 1991.

Kyle, R.A., and Gertz, M.A.: Second malignancies after chemotherapy. In Perry, M.C. (ed.): The Chemotherapy Source Book. (pp. 689–702). Baltimore, Williams & Wilkins, 1992.

Loescher, L., et al.: Surviving adult cancers: Part 1. Physiological effects. Ann. Intern. Med. 111:411–432, 1989.

Nichols, C.R., et al.: Secondary leukemia associated with a conventional dose of etoposide: Review of serial germ cell tumor protocols. J. Natl Cancer Inst. 85:554–558, 1993.

Ortiz, A., et al.: Bladder cancer after cyclophosphamide therapy for lupus nephritis. Nephron 60:378–379, 1992.

Pape, L.H.: Therapy related acute leukemia: An overview. Cancer Nurs. 11:295–302, 1988.

Ruccione, K., and Fergusson, J.: Late effects of childhood cancer and its treatment. Oncol. Nurs. Forum 11(5):54–64, 1984.

Ruccione, K., and Weinberg, K.: Late effects in multiple body systems. Semin. Oncol. Nurs. 5(1):4–13, 1989.

Smith, M.A., et al.: Report of the Cancer Therapy Evaluation Program monitoring plan for secondary acute myeloid leukemia following treatment with epipodophyllotoxins. J. Natl Cancer Inst. 88:554–558, 1993.

Toh, B.T., Gregory, S.A., and Knospe, W.H.: Acute leukemia following treatment of polycythemia vera and essential thrombocythemia with uracil mustard. Am. J. Hematol. 28:58–60, 1988.

Tucker, M.A.: Secondary cancers. In DeVita, V.T., Jr., Hellman, S., and Rosenberg, S.A. (eds.): Cancer: Principles and Practice of Oncology, 4th ed. (pp. 2407–2416). Philadelphia, J.B. Lippincott, 1993.

Tucker, M.A., and Fraumeni, J.F.: Treatment-related cancers after gynecologic malignancy. Cancer 60:2117–2122, 1987.

Valagussa, P., et al.: Absence of treatment induced second neoplasms after ABVD in Hodgkin's disease. Blood 59:488–494, 1982.

Young, D., Canellos, G.P.: Secondary malignancies and cancer therapy. Clin. Oncol. 4:535–557, 1985.

Zarrabi, M.H., and Rosner, F.: Second neoplasms in Hodgkin's disease: Current controversies. Hematol./Oncol. Clin. North Am. 3:303–318, 1989.

Chapter 13

Other Systems Affected by Chemotherapy and Biotherapy

Linda Tenenbaum, R.N., M.S.N., O.C.N.
Debi Leshin, R.N., B.S.N., O.C.N.
Catherine A. Hydzik, R.N., M.S., O.C.N.

Other systems and organs are affected by chemotherapeutic agents and biologic response modifiers (BRMs). These include the renal, respiratory, cardiac, neurological, and hepatic systems. Fluid and electrolyte alterations are **also** noted with some agents. A **flulike syndrome** is common with most BRMs. **Hypersensitivity reactions** and, in some cases, **anaphylaxis** have been reported with some chemotherapeutic agents and BRMs. These alterations and nursing interventions will be discussed in this chapter.

Renal Alterations

Renal complications may be the result of the disease process or of therapy (specific chemotherapeutic agents, BRMs, radiation therapy).

Hyperuricemia

Hyperuricemia is a common occurrence with myeloproliferative disorders (leukemias, lymphomas, multiple myelomas) and disseminated metastatic carcinomas, and may be precipitated or aggravated by chemotherapy. It is the result of increased production or decreased elimination of uric acid, or both.

Other Renal Alterations

The renal system may be affected in other ways by antineoplastic medications, including aldesleukin, bleomycin, cisplatin (and, to a lesser degree, carboplatin), cyclophosphamide, decarbazine, hydroxyurea, ifosfamide, interleukin-2, methotrexate (high-dose), mitomycin-C, paclitaxel, plicamycin, and streptozocin. Each medication acts in a different manner and at different times. Cisplatin, ifosfamide, methotrexate, plicamycin, and streptozocin affect the renal tubules. Renal alterations, manifested by oliguria and an increased creatinine level, are common with interleukin-2. Ifosfamide administered without mesna, or cyclophosphamide may cause hemorrhagic cystitis, which is manifested in 2 to 5 days after administration. The effects of high-dose methotrexate (1 to 15 g/m^2) may be seen 6 to 12 hours after administration. Nitrosoureas have been associated with delayed renal failure, occurring months to years after carmustine and semustine therapy and as long as 2 years after lomustine therapy.

Hemolytic Uremic Syndrome

Hemolytic uremic syndrome (HUS) is associated with administration of mitomycin-C. It is characterized by renal failure and hemolysis and appears to be the result of renal endothelial injury by the drug (Cattell, 1985). The incidence of HUS is dose-related. HUS is rare at doses below 30 mg/m^2. The incidence rate is less than 2% at 50 mg/m^2 and as high as 28% at 70 mg/m^2 or greater (Valavaara and Nordman, 1985). The median time interval between the initiation of mitomycin-C administration and the onset of HUS is 9½ months. Presently, there are no strategies to prevent HUS. Conventional therapy has been ineffective, and the mortality rate exceeds 50% (Hoaglund, 1992). It is recommended that follow-up tests to assess renal function be performed for at least 6 months after administration.

New Developments

In the past decade, we have seen the development of medications that can reduce renal system toxicities. Carboplatin, an analogue, is less nephrotoxic than the parent compound, cisplatin. Mesna (Mesnex), when administered prior to and following ifosfamide, functions as a uroprotective agent, with marked reduction in the incidence of hemorrhagic cystitis (Zalpuski and Baker, 1988). Mesna bonds chemically with acrolein and 4-hydroxy-ifosfamide, the urotoxic metabolites of ifosfamide, to form a nonurotoxic substance, thus reducing the incidence of hemorrhagic cystitis. Some protocols include mesna as a uroprotective agent administered in conjunction with cyclophosphamide as well.

Nursing Measures

Adequate hydration before, during, and after chemotherapy is imperative when administering nephrotoxic or bladder toxic agents. Additional measures that can be taken to reduce renal toxicity include administration of a diuretic prior to cisplatin, alkalinization of the urine to a pH of 7.0 or higher prior to high-dose methotrexate, and administration of citrovorum rescue (leucovorin) until methotrexate reaches nontoxic concentrations (see Chapter 3). When administering high-dose methotrexate with leucovorin rescue, it is imperative that all doses of leucovorin are taken per schedule. If oral leucovorin is to be taken by the patient in the home setting, the nurse must teach the importance of this medication and what actions to take in the event of nausea and vomiting so it will not be omitted.

Many clients receiving chemotherapy are also receiving antimicrobial medications, which may cause alterations in renal function. The nurse should be familiar with toxicities for all medications the patient is receiving. If necessary, the nurse should review product literature or pharmacology text, or consult with a pharmacy or peers.

A plan of care for the client with potential or actual renal impairment related to chemotherapeutic agents can be found in Table 13–4. Specific nursing interventions for each medication can be found in the tables in Chapters 3 and 4, in the "Nursing Interventions" column.

Pulmonary Alterations

Pulmonary toxicity may be caused by some cytotoxic agents. The onset of pulmonary toxicity may be acute or chronic, developing within days, months, or years after therapy. The agent that most commonly causes pulmonary toxicity is bleomycin. The incidence with bleomycin is dose-related; clinically significant pulmonary toxicity reaches an incidence rate of 10% at total doses of 450 U or greater (Blum et al., 1973). The maximum recommended cumulative dose for bleomycin is 400 to 500 U, with a reduction for persons older than 70 years or those who have received concurrent radiation therapy (Hydzig, 1990).

Long-term treatment with busulfan may cause intra-alveolar pulmonary fibrosis and pulmonary dysplasia (Sostman et al., 1977). Manifestations include cough, dyspnea, and low-grade fever. Diminished diffusion capacity and decreased pulmonary compliance may be evident with pulmonary function studies. Onset is within 8 months to 10 years after the initiation of therapy, with the average duration of therapy being 4 years (product information). Treatment includes immediate discontinuation of busulfan. Administration of corticosteroids has been suggested

(Leake, 1963), but this has not been uniformly successful (product literature). The prognosis for busulfan lung syndrome is poor, and many patients have died within 6 months after the diagnosis was established (product literature).

Other drugs that can cause pulmonary toxicity include carmustine, chlorambucil, cyclophosphamide, cytarabine, lomustine, melphalan, mercaptopurine, methotrexate, and procarbazine.

Risk Factors

Some patients are at higher risk for development of pulmonary complications when receiving a medication that is toxic to the lungs. High-risk factors include age older than 60 years, history of smoking, pre-existing pulmonary disease, prior or concurrent radiation therapy to the chest, high-dose oxygen therapy, and renal dysfunction. The specific agent, route of administration, and cumulative dose must be considered as well.

Presenting Signs and Symptoms

Dyspnea is the cardinal symptom and usually the presenting symptom of pulmonary complications. Other findings may include a dry, nonproductive cough, fatigue, fever, low exercise tolerance, rales or rhonchi, restlessness, tachypnea, and confusion. The clinical presentation may be subtle, making detection difficult.

Nursing Measures

The ideal intervention for pulmonary complications is prevention. There is no specific method for treating pulmonary alterations associated with antineoplastic agents, thus the nursing responsibility lies with identifying and assessing the high-risk population to detect problems at an early stage. The high-risk patient must be identified, assessed, and taught to report early pulmonary changes so that therapy can be altered or discontinued if necessary. Treatment may include a course of corticosteroid therapy, with a slow and careful tapering schedule (Stover, 1993).

A plan of care for the client with impaired gas exchange can be found in Table 13–5.

Cardiac Alterations

Cardiotoxicity may occur with administration of anthracycline antibiotics (daunorubicin and doxorubicin) and to a lesser extent with epirubicin, idarubicin, mitoxantrone, and rubidazone. This may be manifested within 1 week after administration as tachycardia, extrasystoles, and/or ST-T wave changes in the electrocardiogram (EKG). Congestive heart failure (CHF) may develop as well, but usually later. Cardiotoxicity is usually dose-related; CHF is rare with lower doses. Anthracycline-induced cardiotoxicity may be potentiated by concomitant administration of cyclophosphamide and/or radiation therapy to the chest. Maximum recommended cumulative doses without radiation, with values if mediastinal radiation has been administered appearing in parentheses, are as follows: doxorubicin, adults—550 mg/m^2 (450 mg/m^2), children—450 mg/m^2 (350 mg/m^2); daunomycin, adults—600 mg/m^2 (500 mg/m^2) (Hydzik, 1990).

Myocardial damage is rare, but has been reported with high doses of cyclophosphamide. Bradycardia, bigeminy, trigeminy, and premature ventricular contractions (PVCs) have been associated with paclitaxel and usually occur up to 8 hours after completion of the infusion. Chest pain was reported in some of these patients as well (McGuire et al., 1991). Arrhythmias, precordial pain, and cardiac failure have been reported with 5-fluorouracil (Collins and Weeden, 1987; Freeman and Constanza, 1988).

Supraventricular tachyarrhythmias may occur with interferon (IFN) as a direct effect, or related to fever (Kirkwood and Ernstoff, 1991). Conduction disturbances associated with IFN-γ include bradycardia with high-grade heart block. Onset may be acute or secondary to the insidious fluid volume deficit that accompanies peripheral vasodilation (Kirkwood and Ernstoff, 1991).

Risk Factors

Persons at increased risk for developing cardiotoxicity from chemotherapy or biologic agents are children, adults older than 50 years, persons with pre-existing heart disease, and persons who have received or are receiving chest or mediastinal irradiation. Scheduling affects risks as well. Clinical studies have reported decreased cardiac toxicity when doxorubicin is administered as a continuous infusion (Casper et al., 1991; Hortobagyi et al., 1989; Pratt et al., 1978; Von Hoff et al., 1982).

Hypotension

Hypotension may occur with aminoglutethamide, altretamine, etoposide, IFNs, interleukin-2 (IL-2), teniposide, and tumor necrosis factor (TNF). **Orthostatic (postural) hypotension** with etoposide or teniposide is usually associated with rapid intravenous administration.

Hypotension associated with the IFNs is more common with IFN-γ than with IFN-α and -β, and usually occurs 1 to 2 hours after administration. One type of IFN-related hypotension is related to peripheral vasodilation and responds well to fluid replacement. Another type is secondary to fever and insidious fluid imbalances and occurs with chronic administration of IFN.

Hypotension associated with IL-2 can be profound and may be accompanied by tachycardia and arrhythmias as part of the **"capillary (or vascular) leak syndrome,"** which is discussed in more detail later in this chapter. Hypotension occurs within several hours after administration of TNF, and has been the dose-limiting toxicity in clinical trials (Creagan et al., 1988; Feinberg et al., 1988; Moldawer and Figlin, 1988).

Nursing Interventions

Hypotension may be ameliorated by prehydrating the patient. With higher drug doses, pressor agents may be required. In the inpatient and office setting, blood pressure should be monitored at periodic intervals.

Orthostatic hypotension that occurs with etoposide or teniposide can be prevented by administering the medication by slow IV drip over a period of at least 30 to 60 minutes. The patient receiving these medications should be taught to arise slowly when moving from sitting to lying or from lying to standing positions.

Hypertension

Episodes of mild hypertension accompanied by tachycardia have occurred shortly after bolus administration of TNF. This may be secondary to an acute febrile reaction. Elevated blood pressure may also be seen with bleomycin, especially with doses greater than 25 U/day and/or in the presence of hyperbilirubinemia (Chabner and Myers, 1993).

Intermediate and Late Cardiac Toxicities

The manifestations described above are acute toxicities, occurring shortly after or within days following administration of cardiotoxic agents. Many arrhythmias are transient. Subacute alterations may appear immediately after the last dose or up to 30 months later, with peak onset at 3 months. CHF may develop weeks, months, or years after therapy. Late presentation of cardiomyopathy occurs 5 or more years after anthracycline therapy (Steinhertz and Yaholam, 1991).

Capillary or Vascular Leak Syndrome

Causes and Initial Manifestations.   Capillary or vascular leak syndrome (CLS, VLS) is a major dose-related and dose-limiting toxicity of IL-2 that involves the cardiac and vascular systems (Siegel and Puri, 1991). Increased capillary permeability results in extravasation of albumin, other proteins, and fluid into the extravascular space. This leads to loss of vascular tone, hypotension, tachycardia, and reduced organ perfusion. Weight gain and pulmonary edema may occur as the result of peripheral edema, along with fluid retention in peritoneal tissues. Other effects include malaise, low-grade fever, and myalgias. Hypotension (systolic blood pressure less than 90 mm Hg, or a 20 mm or greater decrease from baseline) may develop soon after the onset of treatment (Jassak, 1993). Treatment includes plasma protein fraction or albumin, the pressor agents dopamine HCl, phenylephrine HCl, digoxin, or verapamil, diuretics, and oxygen therapy (Creagan, 1992; Jassak, 1993).

New Developments

New analogues of anthracycline, antitumor antibiotics with less cardiotoxicity, and dexrazoxane (ADR-529, Zinecard), a chelating agent, are currently being used in clinical trials. Dexrazoxane (ADR-529) has shown protection against the cardiotoxicity of doxorubicin and may allow for use of higher and more effective doses of anthracyclines (Speyer et al., 1988). Studies have suggested that verapamil, a calcium channel blocker, may function as a cardioprotective agent (Allen, 1992).

Nursing Measures and Diagnostic Assessments

The nurse must assess patients at risk for cardiac manifestations and teach them to recognize and report evidence of early cardiac alterations. Should CHF develop, the patient may be given a low-sodium diet with or without fluid restriction, diuretics, and potassium. Digitalis may be administered if cardiac irregularities are present.

Prior to treatment and throughout the course of therapy, multigated angiographic scanning (MUGA scan) should be done when cardiotoxic agents are administered. This is a noninvasive assessment of the left ventricular ejection fraction (LVEF) and the heart's ability to function as a pump. The LVEF is considered abnormal if it is less than 55% when resting or decreases 5% or more from the resting value when exercising (Goodman, 1989). The patient must be observed for evidence of arrhythmias and CHF (tachycardia, shortness of breath, distended neck veins, ankle edema, hepatomegaly, cardiomegaly). Cardiac enzymes as well as the EKG and echocardiogram should be monitored. Endomyocardial biopsy, an invasive procedure, is the most reliable method for assessing myocardial damage (Pegelow, et al., 1984).

Patient Education

The nurse must teach the patient and significant other to recognize and report evidence of early cardiac alterations. The patient should be taught to space activities and plan rest periods in order to avoid taxing the heart. Should CHF develop, a low-sodium diet with or without fluid restriction may be ordered and must be explained to the patient/ significant other. If digitalis and diuretics are administered, this may warrant additional patient and family education including teaching about medications, actions, and side effects and explaining how to monitor the pulse and recognize side effects. The patient who is receiving medications that may cause postural hypotension should be taught to arise slowly when moving from sitting to lying or from lying to standing positions.

A plan of care for the client with alterations in cardiac status can be found in Table 13–6.

Neurological Alterations

Neurotoxicity is most commonly seen with administration of *Vinca* (plant) alkaloids. It is most common with vincristine and is the dose-limiting toxicity. It is seen less often with vinblastine and vindesine. Neurotoxicity may also occur with α IFN, altretamine, cytarabine, fludarabine, 5-fluorouracil, IL-2, methotrexate, paclitaxel, procarbazine, and TNF.

Clinical Manifestations

The patient with **peripheral neuropathy** may exhibit the following: paresthesias involving the hands and/or feet; pain along the facial trigeminal nerve pathway; loss of deep tendon reflexes (DTRs); and motor weakness. The motor weakness is usually more prominent in the lower extremities and is evidenced by foot drop, a slapping gait, and wrist drop. The neuromuscular side effects associated with vincristine frequently develop in a sequence. Initially, only sensory impairment and paresthesias may occur. With continued treatment neuritic pain and, later, motor difficulties may appear (product literature, vincristine). Pyridoxine may be administered concurrent with altretamine in an effort to minimize peripheral neuropathy.

Central nervous system (CNS) toxicities such as headache and alterations in speech, level of consciousness, and memory have been observed with IL-2 and TNF, and to a lesser degree with α IFN.

Arachnoiditis is associated with intrathecal methotrexate. It occurs 2 to 4 hours after administration and is manifested by fever, vomiting, headache, dizziness, and back pain. Rare manifestations include weakness or paralysis and transient or progressive encephalopathy.

Constipation associated with *Vinca* alkaloids is the result of paralysis of the autonomic nerves that control intestinal motility. This problem is discussed further in Chapter 8.

Ocular Alterations

Presently, there are more than 20 chemotherapeutic agents known to cause eye toxicities (Cloutier, 1992, p. 1251). Radiation therapy to the CNS may be another cause of ocular disorders. Ocular alterations may also be the direct result of primary ocular cancer or metastases. The most common sources of metastases are the breast, lung, genitourinary, or gastrointestinal systems. Less common tumors that can metastasize to the eyes include kidney, thyroid, and prostate tumors, and B-cell lymphomas (Cloutier, 1992, p. 1251). Specific ocular alterations can be found in the "toxicity" columns of the tables in Chapter 3.

Auditory Alterations

Ototoxicity, characterized by progressive, high-frequency hearing loss, is seen with administration of cisplatin. The hearing loss is dose-related and more common in the very young and the very old. The hearing loss is worse in children, and may be exacerbated by concurrent cranial radiation therapy (MacDonald, 1992).

A plan of care for the client with altered neurologic function related to sensory/perceptual alteration or impaired physical mobility can be found in Table 13–7.

Hepatic Alterations

Hepatotoxicity may occur with some chemotherapeutic agents that are metabolized by the liver, but this is rare. It is evidenced by elevation of the hepatic enzymes SGOT (or aspartate aminotransferase [AST]), SGPT (or alanine aminotransferase [ALT]), lactic dehydrogenase (LDH), bilirubin, and alkaline phosphatase. Other manifestations include depression of fibrinogen and other coagulation factors, upper right quadrant abdominal pain, jaundice, hepatomegaly, ascites, lethargy, anorexia, and nausea. Most changes are reversible after the medication is withdrawn. In some cases, dose modification is required.

Many clients receiving chemotherapy are also receiving antimicrobial medications, which may cause alteration in hepatic function. The nurse should be familiar with manufacturers' literature for these medications and their potential toxicities.

Nursing measures include monitoring for and reporting the earliest signs of hepatotoxicity, so that dosage alterations can be made.

Alterations in Fluid and Electrolyte Homeostasis

Fluid and electrolyte alterations may occur with many chemotherapeutic agents. These include imbalances in sodium, potassium, magnesium, phosphates, and body fluids (deficit or excess).

Hypercalcemia may occur with androgens, estrogens, and antiestrogens, and is referred to as "tumor flare." It is more commonly seen as a complication of cancer. Incidence is highest (40% to 50%) in carcinomas of the breast and multiple myeloma, intermediate in non-small cell lung cancer, and rare in small-cell carcinoma of the lung and colon cancer (Warrell, 1993). The elevated blood calcium may be the result of increased parathyroid hormone-like factor (PGE_2), a potent osteoclast stimulator; cytokines known as osteoclast-activating factors (OAFs); immobility; or bone metastases (Lang-Kummer, 1993, p. 651).

Interventions will vary with the extent of hypercalcemia. When possible, the underlying cause should be corrected. Other interventions include encouraging physical activity and ambulation, maintaining hydration with normal saline solution, and administering medications (Table 13–8).

Syndrome of inappropriate antidiuretic hormone (SIADH) may occur with normal doses of cisplatin, cyclophosphamide, or ifosfamide, and with high doses of aminoglutethamide, vinblastine, vincristine, and vindesine. SIADH may also occur in patients with leukemias, lymphomas, small-cell carcinomas of the lung, and other solid tumors.

A plan of care for the client with alterations in fluid and electrolyte homeostasis can be found in Table 13–9.

Flulike Syndrome

Flulike syndrome (FLS) is most commonly seen with BRMs, and has been described in Chapter 4. The nurse must observe for symptoms such as fever, chills, rigor, myalgias, arthralgias, headache, and malaise. Upper respiratory symptoms may or may not accompany FLS.

Hypersensitivity Reactions (HSRs)

HSRs may occur in patients receiving chemotherapy. Drugs that can cause these responses are listed in Table 13–1. The frequency and types of reactions vary, as indicated in Table 13–2.

The nurse who administers chemotherapy and/or biotherapy must be familiar with the risks for HSRs and be able to recognize clinical

Table 13–1 Antineoplastic Agents Causing Hypersensitivity Reactions

MEDICATION	TYPE OF REACTION	FREQUENCY
L-asparaginase	Type I	10–20%
Anthracycline antibiotics	Type I	<1–15% (varies with medication)
Bleomycin	Type I	Case reports
Carboplatin	Type I	Up to 10%
Chlorambucil	Type I	Case reports
Cisplatin		
Intravesical	Type I	Up to 20%
Intravenous	Type I	<5%
Cyclophosphamide	Type I	Case reports
Cytarabine	Type I	Case reports
Dacarbazine	Type I	Case reports
Etoposide	Type I	Case reports
5-Fluorouracil	Type I	Case reports
Ifosfamide	Type I	Case reports
Mechlorethamine		
Topical	Type IV	10–20%
Intravenous	Type I	Case reports
Melphalan (intravenous)	Type I	2–5%
Methotrexate	Type I	Case reports
	Type II	Case reports
	Type III	Case reports
Mitomycin	Type I	Case reports
Mitoxantrone	Type I	Case reports
Paclitaxel (Taxol)	Type I	Up to 10%
Procarbazine	Type I	Up to 15%
	Type III	Case reports
Teniposide	Type I	5–15% (depending on cancer being treated)
Vinca alkaloids	Type I	Case reports

From Perry, M.C. (ed.): *The Chemotherapy Source Book* (p. 564). Baltimore, Williams & Wilkins, 1992. Reprinted with permission.

manifestations. Responses may vary in severity from subacute reactions (mild rash, low-grade fever) to more generalized and severe reactions more commonly seen in patients receiving bleomycin, L-asparaginase, monoclonal antibodies, or paclitaxel. Occasionally, full anaphylaxis, loss of consciousness, or death may occur. An emergency treatment tray (Table 13–3) must be readily accessible when administering agents with the potential to cause HSRs.

Interventions to prevent anaphylaxis include test dosing (with bleomycin, L-asparaginase) or prolonging administration time. A prophylactic regimen that may be administered to prevent or ameliorate anaphylactic reactions with paclitaxel may include an antihistamine (benadryl,

Table 13–2   Types of Hypersensitivity Reactions (Gell and Coombs Classification)

TYPE	MAJOR SIGNS AND SYMPTOMS	MECHANISM
I	Urticaria, angioedema, rash, bronchospasm, abdominal cramping, extremity pain, agitation and anxiety, hypotension	Degranulation caused by antigen interaction with IgE bound to mast cell membrane, and drug binding to mast cell surface. Anaphylactoxins produced by activation of classic or alternative complement pathways. Neurogenic release of vasoactive substances.
II	Hemolytic anemia	Activation of complement by cell-bound antigen and antibody reaction.
III	Tissue injury resulting from deposition of immune complexes in tissues	Antigen-antibody complexes form intravascularly and deposit in or on tissues.
IV	Contact dermatitis, granuloma formation, homograft rejection	Release of lymphokines by reaction of sensitized T lymphocytes with antigen.

From Perry, M.C. (ed.): *The Chemotherapy Source Book* (p. 554). Baltimore, Williams & Wilkins, 1992. Reprinted with permission.

Table 13–3   Emergency Medications and Equipment for Potential Hypersensitivity Reactions to Antineoplastic Agents

Medications:

Epinepherine 1 : 1000 for S.C. injection
Epinepherine 1 : 1000 for I.V. injection
Diphenhydramine (Benadryl) 50 mg for I.V. injection
Hydrocortisone 50 mg for I.V. injection

Equipment:

IV solutions and administration equipment
Oxygen and setup
Suction and setup
Tracheostomy tray
Crash cart

From Galassi, A.: The next generation: Chemotherapy agents for the 1990s [Review]. Semin. Oncol. Nurs. 8:89, 1992. Reprinted with permission.

diphenhydramine), a corticosteroid (dexamethasone), and an H-2 receptor antagonist (cimetidine, ranitidine hydrochloride). Signs and symptoms of HSRs for specific agents are included in appropriate tables in Chapters 3 and 4.

A plan of care for the patient with potential or actual HSRs can be found in Table 13–10.

Chronic Fatigue Syndrome

A problem associated with long-term administration of TNF is **chronic fatigue syndrome**. This begins after several months of therapy, and incidence may be related to the IFN preparation used. Specific mechanisms underlying this disorder are unclear (St. Pierre et al., 1992). At Memorial Sloane-Kettering Cancer Center, researchers reported an incidence rate of 21% after treatment for 12 months with IFN-α-2A, and 44% after treatment for 18 months (Moormeier and Golumb, 1991).

All toxicities of antineoplastic agents are summarized in the tables that follow the introduction to this section (pp. 210–219).

Table 13-4 Plan of Care for the Patient with Potential Renal Function Alteration

PATIENT PROBLEM	EXPECTED OUTCOMES	STANDARD OF PRACTICE
Knowledge deficit related to potential alterations of chemotherapy/biotherapy: • kidney alterations • bladder alterations • electrolyte alterations.	The patient/significant other will: State a potential urinary tract alteration specific to the medication he/she is receiving, or as a risk of his/her disease. Discuss measures that must be taken to prevent renal or urinary complications. State daily fluid intake requirements. Identify/demonstrate measures and alternatives to take or avoid to maintain renal function.	1. Assess level of knowledge. 2. Instruct patient/significant other about kidney or bladder toxicity of specific antineoplastic agents that he/she will receive (see "toxicity" columns of the tables in Chapters 3 and 4). 3. Instruct patient about measures to take or avoid. 4. Provide written learning aids to reinforce teaching. 5. Provide time and climate to allow for questions, discussion, and feedback as needed.
Alteration in renal function related to hyperuricemia.	The patient will: Have a uric acid concentration that is within normal range. Maintain fluid intake of 2,000 to 3,000 ml unless contraindicated.	1. Monitor uric acid levels. **If cardiac status permits:** 2. Hydrate by forcing fluids before, during, and for at least 48 hours after completion of therapy. 3. Increase fluid intake to at least 3,000 ml/day to promote a high fluid flow through renal tubules. **If unable to consume P.O. fluids:** 4. Administer I.V. fluids as prescribed. 5. Assess for adequate diuresis (>100 ml/hr) and report alteration. 6. Administer diuretic agent if prescribed. 7. Administer potential urotoxic I.V. drugs as a dilute and as a continuous infusion over 6 to 8 hours whenever possible.

8. Assess for indications of crystallization of uric acid in urine (e.g., dysuria, frequency, urgency, bladder spasm, or pain) and report.
9. Administer allopurinol (Zyloprim), if ordered, to enhance uric acid excretion.
10. Encourage patient to void frequently, especially before bedtime and during the night when awake, to prevent stasis of urine.
11. Report clinical manifestations of gout (polyarticular pain, joint inflammation, fever, chills).

If prurutis is present:
1. Institute measures to temporarily relieve itching (e.g., add ¼ cup baking soda or Aveeno oatmeal to bath).
2. Assess for and report urticaria and/or rash.
3. Administer antihistamine if ordered.

Potential alteration in renal function related to nephrotoxic and/or urotoxic effects of antineoplastic agents.

The patient will:
Maintain fluid intake of 2,000 to 3,000 ml unless contraindicated.
Maintain urine output of 100 ml/hr or more.
State clinical manifestations of nephrotoxicity, urotoxicity, and fluid volume overload.
Demonstrate ability to assess adequate diuresis.
State measures to be taken if unable to maintain adequate intake and output.

1. Encourage adequate fluid intake. Contact physician if unable to retain P.O. fluid so that I.V. can be initiated.
2. Monitor urine output and report output <100 ml/hr.
3. Report alterations in urine (dark color, sediment).
4. Monitor renal function tests (BUN, creatinine, creatinine clearance) and report alterations.
5. Assess skin turgor and mucous membranes as indicators of hydration status.
6. Avoid bladder irritants (e.g., coffee, tea, alcohol, spices, tobacco).

Table 13–5 Plan of Care for the Patient with Potential Gas Exchange Alteration

PATIENT PROBLEM	EXPECTED OUTCOMES	STANDARD OF PRACTICE
Knowledge deficit related to potential impaired gas exchange secondary to toxicities caused by chemotherapy/biotherapy.	The patient/significant other will: State potential respiratory alterations specific to the medications he/she is receiving. State early signs and symptoms of respiratory alterations. Identify/demonstrate measures that facilitate optimal gas exchange. Discuss potential long-term alterations in pulmonary function and health care maintenance measures. Discuss pre-existing or concurrent factors that contribute to respiratory alterations and ways to minimize these.	1. Assess level of knowledge. 2. Instruct patient/significant other about potential pulmonary toxicity of specific antineoplastic agents that he/she will receive (see "toxicity" columns of the tables in Chapters 3 and 4). 3. Instruct patient about measures that can be taken to maintain maximal pulmonary function. 4. Provide written learning aids to reinforce teaching. 5. Provide time and climate to allow for questions, discussion, and feedback as needed.
Impaired gas exchange related to pulmonary toxicities of chemotherapeutic agents.	The patient will: Maintain adequate oxygenation as reflected by arterial blood gases (ABGs) within normal range and absence of dyspnea or tachypnea. Perform activities of daily living without shortness of breath. Execute measures that promote adequate oxygenation. Demonstrate alternative breathing patterns when necessary. Abstain from activities that may impair pulmonary function.	1. Obtain baseline pulmonary function studies and ABGs as prescribed. 2. Assess respiratory function: a. Quality of respirations (rate, rhythm, depth) and breath sounds. b. Use of accessory muscles, chest wall expansion, pain on inspiration. c. Monitor skin color, peripheral pulses, weakness, fatigue, level of consciousness (LOC), and restlessness. 3. Obtain ABGs and administer oxygen therapy and pulse oximetry as ordered. 4. Instruct and demonstrate diaphragmatic and pursed-lip breathing techniques if indicated. 5. Position patient for maximum aeration and comfort. 6. Instruct patient to limit exposure to respiratory irritants.

a. Encourage client in a nonjudgmental manner to stop or decrease smoking.
b. Avoid exposure to aerosols, perfumes, or inhalants.
c. Arrange for occupational counseling if indicated.

7. Institute measures to facilitate expectoration of pulmonary secretions.
a. Encourage deep breathing and position change every 2 hours.
b. Encourage fluid intake of 3,000 ml daily unless contraindicated.
c. Humidify air.
d. Administer mucolytic agent or expectorant as prescribed.
e. Instruct patient on how to deep breathe, cough, and expectorate secretions.
f. Use suction as prescribed when indicated.

8. Monitor respirations when administering medications that may compromise respiratory status (e.g., narcotics, sedatives, tranquilizers, muscle relaxants).

9. Maintain optimal nutritional status.

10. Encourage client to alternate periods of rest and activity.

Potential altered health maintenace related to long-term pulmonary toxic effects of antineoplastic agents.	The patient will: Describe long-term pulmonary toxic effects of antineoplastic agents. Discuss measures to maintain optimal long-term health. List resources, e.g. American Lung Association, to aid with long-term adaptation to altered respiratory function.

1. Teach patient about potential long-term toxicities of specific agent(s) he/she has taken (e.g., pneumonitis, pulmonary fibrosis).

2. Instruct and encourage patient to see physician to obtain physical examination semi-annually or more frequently if indicated.

3. Instruct patient to recognize and report early signs and symptoms of long-term pulmonary toxicities.

Table 13–6 Plan of Care for the Patient with Potential Cardiac Status Alteration

PATIENT PROBLEM	EXPECTED OUTCOMES	STANDARD OF PRACTICE
Knowledge deficit related to potential cardiac alterations related to toxicities of chemotherapy/biotherapy.	The patient/significant other will: State potential cardiac alterations specific to the medication they are receiving. State early signs and symptoms of cardiac alterations. Discuss potential long-term alterations in cardiac status and health care maintenance measures.	1. Assess level of knowledge. 2. Instruct patient/significant other about potential cardiac toxicity of specific antineoplastic agents that he/she will receive (see "toxicity" columns of the tables in Chapters 3 and 4). 3. Instruct patient about signs and symptoms that must be reported to health care personnel. 4. Provide written learning aids to reinforce teaching. 5. Instruct patient about potential cumulative effects of more than one cardiotoxic medication, or a cardiotoxic medication and radiation therapy to the chest region. 6. Provide time and climate to allow for questions, discussion, and feedback as needed.
Potential alteration in cardiac output related to toxicities of antineoplastic and/or biologic agents: • dysrhythmias • hypotension • hypertension • capillary leak syndrome • congestive heart failure.	The patient will: State potential cardiac alterations specific to the medication he/she is receiving. State measures to recognize cardiac toxicities. Demonstrate ability to self-assess pulses. List signs and symptoms of hypotension or hypertension as applicable. Discuss system-specific side effects that may be associated with capillary leak syndrome. State three early manifestations of congestive heart failure.	1. Obtain baseline cardiac function studies as ordered (e.g., EKG, MUGA scan, echocardiogram). 2. Assess cardiac function: a. Rate and quality of apical pulse. b. Blood pressure. c. Skin color and turgor, capillary refill, peripheral pulses, and mental status. d. Peripheral or periorbital edema. 3. Instruct patient to report feelings of palpitation, pulse irregularity, or sensation of skipped beats or fluttering in chest. 4. Monitor electrolytes and cardiac enzymes and report alterations. 5. Attach patient to cardiac monitor if ordered.

If patient is receiving a medication that may cause hypotension (e.g., etoposide, IL-2, interferons, TNF):

1. Monitor B/P in lying, sitting, and standing positions.
2. Teach client to arise gradually when moving from lying to sitting or sitting to standing positions.

Should CHF develop:

1. Assess lung sounds, B/P, apical and peripheral pulses, EKG, respiratory rate, and alterations in breathing pattern.
2. Place in a position that facilitates breathing (e.g., Fowler's or semi-Fowler's).
3. Administer diuretic and cardiac glycoside as ordered.
4. Limit fluid intake to 1,000 ml/24 hr.
5. Monitor I & O.
6. Maintain bedrest if ordered.

If patient is receiving a medication that may cause capillary leak syndrome (CLS) (e.g., IL-2):

1. Instruct patient to report early signs and symptoms (e.g., dizziness, dyspnea, edema, tachycardia).
2. Monitor B/P and pulses.
3. Assess patient for tachydysrhythmias and signs of "third spacing" (hypotension peripheral or pulmonary edema, ascites).

Should CLS develop:

1. Place patient in supine position if B/P is lowered.
2. Administer vasopressors, albumin, and other parenteral medications as ordered.
3. Attach patient to cardiac monitor and report alterations.
4. Monitor B/P and report alterations.

(Continued)

Table 13–6 Plan of Care for the Patient with Potential Cardiac Status Alteration (Continued)

PATIENT PROBLEM	EXPECTED OUTCOMES	STANDARD OF PRACTICE
Potential altered health maintenance related to long-term cardiac toxic effects of antineoplastic agents.	The patient will: Describe long-term cardiac effects of antineoplastic agents. Discuss measures to maintain optimal long-term health.	1. Teach patient about potential long-term toxicities of specific agent(s) he/she has taken (e.g., CHF, MI, decreased cardiac ejection fraction). 2. Instruct and encourage patient to obtain physical examination semi-annually or more frequently if indicated. 3. Instruct patient to recognize and report early signs and symptoms of long-term cardiac toxicities.

Table 13–7 Plan of Care for the Patient with Potential Neurologic Function Alteration

PATIENT PROBLEM	EXPECTED OUTCOMES	STANDARD OF PRACTICE
Knowledge deficit related to potential neurologic alterations of chemotherapy/biotherapy.	The patient/significant other will: State potential neurologic alterations specific to the medication he/she is receiving. Discuss safety measures that must be taken should neurologic alterations occur. Teach patient signs and symptoms to report.	1. Assess level of knowledge. 2. Instruct patient/significant other about potential neurologic toxicities of specific antineoplastic agents that he/she will receive (see "toxicity" columns of the tables in Chapters 3 and 4). 3. Instruct patient about measures to take or avoid. 4. Provide written learning aids to reinforce teaching. 5. Provide time and climate to allow for questions, discussion, and feedback as needed.

Sensory/perceptual alterations related to neurological toxicities of chemotherapy/biotherapy.	The patient will: List signs and symptoms of sensory/perceptual alterations. Perform daily self-care tasks independently or with minimal assistance. Recognize and report early signs and symptoms of sensory/perceptual alterations.	1. Perform baseline neurologic assessment, and re-evaluate frequently, based on drug regimen.
		  a. Level of consciousness (LOC).
		  b. Pupillary size and reaction.
		  c. Gait.
		  d. Sensation in extremities.
		  e. Gross motor skills/mobility.
		  f. Fine motor skills.
		  g. Bowel and bladder function.
		  h. Deep tendon reflexes (DTRs).
		  i. Pain.
		  j. Speech alterations.

(Continued)

Table 13–7 Plan of Care for the Patient with Potential Neurologic Function Alteration (Continued)

PATIENT PROBLEM	EXPECTED OUTCOMES	STANDARD OF PRACTICE
		2. Assess for and report neurological changes caused by specific agents (see toxicities for individual drugs in Chapters 3 and 4).
		3. Assess for headache, vertigo, slurred speech, or hoarseness.
		4. Encourage and assist with mobility.
		For patient receiving *Vinca* alkaloids:
		1. Assess bowel sounds frequently.
		For patients receiving drugs that may alter the senses:
		1. Assess for changes in the senses (hearing, vision, touch, taste, smell).
		2. Discuss effect(s) of medications on sensory perceptions.
		3. Institute safety measures if neurologic deficit is present, and instruct patient/family regarding safety in the home environment.
		4. Instruct patient and significant other to perform range of motion (ROM) exercises to all extremities.
		5. Consult physical therapist to develop exercise program and provide physical aides if needed.
		6. Instruct patient to limit use of sensory-altering substances (e.g., alcohol, tranquilizers, narcotics, sedatives, barbiturates, recreational drugs).
		7. Utilize appropriate methods to prevent constipation (e.g., adequate hydration, high fiber diet, stool softener).

8. Administer pyridoxine and monitor its effectiveness as this may possibly decrease neurotoxicity.

For patient receiving cisplatin:
1. Obtain baseline audiometric assessment.
2. Assess for and report alteration in hearing.

Should hearing loss occur:
1. Speak clearly and loud enough for the patient to understand.
2. Use written communication in addition to or instead of verbal communication.

Potential altered health maintenance related to long-term neurosensory alterations of antineoplastic agents.

The patient will:
Describe potential long-term neurosensory alterations of antineoplastic agents. Discuss measures and adaptations necessary to maintain optimal long-term health and functioning, including community resources.

Long-term health maintenance:
1. Teach patient about potential long-term toxicities of specific agent(s) he/she has taken (e.g., cataracts, glaucoma, hearing loss).
2. Encourage patient to obtain physical examination semi-annually or more frequently if indicated.
3. Instruct patient to recognize and report early signs and symptoms of long-term neurologic, ophthalmologic, or ototoxicities.
4. Teach patient about adaptive and supportive measures that can be taken should a long-term neurosensory alteration occur.
5. Facilitate access to community resources (e.g., home care, social services, vocational rehabilitation).

Table 13-8 Treatment of Cancer-Related Hypercalcemia

AGENT*	DOSAGE	COMMENTS
Tumor ablation	Tumor-specific	The only definitive approach to long-term resolution of hypercalcemia.
Normal saline solution	5–8 L I.V. in first 24 hr, then 3 L/day	Vigorous saline hydration is an integral part of hypercalcemia therapy. Restores plasma volume, ↑ renal Ca^+ excretion. Continue until Ca^+ <12.0 mg/dl. May require cardiac and central venous pressure (CVP) monitoring with compromised cardiovascular or renal function.
Furosemide (Lasix)	Diuretic dose—20 mg q 4–6 hr; calciuretic dose—80–100 mg q 1–2 hr	Diuretic dose to control overhydration; calciuretic dose requires intensive care unit (ICU) monitoring and replacement of fluid and electrolyte losses.
Bisphosphonates		
Etidronate disodium (Didronel)	7.5 mg/kg/d I.V. over 2–4 hr × 3–7 days, then 5–10 mg/kg/d P.O. for up to 3 months	For mild or moderate hypercalcemia. Inhibits osteoclast bone resorption. When effective, calcium level will normalize in 3–5 days. Contraindicated in renal failure, administer with saline hydration. Adverse effects include taste perversions, nausea, fever, fluid overload, hypomagnesemia, hypophosphatemia, occasional nephropathy. Osteomalacia may occur with long-term use.
Pamidronate disodium (Aredia)	60–90 mg in 1000 ml I.V. fluid as a single dose over 3–24 hr	For moderate to severe hypercalcemia. Inhibits bone resorption. Onset of action 24–48 hr. Longer duration of action. Adverse effects include taste perversions, nausea, anorexia, fever, lethargy, hypocalcemia, hypomagnesemia, hypophosphatemia, I.V. site reactions, EKG alterations.

Drug	Dosage	Comments
Calcitonin (Calcimar, Miacalcin)	2–8 IU/kg q 12 hr I.M. or S.C. (usually administered in combination with hydrocortisone)	Nausea, with or without emesis (most evident when treatment started, less common with continued therapy). Local inflammation at injection site. Allergic reactions (rare).
Corticosteroids (e.g., prednisone)	P.O. 40–100 mg/day in divided doses administered q 6 hr (usually administered in combination with calcitonin)	Hyperglycemia, sodium and fluid retention, gastritis. Administer with food to minimize gastritis.
Plicamycin (Mithracin)	10–50 μg/kg (maximum 1500 μg) as single I.V. dose over 4 hr. May repeat in 48 hr	For moderate to severe hypercalcemia. Onset of action within 24–48 hr. Adverse effects include thrombocytopenia, bleeding syndrome (usually begins with epistaxis), hypocalcemia, hypophosphatemia, hypokalemia, hepatic, renal toxicity, nausea, and vomiting. Extravasation may cause cellulitis at site.
Phosphate (Neutra-Phos)	P.O. 1–3 g/dl in divided doses	For mild or moderate hypercalcemia. Prevents intestinal Ca^{++} absorption and inhibits bone matrix reabsorption. Dose-limiting toxicity—diarrhea usually occurs at 2 g/dl. Chronic administration accompanied by loss of effectiveness. Contraindicated with renal failure or serum phosphorous level >3.8 mg/dl.
Gallium nitrate (Ganite)	100–200 mg/m²/day as a continuous I.V. infusion for up to 5–7 days	For moderate to severe hypercalcemia. Inhibits osteoclast bone resorption. Median duration of response 6 days. More effective than calcitonin or etidronate in achieving normocalcemia. Adverse effects include asymptomatic hypophosphatemia and nephrotoxicity. Five-day continuous infusion limits outpatient use.

*The prostaglandin inhibitors have been omitted due to their general lack of efficacy in most cases of malignant hypercalcemia. Investigational agents have not been included.

Adapted from Lang-Kummer, J.: Hypercalcemia. In Groenwald, S.L., et al. (eds.): *Cancer Nursing: Principles and Practice*, 3rd ed. (p. 655). Boston, MA, Jones and Bartlett, 1993; Warrell, R.P.: Metabolic emergencies. In DeVita, V.T., Jr., Hellman, S., and Rosenberg, S.A. (eds.): *Cancer: Principles and Practice of Oncology* (p. 2131). Philadelphia, J.B. Lippincott; and product literature.

Table 13–9 Plan of Care for the Patient with Potential Altered Fluid/Electrolyte Status

PATIENT PROBLEM	EXPECTED OUTCOMES	STANDARD OF PRACTICE
Knowledge deficit related to potential fluid/electrolyte alterations secondary to chemotherapy/biotherapy: • syndrome of inappropriate antidiuretic hormone (SIADH) (hyponatremia) • hypomagnesemia • hypercalcemia • hypokalemia • hypernatremia	The patient/significant other will: State potential fluid/electrolyte alterations specific to the medication(s) he/she is receiving. State early signs and symptoms of fluid/electrolyte alterations. Describe interventions that can be taken to prevent or correct a specific alteration in fluid/electrolyte homeostasis. Discuss dietary modifications that are necessary with a specific alteration in fluid/electrolyte status.	1. Assess level of knowledge. 2. Instruct patient/significant other about potential fluid/electrolyte alterations of specific antineoplastic agents that he/she will receive (see "toxicity" columns of the tables in Chapters 3 and 4). 3. Instruct patient about signs and symptoms to report to health care personnel. 4. Provide written learning aids to reinforce teaching. 5. Provide time and climate to allow for questions, discussion, and feedback as needed.

Potential alteration in fluid/electrolyte balance related to toxicities of antineoplastic and/or biologic agents:
• SIADH (hyponatremia)
• hypomagnesemia
• hypercalcemia
• hypokalemia
• hypernatremia
	The patient will:
	State potential fluid/electrolyte alterations specific to the medication he/she is receiving.
	State measures to recognize fluid/electrolyte toxicities. Describe dietary alterations necessary with specific fluid/electrolyte alterations.
	Recognize early signs and symptoms of fluid/electrolyte imbalances specific to the medication(s) he/she is receiving. Maintain appropriate fluid intake.
	State three early manifestations of CHF.
	State purposes of and comply with medication regimen for correction of specific electrolyte imbalance, if applicable.
		1. Obtain baseline fluid/electrolyte studies.
		For patients receiving cisplatin, cyclophosphamide, and other medications that may cause SIADH:
		1. Assess for:
		  a. Excessive retention of water (edema, weight gain).
		  b. Decreased serum osmolality (<280 mOs/kg).
		  c. Hyponatremia (serum Na^+ <135 mE/L).
		  d. ↑ excretion of urinary Na^+ (>20 mEq/L).
		2. If SIADH is present:
		  a. Restrict fluid intake to 500 ml/24 hr.
		  b. Discontinue drug causing SIADH.

c. Administer hypertonic saline, with or without furosemide.

d. Monitor blood electrolytes and administer electrolyte replacement therapy as indicated.

e. Encourage consumption of high-sodium foods, unless contraindicated by cardiac or renal status.

For patients receiving cisplatin or other medications that may cause hypomagnesemia:

1. Assess blood magnesium level (normal = 1.5–2.5 mEq/L) and report reduction.

2. Assess for signs or symptoms of hypomagnesemia (e.g., dizziness, paresthesias, cardiac arrhythmias).

3. Continue to monitor patient's status, laboratory values, and EKG, and report alterations.

4. Assess patient who is taking digoxin for toxicity as magnesium deficit enhances the action of digoxin.

For patients receiving androgens, antiestrogens, and other medications that may cause hypercalcemia:

1. Assess blood calcium level (normal = 9–11 mg/dL) and report increase.

2. Assess for signs or symptoms of hypercalcemia (e.g., nausea, vomiting, anorexia, constipation, gastrointestinal (GI) pain, lethargy, confusion, polyuria, paresthesias, positive Trousseau's and/or Chovstek's signs, increased muscular irritability).

(Continued)

Table 13–9 Plan of Care for the Patient with Potential Altered Fluid/Electrolyte Status (Continued)

PATIENT PROBLEM	EXPECTED OUTCOMES	STANDARD OF PRACTICE

		3. Discourage intake of foods high in calcium (e.g., dairy products, sardines).
		4. Encourage intake of foods with high oxylate level (e.g., spinach, rhubarb), as they combine with and aid in the elimination of calcium via the GI tract.
		5. Encourage exercise and activity program to maintain muscle tone and promote reabsorption of calcium.
		6. Administer I.V. fluids and medications as prescribed to reduce calcium levels (see Table 13–8).
		7. Encourage consumption of foods high in magnesium (e.g., cocoa, chocolate, molasses, nuts, fish, seafood).
		8. Assess for positive Trousseau's and/or Chovstek's signs, which occur with severe hypomagnesemia.
		9. Administer magnesium supplement if ordered.
		
		If patient is taking plicamycin, cisplatin corticosteroids, or other medications that may cause hypokalemia:
		1. Assess serum potassium levels (normal = 3.5–5.0 mEq/L) and report alterations.
		2. Monitor vital signs and report the following:
		   a. Tachycardia.
		   b. Weak or irregular pulse.
		   c. Hypotension.

3. Monitor EKG and report arrhythmias.
4. Assess for and report other signs or symptoms of hypokalemia (e.g., muscle weakness, flaccid paralysis, anorexia, nausea, vomiting, paralytic ileus).

If hypokalemia is present (K+ 3.5 mEq/L):
1. Assess for increased neuromuscular excitability.
2. Assess bowel sounds, as paralytic ileus may occur.
3. Continue to monitor vital signs and EKG and report alterations.
4. Observe for signs of metabolic acidosis, which is frequently associated with hypokalemia (e.g., pH > 7.45, bicarbonate > 26 mEq/L, $pACO_2 > 42$ mm Hg, depressed respirations, paresthesias).

If patient is taking corticosteroids, androgens, estrogens, antiestrogens, progestins, or other medications that may cause hypernatremia:
1. Assess laboratory values for serum sodium (normal = 135–145 mEq/L).
2. Assess patient for signs and symptoms of hypernatremia (e.g., irritability, oliguria, edema, weight gain, elevated serum sodium).

If serum sodium is elevated:
1. Assess blood pressure and report elevations.
2. Monitor central venous pressure, if prescribed, and report elevation.
3. Maintain accurate intake and output.

(Continued)

Table 13–9 Plan of Care for the Patient with Potential Altered Fluid/Electrolyte Status (Continued)

PATIENT PROBLEM	EXPECTED OUTCOMES	STANDARD OF PRACTICE
		4. Monitor daily weight.
		5. Assess for and report signs or symptoms of CHF (e.g., edema, shortness of breath, distended neck veins, hypertension).
		6. Assess respirations.
		If elevated serum sodium is accompanied by edema:
		1. Place patient in Fowler's or semi-Fowler's position if necessary to facilitate breathing.
		2. Place patient on low-sodium diet.
		3. Administer low sodium fluids P.O. or I.V. unless contraindicated by cardiac or renal status.
		4. Administer antihypertensive agent, diuretic, and potassium supplement, if ordered.
		5. Assess for altered sensorium or seizures that may occur secondary to cerebral edema.
		6. Implement seizure precautions.

Table 13–10 Plan of Care for the Patient with a Potential Hypersensitivity Reaction

PATIENT PROBLEM	EXPECTED OUTCOMES	STANDARD OF PRACTICE
Knowledge deficit related to potential hypersensitivity reaction to antineoplastic agent(s).	The patient/significant other will: State at least three manifestations of a hypersensitivity reaction specific to the medication they are receiving. Discuss measures that must be taken to control and/or limit a hypersensitivity reaction.	1. Assess level of knowledge. 2. Instruct patient/significant other about potential for hypersensitivity reaction to specific antineoplastic agent(s) that he/she will receive (see "toxicity" columns of the tables in Chapters 3 and 4). 3. Instruct patient about measures to take should any manifestation of a hypersensitivity reaction be noted. 4. Provide written learning aids to reinforce teaching. 5. Provide time and climate to allow for questions, discussion, and feedback as needed.
Potential for injury related to hypersensitivity reaction to antineoplastic agent(s).	The patient will: Develop and maintain a written allergy history. State at least three signs and symptoms of a hypersensitivity reaction to medications he/she is receiving. The patient/significant other will: Demonstrate knowledge of emergency measures to be taken should signs and symptoms occur. Maintain a patent airway.	1. Obtain allergy history from patient. 2. Obtain baseline vital signs before chemo/biotherapy and monitor during therapy (every 15 minutes if I.V. antineoplastic agent administered). 3. Administer test dose (for L-asparaginase, bleomycin) and observe results before administering full dose. 4. Have emergency medications and equipment on hand (see Table 13–8). Premedicate with diphenhydramine and/or hydrocortisone if prescribed. 5. If administering the drug by infusion, run slowly if indicated in drug literature.

(Continued)

Table 13–10 Plan of Care for the Patient with a Potential Hypersensitivity Reaction *(Continued)*

PATIENT PROBLEM	EXPECTED OUTCOMES	STANDARD OF PRACTICE
		6. Monitor patient for signs or symptoms of hypersensitivity reaction when administering cytotoxic agent (e.g., hypotension, restlessness, agitation, bronchospasm, laryngospasm).
		Should signs of hypersensitivity be noted during I.V. administration of cytotoxic agent:
		1. Immediately stop infusion and maintain I.V. at keep vein open rate.
		2. Call for help.
		3. Maintain a patent airway and anticipate the need for emergency intubation or CPR.
		4. Obtain vital signs.
		5. Notify physician.
		6. Administer emergency medication(s) as prescribed (see Table 13–9).
		7. Continue to monitor vital signs.
		8. If hypotensive, place in recumbent or Trendelenberg position and maintain maximum rate of infusion of normal saline solution unless contraindicated.
		9. Administer supplemental oxygen if necessary.
		10. Reassure patient and, if present, significant other.
		11. Document incident in patient's medical record.

References

Allen, A.: The cardiotoxicity of chemotherapeutic drugs. In Perry, M.C. (ed.): *The Chemotherapy Source Book* (pp. 582–597). Baltimore, Williams & Wilkins, 1992.

Blum, R.H., Carter, S.G., Agre, K.: A clinical review of bleomycin: A new antineoplastic agent. Cancer *31*:903–914, 1973.

Casper, E.S., et al.: A prospective randomized trial of adjuvant chemotherapy with bolus versus continuous infusion of doxorubicin in patients with high-grade extremity soft tissue sarcoma and analysis of prognostic factors. Cancer *68*:1221–1229, 1991.

Cattell, V.: Mitomycin-induced hemolytic uremic kidney: An experimental model in the rat. Am. J. Pathol. *121*:88–95, 1985.

Chabner, B.A., and Myers, C.E.: Antitumor antibiotics. In DeVita, V.T., Jr., Hellman, S., and Rosenberg, S.A. (eds.): *Cancer: Principles and Practices of Oncology*, 4th ed. (pp. 374–384). Philadelphia, J.B. Lippincott, 1993.

Cloutier, A.O.: Ocular side effects of chemotherapy: Nursing management. Oncol. Nurs. Forum *19*:1251–1259, 1992.

Collins, C., and Weeden, P.L.: Cardiotoxicity of 5-fluorouracil. Cancer Treat. Rep. *71*:733–736, 1987.

Creagan, E.T.: Biologics. In Perry, M.C. (ed.): *The Chemotherapy Source Book* (pp. 430–438). Baltimore, Williams & Wilkins, 1992.

Creagan, E.T., et al.: A phase I clinical trial of recombinant human tumor necrosis factor. Cancer *62*:2467–2471, 1988.

Feinberg, B., et al.: A phase I trial of intravenously-administered recombinant human tumor necrosis factor-alpha in cancer patients. J. Clin. Oncol. *6*:1328–1334, 1988.

Freeman, N.J., and Constanza, M.E.: 5-Fluorouracil-associated cardiotoxicity. Cancer *11*: 36–45, 1988.

Galassi, A.: The new generation: New chemotherapy agents for the 1990s. Semin. Oncol. Nurs. *8*:83–94, 1992.

Goodman, M.: Managing the side effects of chemotherapy. Semin. Oncol. Nurs. *5*(Suppl. 1):29–52, 1989.

Hoaglund, H.C.: Hematologic complications of cancer therapy. In Perry, M.C. (ed.): *The Chemotherapy Source Book* (pp. 498–507). Baltimore, Williams & Wilkins, 1992.

Hortobagyi, G.N., et al.: Decreased cardiac toxicity of doxorubicin administered by continuous infusion in combination chemotherapy for metastatic breast cancer. Cancer *63*: 37–45, 1989.

Hydzik, C.A.: Late effects of chemotherapy: Implications for patient management and rehabilitation. Nurs. Clin. North Am. *25*:423–446, 1990.

Jassak, P.F.: Biotherapy. In Groenwald, S.L., et al. (eds.): *Cancer Nursing: Principles and Practice*, 3rd ed. (pp. 366–392). Boston, Jones and Bartlett, 1993.

Kirkwood, J.M., and Ernstoff, M.S.: Cutaneous melanoma. In DeVita, V.T., Jr., Hellman, S., Rosenberg, S.A. (eds.): *Biologic Therapy of Cancer*, 4th ed. (pp. 311–333). Philadelphia, J.B. Lippincott, 1991.

Lang-Kummer, J.M.: Hypercalcemia. In Groenwald, S.L., et al. (eds.): *Cancer Nursing: Principles and Practice*, 3rd ed. (pp. 644–661). Boston, Jones and Bartlett, 1993.

Leake, E., Smith, W.G., and Woodliff, H.H.: Diffuse interstitial pulmonary fibrosis after busulphan therapy. Lancet *2*:432–434, 1963.

MacDonald, D.R.: Neurotoxicity of chemotherapeutic agents. In Perry, M.C. (ed.): *The Chemotherapy Source Book* (pp. 666–677). Baltimore, Williams & Wilkins, 1992.

McGuire, W.P., et al.: Taxol: A unique antineoplastic agent with significant activity in advanced ovarian epithelial neoplasma. Ann. Intern. Med. *111*:273–279, 1991.

Moldawer, N.P., and Figlin, R.A.: Tumor necrosis factor: Current clinical status and implications for nursing management. Semin. Oncol. Nurs. *4*:120–125, 1988.

Moormeier, J.A., and Golumb, H.M.: Interferons: Clinical applications. In DeVita, V.T., Jr., Hellman, S., and Rosenberg, S.A. (eds): *Biologic Therapy of Cancer*, 4th ed. (pp. 275–289). Philadelphia, J.B. Lippincott, 1991.

Pegelow, C.H., et al.: Endomyocardial biopsy to monitor anthracycline therapy in children. J. Clin. Oncol. 2:443–446, 1984.

Pratt, C.B., Ransom, J.L., and Evans, W.E.: Age-related adriamycin cardiotoxicity in children. Cancer Treat. Rep. 62:1381–1385, 1978.

Siegel, J.P., and Puri, R.K.: Interleukin-2 toxicity. J. Clin. Oncol. 9:694–704, 1991.

Sostman, H.D., et al.: Cytotoxic drug-induced lung disease. Am. J. Med. 62:608–615, 1977.

Speyer, J.L., et al.: Protective effect of the bispiperazinedione (ICRF-187) against doxorubicin-induced cardiac toxicity in women with advanced breast cancer. N. Engl. J. Med. 319:745–752, 1988.

Steinhertz, L.J., and Yaholam, J.: Cardiac toxicity 4–20 years after completing anthracycline therapy. JAMA 266:1672–1677, 1991.

Stover, D.A.: Adverse effects of treatment: Pulmonary toxicity. In DeVita, V.T., Jr., Hellman, S., and Rosenberg, S.A. (eds.): *Cancer: Principles and Practices of Oncology*, 4th ed. (pp. 2362–2370). Philadelphia, J.B. Lippincott, 1993.

St. Pierre, B.A., Kasper, C.E., and Lindsey, A.: Fatigue mechanisms in patients with cancer: Effects of tumor necrosis factor and exercise on skeletal muscle. Oncol. Nurs. Forum 19(3):419–425, 1992.

Valavaara, R., and Nordman, E.: Renal complications of mitomycin-C, with special reference to the total dose. Cancer 55:47–50, 1985.

Von Hoff, D.D., et al.: Risk factors for doxorubicin-induced congestive heart failure. Ann. Intern. Med. 91:710–717, 1982.

Warrell, R.P., Jr.: Metabolic emergencies. In DeVita, V.T., Jr., Hellman, S., and Rosenberg, S.A. (eds.): *Cancer: Principles and Practices of Oncology*, 4th ed. (pp. 2128–2141). Philadelphia, J.B. Lippincott, 1993.

Zalpuski, M., and Baker, L.H.: Ifosfamide. J. Natl Cancer Inst. 80:556–566, 1988.

Recommended Readings

General References

American Nurses Association: *ANA/ONS Standards of Oncology Nursing Practice*. Kansas City, MO, American Nurses Association, 1987.

Brophy, L., and Sharp, E.: Physical symptoms of combination biotherapy: A quality-of-life issue. Oncol. Nurs. Forum 18:23–40, 1991.

Cunningham, M.: Nonhematologic toxicities of selected chemotherapeutic agents used in treatment of adult leukemia. Semin. Oncol. Nurs. 6:67–75, 1990.

Dorr, R.T.: *Ifosfamide and Cyclophosphamide—Review and Appraisal*. Princeton, NJ, Bristol-Myers Squibb, 1992.

Goodman, M.: Managing the side effects of chemotherapy. Semin. Oncol. Nurs. 5(Suppl. 1):29–52, 1992.

Gootenberg, J.E., and Pizzo, P.A.: Optimal management of acute toxicities of therapy. Pediatr. Clin. North Am. 38:269–297, 1991.

Loescher, L., et al.: Surviving adult cancers: Part 1: Physiological effects. Ann. Intern. Med. 111:411–432, 1989.

Perry, M.C. (ed.): *The Chemotherapy Source Book*. Baltimore, Williams & Wilkins, 1992.

Skelton, J., and Pizzo, P.: Problems of intensive therapy in childhood cancer. Cancer 58:488–503, 1986.

Ulrich, S., Canale, S.W., and Wendell, S.A.: *Nursing Care Planning Guides: A Nursing Diagnosis Approach.* Philadelphia, W.B. Saunders, 1990.

Cardiotoxicity

Arnold, A.Z., et al.: Right heart failure after chemotherapy. Cleve. Clin. J. Med. *58:*357–360, 1991.

Azar, J.J., and Theriault, R.L.: Acute cardiomyopathy as a consequence of treatment with interleukin-2 and interferon-α in a patient with metastatic carcinoma of the breast. Am. J. Clin. Oncol. *14:*530–533, 1991.

Doroshow, J.H.: Doxorubicin-induced cardiac toxicity. N. Engl. J. Med. *324:*843–845, 1991.

Doz, F., et al.: Experimental basis for increasing the therapeutic index of carboplatin in brain tumor therapy by pretreatment with WR compounds. Cancer Chemother. Pharmacol. *28:*308–310, 1991.

Goorin, A.M.: Initial congestive heart failure after doxorubicin chemotherapy for childhood cancer. J. Pediatr. *116:*144–147, 1990.

Konig, J., Palmer, P., and Franks, C.F.: Cardioxane-ICRF-187: Towards anticancer drugs specificity through selective toxic reduction. Cancer Treat. Rev. *18:*1–19, 1991.

Lipshultz, S.E., et al.: Late cardiac effects of doxorubicin therapy for acute lymphoblastic leukemia in childhood. N. Engl. J. Med. *324:*808–815, 1991.

Rowinsky, E.K., et al.: Cardiac disturbance during the administration of taxol. J. Clin. Oncol. *9:*1704–1712, 1991.

Speyer, J.L., et al.: ICRF-187 permits longer treatment with doxorubicin in women with breast cancer. J. Clin. Oncol. *10:*117–127, 1992.

Steinhertz, L.J., and Yaholam, J.: Cardiac complications of cancer therapy. In DeVita, V.T., Jr., Hellman, S., and Rosenberg, S.A. (eds.): *Cancer: Principles and Practices of Oncology,* 4th ed. (pp. 2370–2385). Philadelphia, J.B. Lippincott, 1993.

Fluid and Electrolyte Alterations

Body, J.J.: Medical treatment of tumor-induced hypercalcemia and tumor-induced osteolysis: Challenges for future research. Supportive Care in Cancer 1(1):26–33, 1993.

Conrad, K.J.: Cerebellar toxicities associated with cytosine arabinoside: A nursing perspective. Oncol. Nurs. Forum 13(5):57–59, 1986.

Gucalp, R., et al.: Comparative study of pamidronate disodium and etidronate disodium in the treatment of cancer-related hypercalcemia. J. Clin. Oncol. *10:*134–142, 1990.

Mahon, S.M.: Nursing considerations in hypercalcemia of malignancy. Oncol. Update 12–14, 1992.

Mahon, S.M.: Symptoms as clues to calcium levels. Am. J. Nurs. *87:*354–356, 1987.

Mahon, S.M., and Casperson, D.S.: Pathophysiology of hypokalemia in patients with cancer: Implications for nurses. Oncol. Nurs. Forum 20(6):919–946, 1996.

McDermott, K.C., Almadrones, L.A., and Bajorunas, D.R.: The diagnosis and management of hypomagnesemia: A unique treatment approach and case report. Oncol. Nurs. Forum *18:*1145–1152, 1991.

Metheny, N.M.: *Fluid and Electrolyte Balance, Nursing Considerations.* Philadelphia, J.B. Lippincott, 1987.

Muscari-Lin, E., and Polomano, C.: Fluid and electrolyte imbalance. In Daeffler, R.J., and Petrosino, B.M.: *Manual of Oncology Nursing Practice* (pp. 131–141). Rockville, MD, Aspen, 1990.

Poe, C., and Taylor, L.M.: Syndrome of inappropriate antidiuretic hormone: Assessment and nursing implications. Oncol. Nurs. Forum *16:*373–381, 1989.

Ralston, S.H., et al.: Cancer-associated hypercalcemia: Morbidity and mortality. Ann. Intern. Med. 112:499–504, 1991.

Terry, J.: The other electrolytes: Magnesium, calcium and phosphorous. J. Intravenous Nurs. 1(14):167–176, 1991.

Theriault, R.L.: Management of hypercalcemia in breast cancer. Oncology 4(2):43–46, 1990.

Todd, P.A., and Fitton, A.: Gallium nitrate: A review of the pharmacological properties and therapeutic potential in cancer related hypercalcemia. Drugs 261–273, 1991.

Warrell, R.P., et al.: Gallium nitrate inhibits calcium resorption from bone and is effective treatment for cancer-related hypercalcemia. J. Clin. Invest. 73:1487–1490, 1984.

Yarnell, R.P., and Craig, M.P.: Detecting hypomagnesemia: The most overlooked electrolyte imbalance. Nursing 21(7):55–57, 1991.

Hepatotoxicity

Perry, M.C.: Hepatotoxicity and chemotherapeutic agents. In Perry, M.C. (ed.): *The Chemotherapy Source Book* (pp. 635–647). Baltimore, Williams & Wilkins, 1992.

Hypersensitivity Reactions, Flu-like Syndrome

Hammond, E.: Anaphylactic reactions to chemotherapeutic agents. J. Assoc. Pediatr. Oncol. Nurses 5(3):16–19, 1988.

Haeuber, D.: Recent advances in the management of biotherapy-related side effects: Flu-like syndrome. Oncol. Nurs. Forum 16(suppl. 6):35–41, 1989.

Moeser, L.C.: Anaphylaxis: A preventable complication of home infusion therapy. J. Intravenous Nurs. 14:108–112, 1991.

Oncology Nursing Society: *Cancer Chemotherapy Guidelines, Recommendations for the Management of Extravasation and Anaphylaxis*. Pittsburgh, PA, Oncology Nursing Society, 1992.

Reiger, P.T.: Management of cancer-related fatigue. Dimens. Oncol. Nurs. 2(3):5–8, 1988.

Weiss, R.B.: Hypersensitivity reactions. In Perry, M.C. (ed.): *The Chemotherapy Source Book* (pp. 553–569). Baltimore, Williams & Wilkins, 1992.

Weiss, R.B., and Baker, J.R.: Hypersensitivity reactions from antineoplastic agents. Cancer Metastasis Rev. 6:413–432, 1987.

Weiss, R.B., et al.: Hypersensitivity reactions from taxol. J. Clin. Oncol. 8:1263–1268, 1990.

Neurotoxicity/Ototoxicity/Ocular Toxicity

Baker, W.J., et al.: Cytarabine and neurologic toxicity. J. Clin. Oncol. 9:679–693, 1991.

Cameron, J.C.: Ifosamide neurotoxicity: A challenge for nurses, a potential nightmare for patients. Cancer Nurs. 16(1):40–46, 1993.

Gregg, R.W., et al.: Cisplatin neurotoxicity: The relationship between dosage, time, and platinum concentration in morphologic evidence of toxicity. J. Clin. Oncol. 10:795–803, 1992.

Hayback, P.J.: Tuning in to ototoxicity: The inside story. Nursing 93, 23(6):34–41, 1993.

Holden, S., and Felde, G.: Nursing care of patients experiencing cisplatin-related peripheral neuropathy. Oncol. Nurs. Forum 14(1):13–19, 1987.

Lundquist, D.M.: Documentation of neurotoxicity resulting from high-dose cytosine arabinoside. Oncol. Nurs. Forum 20(9):1409–1413, 1993.

Macdonald, D.R.: Neurologic complications of chemotherapy. Neurol. Clin. N. Am. 9(4):955–967, 1991.

Miller, L.J., and Eaton, V.E.: Ifosfamide-induced neurotoxicity: A case report and review of the literature. Ann. Pharmacother. 26:183–187, 1992.

Mollman, J.E., et al.: Cisplatin neuropathy: Risk factors, prognosis, and protection by WR-2721. Cancer 61:2192–2195, 1988.

Ostchega, Y., Donohue, M., and Fox, N.: High-dose cisplatin-related peripheral neuropathy. Cancer Nurs. 11:23–32, 1988.

Sherwood, G.D.: Altered sensory perception. In Daeffler, R.J., and Petrosino, B.M.: *Manual of Oncology Nursing Practice* (Chapter 21). Rockville, MD, Aspen, 1990.

Smedley, H., et al.: Neurological effects of recombinant human interferon. Br. Med. J. 286:262–264, 1983.

Young, S.B.: Nursing considerations in caring for the child with vincristine-induced neurotoxicities. J. Pediatr. Oncol. Nurs. 7:9–13, 1990.

Pulmonary Toxicity

Gift, A.G.: Dyspnea. Nurs. Clin. North Am. 25:955–965, 1990.

Haylock, P.J.: Breathing difficulty: Changes in respiratory function. Semin. Oncol. Nurs. 3:293–298, 1987.

Kreisman, H., and Wolcove, N.: Pulmonary toxicity of antineoplastic therapy. In Perry, M.C. (ed.): *The Chemotherapy Source Book* (pp. 598–619). Baltimore, Williams and Wilkins, 1992.

Limper, A.H., and McDonald, J.A.: Delayed pulmonary fibrosis after nitrosourea therapy. N. Engl. J. Med. 323:407–409, 1990.

O'Driscoll, B.R., et al.: Active lung fibrosis up to 17 years after chemotherapy with carmustine. N. Engl. J. Med. 323:378–382, 1990.

Wickham, R.: Pulmonary toxicity secondary to cancer treatment. Oncol. Nurs. Forum 13(5):69–76, 1986.

Renal Toxicity

Evans, S.: Nursing measures in the prevention and treatment of renal cell damage associated with cisplatin administration. Cancer Nurs. 14:91–97, 1991.

Hantel, A., Donehower, R.C., Rowinsky, E.K., et al.: Phase I study and pharmacodynamics of piroxantrone (NSC-349174), a new anthrapyrazole. Cancer Res. 50:3284–3288, 1990.

Held, J., and Volpe, H.: Bladder preserving combined modality therapy for invasive bladder cancer. Oncol. Nurs. Forum 18:1849–1857, 1991.

Lydon, A.: Nephrotoxicity of cancer treatment. Oncol. Nurs. Forum 13(2):68–77, 1986.

Patterson, W.P., and Reams, G.P.: Renal and electrolyte abnormalities due to chemotherapy. In Perry, M.C. (ed.): *The Chemotherapy Source Book* (pp. 648–665). Baltimore, Williams & Wilkins, 1992.

Russo, P.: Urologic emergencies. In DeVita, V.T., Jr., Hellman, S., and Rosenberg, S.A. (eds.): *Cancer: Principles and Practices of Oncology*, 4th ed. (pp. 2159–2169). Philadelphia, J.B. Lippincott, 1993.

Vascular Access

Successful treatment of the client with cancer requires safe and repeated access to the vascular system for the delivery of chemotherapy, biological response modifiers, fluids, nutrition, blood components, and antibiotics. Administration of a course of chemotherapy may last weeks or months and can have sclerosing effects on peripheral blood vessels. These effects can, in part, be avoided when chemotherapy is administered via a vascular access device (VAD).

Vascular access may be established by using one of the following devices: peripheral venous catheters, tunneled or nontunneled central venous catheters, peripherally inserted central catheters (PICCs), and implantable infusion ports. Continuous infusion chemotherapy can be delivered via a vascular access catheter or port and a portable infusion pump.

Advantages of Vascular Access

1. Permits repeated administration of chemotherapy without repeated venipuncture when multiple or prolonged courses of treatment are anticipated.
2. Allows for administration of chemotherapy by continuous infusion into a larger vein, with better dilution, without repeated venipunctures.
3. Allows for blood sampling without repeated venipunctures.

4. Averts discomfort of multiple needle sticks that may be required for venipuncture.
5. Reduces pretreatment anxiety.
6. Minimizes risk of extravasation.
7. Prevents peripheral vein sclerosis.
8. Permits venous access when peripheral veins have become sclerosed and can no longer accommodate intravenous administration.
9. Maintains ready access to a vein.
10. Provides a more conveniently accessible access route for administration of chemotherapy in outpatient and home care settings.
11. Provides a route for direct infusion of chemotherapeutic and/or biologic agents into an organ (e.g., liver) or region (e.g., peritoneum).

Each of the next four chapters in this book will further describe the four main modes for vascular access—central venous catheters (CVCs); peripherally inserted central catheters (PICCs); implanted ports; and ambulatory infusion pumps (external or implanted).

Recommended Readings

Camp-Sorrell, D.: Advanced central venous access: Selection, catheters, devices and nursing management. J. Intravenous Nurs. 13:361–370, 1990.

Carter, P., et al.: *Access Device Guidelines: (Modules)*. Pittsburgh, Oncology Nursing Society, 1989.

Hadaway, L.: Evaluation and use of advanced I.V. technology: Part I: Central venous access devices. J. Intravenous Nurs. 12:73–82, 1989.

Kwan, J.W.: High-technology I.V. infusion devices. Am. J. Hosp. Pharm. 46:320–335, 1989.

Kwan, J.W.: Drug delivery technology. Cancer Bull. 42:383–390, 1990.

Marcoux, A., Fisher, S., and Wong, D.: Central venous access devices in children. Pediatr. Nurs. 16:123–133, 1990.

Mirro, J., et al.: A prospective study of Hickman/Broviac catheters and implanted ports in pediatric oncology patients. J. Clin. Oncol. 213:222, 1989.

Schulmeister, L.: An overview of continuous infusion chemotherapy. J. Intravenous Nurs. 15:315–321, 1992.

Wickham, R.S.: Advances in venous access devices and nursing management. Nurs. Clin. North Am. 25:345–364, 1990.

Wickham, R., Purl, S., and Walker, D.: Long-term central venous catheters: Issues for care. Semin. Oncol. Nurs. 133–147, 1992.

Chapter 14

Central Venous Access Devices

Linda Tenenbaum, R.N., M.S.N., O.C.N.
Dixie Brennan Scelsi, R.N., M.S., M.S.N.

Central venous access devices (VADs) are placed with the termination tip in the largest central vein—the superior vena cava. Most are inserted under sterile techniques via the subclavian or jugular vein. An external portion ("pigtail") allows access to the line(s) for insertion of medication or blood products, or withdrawal of blood specimens. VADs are used for continuous or intermittent administration of intravenous (I.V.) fluids. Because the VAD termination site is in a large central vein, hyperosmolar medications and solutions can be safely administered, and rapid dilution and dispersion of irritating drugs will occur. In the patient with cancer, hyperalimentation solutions, chemotherapeutic agents, pain medications, antibiotics, antiemetics, and blood components are administered via a VAD.

Types of Central VADs

Short-term (Nontunneled) Catheters

The short-term central catheter for an adult is 15- to 19-gauge in size. The catheter may be placed for a trial course of chemotherapy prior to insertion of a long-term VAD. The usual duration of placement for short-term catheters is 46 to 60 days. In some situations, however, they have been left in place for a longer period of time (if there have been no complications).

Short-term VADs have no cuff and do not pass through a subcutaneous tunnel. This places the patient with this type of device at increased risk for infection and/or catheter-related sepsis.

Long-term (Tunneled) VADs

Long-term (tunneled) VADs are inserted when a prolonged course of parenteral therapy is anticipated. They are made of medical grade silicone or polyurethane, or a similar material. All are radiopaque. Most are available in single, double, and triple lumen form (Figs. 14–1 and 14–2). The catheter is surgically implanted via the subclavian or jugular vein, with the tip terminating in the superior vena cava, near the right atrium (Fig. 14–3). This procedure may be done under local anesthesia. A portion of the catheter passes through the subcutaneous tissue of the chest wall and exits to the right or left of the midline of the chest wall. A cuff made of Dacron or a similar material forms a seal around the catheter. The cuff is positioned at least 2 cm above the exit site (Weiner et al., 1992). The cuff aids in stabilizing the catheter and reducing the risk of infection by providing a barrier to retrograde migration of microorganisms.

When access to the superior vena cava is not possible (e.g., tortuous vessels, tumor(s) in the chest wall or mediastinum), the cathether may be introduced via the femoral vein and advanced via the inferior vena cava. The cuffed portion of the catheter is tunneled through tissue in the medial aspect of the upper thigh region. The proximal (external) portion of the catheter may be secured to the skin by a suture tied around the catheter. Commercially available long-term VADs are listed in Table 14–1.

Peripherally Inserted Central Catheters (PICCs)

An alternative to central venous catheters is the PICC, which is discussed in detail in Chapter 15.

General Considerations for Catheter Care

VADs require meticulous care to prevent infection and other complications. Specific protocols should be established in each facility or agency for indications; dressing change; site care; medication adminis-

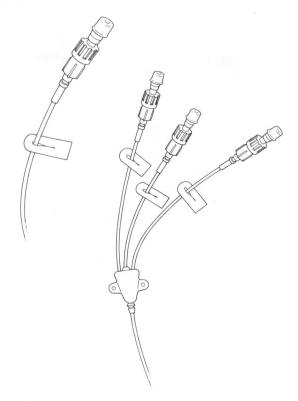

Figure 14–1. Single and triple lumen long-term vascular access catheters. (Original art by Craig L. Kiefer, Naperville, IL.)

tration; irrigation; use of I.V. sets, caps, and other related equipment; and personnel authorized to administer care.

Short-term Central Catheters

Short-term central catheters require a sterile dressing change daily or as otherwise indicated by agency policy. Because these catheters are not tunneled subcutaneously, there is a greater risk for infection. The site is usually cleansed with povidone-iodine, and a dry sterile dressing or transparent dressing is applied. In some cases, self care may not be possible because of the location of the catheter's exit site. Should this occur, dressing changes must be done by the nurse in the office, clinic, or home setting or by a family member who has been taught the sterile dressing procedure. Many of the procedures for care of long-term catheters can be applied to care of short-term catheters as well.

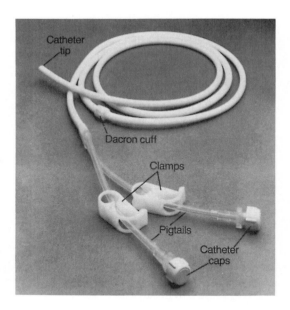

Figure 14–2. Double lumen long-term vascular access catheter (Chemo-Cath). (Courtesy of HDC Corporation, San Jose, CA.)

Long-term Central Catheters

Initial care includes a dressing change at the insertion and exit sites daily or as ordered by the physician. Care of the exit site is the same as for the short-term central catheter. In addition, a smaller dressing is placed at the insertion site and left in place, with routine dressing changes until this incision is healed and sutures are removed.

Procedures for Catheter Care

Site Care and Dressing Changes

Site care and sterile dressing changes should be performed according to institutional policies. The equipment used by most facilities is included in Table 14–2.

1. Agency policy should state which nurses are authorized to care for central catheters.
2. Assess catheter exit site for erythema, drainage, tenderness, warmth and/or inflammation, and positioning.
3. Assess exit site for dilation of blood vessels, which may indicate thrombosis.

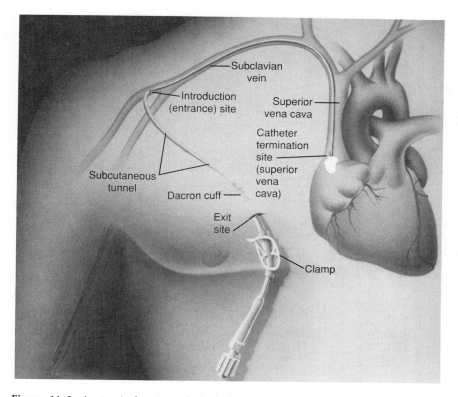

Subclavian
vein

Introduction
(entrance) site

Superior
vena cava

Catheter
termination
site
(superior
vena
cava)

Subcutaneous
tunnel

Dacron cuff

Exit
site

Clamp

Figure 14–3. Anatomic location of single lumen long-term vascular access catheter (Infuse-A-Cath).

4. Should the catheter become dislodged, immediately apply an occlusive dressing to the exit site and notify the physician.
5. Should the catheter break, follow manufacturer's directions for repair.
6. Check position and integrity of the catheter. (*Note:* Most catheters are marked at 10-cm intervals, making inspection and documentation easier.)

Catheter Irrigation

1. To prevent accidental needle sticks, enter the catheter hub or extension tubing hub with a needle-free IV access device or a protected needle whenever possible.
2. Silastic catheters must be irrigated on a regular basis to maintain patency and prevent occlusion.

Table 14–1 Long-term (Tunneled) Central Venous Catheters*

NAME (COMPANY)	CATHETER MATERIAL, CUFF MATERIAL	OUTER DIAMETER (FR)	LENGTH (CM)	INNER (LUMEN) DIAMETER IN MM (ADAPTOR COLOR)	MAXIMUM TOLERATED PSI
Single Lumen					
Broviac (Bard)	Silicone, dacron	2.7	71	0.5	25
Broviac (Bard)	Silicone, dacron	4.2	71	0.7	25
Broviac (Bard)	Silicone, dacron	6.6	90	1.0	25
ChemoCath (HDC)	Silicone, dacron	4.0	71	0.6	40
ChemoCath (HDC)	Silicone, dacron	6.6	92	1.0	40
ChemoCath (HDC)	Silicone, dacron	9.6	92	1.6	40
Cook Catheter (Cook Critical Care)	Silicone, dacron	3	55	0.55	100
Cook Catheter (Cook Critical Care)	Silicone, dacron	4	65	0.66	100
Cook Catheter (Cook Critical Care)	Silicone, dacron	6.5	90	1.0	100
Cook Catheter (Cook Critical Care)	Silicone, dacron	9.5	90	1.6	100
Groshong (Bard)	Silicone, dacron + Vitacuff	3.5	35	0.7	25
Groshong (Bard)	Silicone, dacron + Vitacuff	5.5	40	1.1	25
Groshong (Bard)	Silicone, dacron + Vitacuff	7.0	50	1.3	25
Groshong (Bard)	Silicone, dacron + Vitacuff	8.0	50	1.5	25

Groshong (Bard)	Silicone, dacron + Vitacuff	8.0	65	1.5	25
Harborin (Harbor)	Polyurethane, dacron	7.0	50	1.5	50
Hemed (Gish)	Silicone, dacron	4.0	90	0.6 (green)†	40
Hemed (Gish)	Silicone, dacron	6.6	90	1.0 (blue)	40
Hemed (Gish)	Silicone, dacron	9.5	90	1.6 (white)	40
Hickman (Bard)	Silicone, Vitacuff	9.6	90	1.6	25
OmegaCath (Norfolk)	Silicone, dacron	5.0	78	0.9 (red)	40
OmegaCath (Norfolk)	Silicone, dacron	7.0	90	1.1 (red)	40
OmegaCath (Norfolk)	Silicone, dacron	9.0	90	1.5 (red)	40
Quinton (Quinton)	Silicone, felt	4.0	84	0.75	40
Quinton (Quinton)	Silicone, felt	7.0	94	1.0	40
Quinton (Quinton)	Silicone, felt	10.0	94	1.5	40
Ventra (Pharmacia Deltec)	Silicone, dacron	7.0	72.5	1.2	40
Ventra (Pharmacia Deltec)	Silicone, dacron	9.0	72.5	1.5	40

Dual Lumen (Note: Proximal lumen on first line; distal lumen on second line.)

ChemoCath (HDC)	Silicone, dacron	7.0	71	0.7 (white) / 1.0 (red)	40 / 40
ChemoCath (HDC)	Silicone, dacron	9.6	92	0.7 (white) / 1.3 (red)	40 / 40
ChemoCath (HDC)	Silicone, dacron	12.0	92	1.6 (white) / 1.6 (red)	40 / 40
Cook Catheter (Cook Critical Care)	Silicone, dacron	7.0	65	0.66 (blue) / 1.0 (yellow)	100 / 100
Cook Catheter (Cook Critical Care)	Silicone, dacron	9.0	80	0.99 (blue) / 1.2 (yellow)	100 / 100
Cook Catheter (Cook Critical Care)	Silicone, dacron	12.0	90	1.0 (blue) / 1.6 (yellow)	100 / 100

(Continued)

417

Table 14–1 Long-term (Tunneled) Central Venous Catheters* (Continued)

NAME (COMPANY)	CATHETER MATERIAL, CUFF MATERIAL	OUTER DIAMETER (FR)	LENGTH (CM)	INNER (LUMEN) DIAMETER IN MM (ADAPTOR COLOR)	MAXIMUM TOLERATED PSI
Groshong (Bard)	Silicone, dacron + Vitacuff	9.5	60	1.1 (white) / 1.3 (red)	25 / 25
Groshong (Bard)	Silicone, dacron + Vitacuff	9.5	67.5	1.1 (white) / 1.3 (red)	25 / 25
Harborin (Harbor)	Polyurethane, dacron	9.5	50	1.4 / 1.4	50 / 50
Hemed (Gish)	Silicone, dacron	7.0	90	0.6 (green)† / 1.0 (blue)	40 / 40
Hemed (Gish)	Silicone, dacron	11.0	90	1.0 (blue) / 1.6 (white)	40 / 40
Hemed (Gish)	Silicone, dacron	14.0	90	1.6 (white) / 1.6 (white)	40 / 40
Hemed (Gish)	Silicone, dacron	9.0	90	1.3 (purple) / 1.3 (purple)	40 / 40
Hickman (Bard)	Silicone	7.0	65	0.8 (white) / 1.0 (red)	40
Hickman (Bard)	Silicone	9.0	90	0.7 (white) / 1.3 (red)	40 / 40
Hickman (Bard)	Silicone	12.0	90	1.6 (white) / 1.6 (red)	40 / 40
Leonard (Bard)	Silicone	10.0	90	1.3 (white) / 1.3 (red)	40 / 40
OmegaCath (Norfolk)	Silicone, dacron	10.5	90	1.0 (red) / 1.0 (white)	40 / 40

Catheter (Manufacturer)	Material				
Quinton (Quinton)	Silicone, felt	9.0	90	1.1	40
				1.1	40
Quinton (Quinton)	Silicone, felt	12.0	102	1.5	40
				1.5	40
Quinton (Quinton)	Silicone, felt	13.5	95	1.2 × 3.0	40
				1.2 × 3.0	40
Ventra (Pharmacia Deltec)	Silicone, dacron	9.0	72.5	0.4	40
				1.2	40

Triple Lumen (*Note: Proximal lumen on first line; middle lumen on second line; distal lumen on third line.*)

Catheter (Manufacturer)	Material				
Cook Catheter (Cook Critical Care)	Silicone, dacron	8.0	90	1.1 (yellow)	100
				0.74 (red)	100
				0.74 (blue)	100
Hemed (Gish)	Silicone, dacron	12.5	90	1.0 (blue)	40
				1.0 (blue)	40
				1.6 (white)	40
Hickman (Bard)	Silicone with Vitacuff	12.5	90	1.0 (white)	40
				1.0 (red)	40
				1.5 (blue)	40
Quinton (Quinton)	Silicone, felt	12.0	90	1.0 (white)	40
				1.1 (blue)	40
				1.25 (red)	40
Ventra (Pharmacia Deltec)	Silicone, dacron	11.0	72.5	0.9	40
				0.9	40
				1.3	40

*NOTE: Priming volume varies for each catheter. A minimum of 2 to 3 ml should be used to flush each line.
†Manufacturer recommends that blood not be drawn from this size lumen.

Table 14–2 Equipment for Catheter Care (Site Care, Accessing, Flushing, Medication Administration, Blood Sampling)

- Povidone-iodine swabsticks*
- Alcohol swabsticks*
- Clean gloves
- Sterile gloves*
- Sterile drape*
- Sterile needles and I.V. extension tubing with clamp for safety; a "needleless" or encased needle should be used.
- 10-ml syringe(s) with 2.5 to 6 ml of normal saline for injection
- 10-ml syringe with 5 ml of heparinized saline for injection (100 U/ml)
- Syringe(s) with medications(s). NOTE: The syringe should be 10 ml or larger, regardless of the amount of medication. If multiple medications are being administered in sequence, additional 10-ml syringes with 5 ml of saline will be required for flushing between medications.
- I.V. solution bag and tubing (for drip administration)
- Dressing (gauze and tape, or transparent film dressing)*
- Disposal container for old dressing (if not in dressing kit)
- Accessible sharps container for disposal of needles

*NOTE: May exist in a central venous catheter dressing kit.

3. When a continuous infusion is administered, the central catheter should be irrigated once daily.
4. When administering intermittent medications, the line should be irrigated before and after each solution to prevent medication interactions and remove infusate residues, which may obstruct or damage the catheter.
5. Infusion of normal saline solution is essential before and after administration of blood products to maintain patency in the line.
6. Irrigate according to the physician's order or the irrigation procedure in an institution. Some procedures require the use of saline only, but most require heparinization.

Additional Measures for Multiple Lumen Catheters

In addition to the general principles mentioned above, the following measures specific to the care of triple lumen catheters should be followed:

1. The uses for each pigtail should be designated and clearly marked.
2. Each lumen should be irrigated regularly.
3. Catheter pigtails should be secured to avoid kinking or tension on the catheter.

Groshong Catheter

The Groshong catheter requires no heparinization. A three-position slit valve near the tip of the catheter opens outward during infusion of solutions, inward during blood sampling, and closes automatically when not in use (Fig. 14–4). The following measures are recommended by the manufacturer for proper maintenance of the Groshong catheter:

1. Irrigate the catheter with 5 ml of normal saline or other isotonic solution to remove infusate residues every 7 days (when not in use), or after each installation or infusion.
2. Irrigate the catheter with 20 ml of normal saline preceding and following blood sampling or transfusion of blood components, or when blood is observed in the catheter.
3. Irrigate the catheter with 30 ml of normal saline or any isotonic solution before and after administration of hyperalimentation (TPN) solutions.
4. When irrigating after blood sampling or infusion of TPN, attach the syringe directly to the catheter hub. Do not use a needle through an injection cap.

Routine Heparinization

Heparin is routinely instilled into central venous catheters to maintain patency. The number of units, concentration, and amount instilled vary, and may be specified in the institutional procedure. Heparinized saline (100 U/ml) is the most commonly used concentration. Current studies are underway to investigate the role of heparin versus normal saline solution for maintenance of catheter patency (Danek and Norris, 1992; Goode, 1991; Hamilton et al., 1988).

The volume used in flushing the catheter should be sufficient to equal

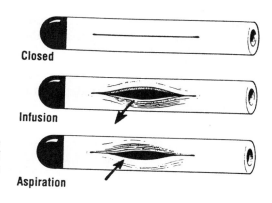

Closed

Infusion

Aspiration

Figure 14–4. Three-way slit valve of Groshong catheter. (Courtesy of Bard Access System, Salt Lake City, UT.)

the filling volume of the catheter, plus an additional 1 to 2 ml to completely flush the line. This ranges from 2 to 5 ml for each lumen of the catheter.

Prevention of Air Embolus

The termination site of the catheter tip (superior vena cava) requires that precautions be taken to prevent air from entering the line during irrigation, medication administration, or I.V. infusion. This includes:

1. Proper clamping of the catheter to ensure that no air is introduced.
2. Purging all air from syringes used for irrigation and medications.
3. Purging all air from I.V. lines.
4. Closure of the catheter clamp as the final ½ ml of solution is being introduced.
5. Clamping the catheter prior to removing the cap or attaching I.V. tubing or syringe for medication administration.*

Capping the Catheter Hub

1. Apply a sterile injection cap or injection port when the central venous cathether is not being used for continuous infusion.
2. A cap or port with a Luer-Lok should always be used for connections.
3. Change the injection cap daily or as specified in hospital or agency policy.
4. Change the cap at the time of irrigation or medication administration to minimize unnecessary handling and opening of the system.

Blood Specimen Withdrawal

Hospital or agency policies for drawing blood from a central catheter should be established. The registered nurse or a member of the I.V. therapy team is usually responsible for performing this procedure.

1. Interrupt I.V. solution flow for at least 1 minute prior to blood sampling to ensure that the specimen contains no infusate.
2. Irrigate the catheter and, when indicated, heparinize after blood sampling.

---

*NOTE: Routine clamping is not required or recommended under normal conditions with the Groshong CV catheter. However, it should be clamped during emergencies such as connector separation or damage to the catheter's external segment.

3. The Groshong catheter must be irrigated with 20 ml of normal saline solution and requires no heparinization.

Accidental Rupture of Silicone Catheters

Silicone catheters may rupture when subjected to excess pressures. Rupture and possible embolization of the catheter or a portion of it may occur when the pressures are too high within the system. This can occur with clots in the catheter, administration of bolus injections while viscous solutions (TPN, lipids) are flowing, or use of a small syringe (TB, 2 or 3 cc). The maximum pressure per square inch (PSI) when administering fluid through a catheter is indicated in Table 14–1.

Patient Education

Dressing changes may be done by the patient or a family member in the home setting, thus the sterile dressing procedure must be taught. The client and family member (when indicated) must be familiar with the following procedures as indicated:

1. Dressing change (A second dressing at the exit site is also necessary with long-term catheters until the site is healed.).
2. Irrigation (via injection cap, extension set, or T-connector with heparinized saline or normal saline).
3. Use of injection caps, extension sets with clamps, or T-connectors.
4. Changing the injection cap, extension set, or I.V. set.
5. Prevention of air embolus by:
   a. Careful handling (purging of air from syringes and tubings, proper clamping).
   b. Use of the Valsalva maneuver when changing extension sets, injection caps, or T-connectors.
6. Emergency measures that must be taken in the event of a break in the catheter.

Self care is best accomplished when the exit site for the catheter is located near the midline of the anterior chest wall. This gives the client easy access to the exit site and hub of the catheter. The exit site is dressed daily or as otherwise specified by the physician.

Good handwashing and proper procedures for sterile dressing changes are taught to the client and (when indicated) a responsible family member. Further information on patient education and sample teaching aids can be found in Chapter 18.

Management of Special Problems

Catheter Occlusion by Fibrin or Plasma Proteins

The VAD may, on occasion, become occluded by fibrin clots and other plasma proteins. Catheter occlusion may be a serious potential complication. Superior vena cava syndrome may occur if a clot occludes the superior vena cava (Bagnall-Reeb et al., 1992.) Initial nursing measures to be taken when this occurs include:

1. Checking all clamps to assure that they are open.
2. Checking the catheter to make sure there are no kinks.
3. Having the client change position (turn, sit up, raise arms).
4. Gently aspirating/irrigating the catheter, using caution to avoid dislodging a clot.

If none of the above steps restores flow, attempts per hospital or agency policy should be made to clear the catheter using heparinized saline. If the infusion is still slow, or if blood cannot be withdrawn after heparinization, urokinase (Abbokinase Open-Cath) may be used to restore patency of the catheter lumen (see Chapter 18).

Repairing the Damaged Catheter

Should the long-term VAD become damaged or cut more than 4 cm from the exit site, the manufacturer's instructions for repair should be followed. Repair procedures may vary somewhat. Repair kits are available for each type of catheter and may be given to the client by the physician, along with instructions for use. Catheter repair for most brands using the repair kit requires that the following measures be taken:

1. Liberally swab the catheter with alcohol and povidone-iodine around the damaged region.
2. Trim the damaged catheter ends.
3. Splice the catheter or insert a connector.
4. Cover the area with a protective sleeve.
5. Secure the protective sleeve with a specially prepared surgical adhesive.

In an emergency situation, when a connector or repair kit is not available, a 14-gauge, 2-inch over-the-needle catheter (angiocath) or a blunt needle may be used for temporary repair as follows:

1. Clamp the cathether close to the chest wall.
2. Cleanse and trim the end of the damaged catheter.
3. Remove connector sleeve (if one is present).

4. Carefully insert the angiocath or blunt needle into the catheter.
5. If an over-the-needle cathether has been inserted, remove and discard the stylet.
6. Tape connection securely.
7. Attach a short I.V. extension set or injection cap to the hub of the needle or angiocath and tape in place. (This step is optional.)
8. Irrigate with heparinized saline solution.

The angiocath or blunt needle will provide temporary access to the catheter until a repair kit can be obtained.

Note: The entire catheter may need replacement if the break is at the main junction of the pigtail(s) and catheter stem. Immediate action to be taken in the event of a catheter break in this area is to clamp the catheter and notify the physician.

References

Bagnall-Reeb, H., Ryder, M., and Anglim, M.A.: Central Venous Access Device Occlusions: Independent Study Module. Abbott Park, IL, Abbott Laboratories, 1992.

Danek, G.D., and Norris, E.M.: Pediatric catheters: Efficacy of saline flush. Pediatr. Nurs. 18:111–113, 122–123, 1992.

Goode, C.J.: A meta-analysis of effects of heparin flush and saline flush: Qualitative and cost implications. Nurs. Res. 40:324–330, 1991.

Hamilton, R.A., et al.: Heparin sodium versus 0.9% sodium chloride injection for maintaining patency of indwelling intermittent infusion devices. Clin. Pharmacol. 7:439–443, 1988.

Weiner, E.S., et al.: The CCSG prospective study of venous access device: An analysis of insertions and causes for removal. J. Pediatr. Surg. 27:155–164, 1992.

Recommended Readings

Alberts, D.S., and Servetar, E.M.: A case report of Twiddler's syndrome in a pediatric patient. J. Pediatr. Oncol. Nurs. 9:25–28, 1992.

Andrews, P.: Increased dwell time with the Landmark® midline catheter: Clear indication of a technique-related learning curve. J. Vasc. Access Nurs. 1(2):14–19, 1991.

Baranowski, L.: Central venous access devices: Current technologies, uses, and management strategies [Review]. J. Intravenous Nurs. 16(3):167–194, 1993.

Bern, M., et al.: Very low doses of warfarin can prevent thrombosis in central venous catheters. Ann. Intern. Med. 112:423–428, 1990.

Bosserman, G., et al.: Multidisciplinary approach to management of vascular access devices. Oncol. Nurs. Forum 17:879–886, 1990.

Brown-Smith, J., Stoner, M., and Barley, Z.: Tunneled catheter thrombosis: Factors related to incidence. Oncol. Nurs. Forum 17:543–549, 1990.

Camp, L.D.: Care of the Groshong catheter. Oncol. Nurs. Forum 15:745–749, 1988.

Cassidy, F., et al.: Noninfectious complications of long-term central venous catheters. Am. J. Radiol. 149:671–675, 1987.

Central venous catheter complications: A nursing perspective. J. Vasc. Access Nurs. *1*(3): 27–28, 1991.

Conly, J.M., Grieves, K., and Peters B.: A prospective, randomized study comparing transparent and dry gauze dressings for central venous catheters. J. Infect. Dis. *159:* 310–319, 1989.

Cunliffe, M.T., and Palomano, R.: How to clear cathether clots with urokinase. Nursing *16*(12):40–43, 1986.

Eisenberg, P.G., Howard, P., and Gianino, M.S.: Improved long-term management of central venous catheters with a new dressing technique. J. Intravenous Nurs. *13:*279–284, 1990.

Freiberger, D., Bryant, J., and Marino, B.: The effects of different central venous line dressing changes on bacterial growth in a pediatric oncology population. J. Pediatr. Oncol. Nurs. *9*(1):3–7, 1992.

Goodwin, M.: Central venous catheter tip malposition following optimal placement in the superior vena cava. J. Vasc. Access Nurs. *1*(3):18–21, 1991.

Gullatte, M.: Nursing management of external venous catheters. Adv. Clin. Care *5*(4): 12–17, 1990.

Haire, D., et al.: Obstructed central venous catheters: Restoring function with a 12-hour infusion of low dose urokinase. Cancer *66:*2279–2285, 1990.

Hadaway, L.: Evaluation and use of advanced IV technology: Part I. Central venous access devices. J. Intravenous Nurs. *12*(2):73–82, 1989.

Howard, P., and Gianino, M.S.: Improved long-term management of central venous catheters with a new dressing technique. J. Intravenous Nurs. *13:*279–284, 1990.

Howard, P., Gianino, S., and Eisenberg, P.: Dressing a central venous catheter: A better way. Nursing 92, *22*(3):60–61, 1992.

Jones, P.M.: Indwelling central venous catheter-related infections and two different procedures of catheter care. Cancer Nurs. *10*(3):123–130, 1987.

Keegan-Wells, D., and Stewart, J.L.: The use of venous access devices in pediatric oncology nursing practice. J. Ped. Oncol. Nurs. *9*(4):159–169, 1992.

Kelly, C., Dumenko, L.S., McGregor, S.E., and McHutchion, M.E.: A change in flushing protocols of central venous catheters. Oncol. Nurs. Forum *19:*599–605, 1992.

Klappers-Klunne, M.C., et al.: Complications from long-term indwelling central venous catheters in hematologic patients with special reference to infection. Cancer *64:*1747–1752, 1989.

Lum, P., and Soski, M.: Management of malpositioned inserted central venous catheters. J. Intravenous Nurs. *12:*356–365, 1989.

Marcoux, C., Fisher, S., and Wong, D.: Central venous access devices in children. Pediatr. Nurs. *16:*123–133, 1990.

McAfee, T., Garland, L.R., and McNabb, T.S.: How to safely draw blood from a vascular access device. Nursing *20*(11):42–43, 1990.

Mirro, J., et al.: A prospective study of Hickman/Broviac catheters and implanted ports in pediatric oncology patients. J. Clin. Oncol. *7*(2):214–222, 1989.

Moss, J.F., et al.: Central venous thrombosis related to the silastic Hickman-Broviac catheter in an oncologic population. J. Parenter. Enteral Nutr. *13:*397–400, 1989.

Oncology Nursing Society: *Oncology Nursing Society: Access Device Guidelines: Recommendations for Nursing Education and Practice—Module 1. Central Venous Catheters.* Pittsburgh, PA, Oncology Nursing Society, 1989.

Peterson, F.Y., and Kirchhoff, K.T.: Analysis of the research about heparinized versus non-heparinized intravascular lines. Heart Lung *20:*631–642, 1991.

Petrosino, B., Becker, H., and Christian, B.: Infection rates in central venous catheter dressings. Oncol. Nurs. Forum *15:*709–717, 1988.

Rasor, J.: Review of catheter-related infection rates: Comparison of conventional catheter materials with Aquavene. J. Vasc. Access Nurs. *1*(3):8–16, 1991.

Robertson, J.: Changing central venous catheter lines: Evaluation of a modification to clinical practice. J. Pediatr. Oncol. Nurs. 8:173–179, 1991.

Schatten, K.: Cardiovascular catheter polymer materials. J. Vasc. Access Nurs. 1(2):20–21, 1991.

Servetar, E.M.: A case report of Twiddler's syndrome in a pediatric patient. J. Pediatr. Oncol. Nurs. 9:25–28, 1992.

Shirnan, J.C., et al.: A comparison of transparent dressing and dry sterile gauze dressings for long-term central catheters in patients undergoing bone marrow transplant. Oncol. Nurs. Forum 18:1349–1356, 1991.

Smeed, C.: Use of midline catheter in PWA's. AIDS Patient Care 4(3):34–37, 1990.

Sohl, L., Nze, R.: Working with triple lumen central venous catheters. Nursing 18:50–55, 1988.

Speer, E.W.: Central venous catheterization: Issues associated with the use of single- and multiple-lumen catheters. J. Intravenous Nurs. 13:30–39, 1990.

Tillman, K.R.: Venous access devices: Guidelines for handling. Home Healthcare Nurse 9(55):13–17, 1991.

Viall, C.D.: Your complete guide to central venous catheters. Nursing 90 20(2):34–41, 1990.

Wickham, R.: Advances in venous access devices and nursing management strategies. Nurs. Clin. North Am. 25:345–364, 1990.

Wickham, R.: Techniques for long-term venous access. In Nursing Management of the Patient Receiving Chemotherapy (pp. 9–20). Atlanta, American Cancer Society, 1988.

Chapter 15

Peripherally Inserted Central Catheters

Joseph Brown, R.N., B.S.N., C.R.N.I.

Access to the peripheral venous system has changed very little since its development in the early 1900s. It was the preferred choice for intravenous (I.V.) therapy until the development of the subclavian approach for central venous access in 1952. Long-term peripheral venous access has been attempted with varying degrees of success over the past 40 years. In the early 1970s, the Intrasil, developed by Travenol Laboratories, saw extensive use in the oncology setting at M.D. Anderson Hospital. While the device established the viability of long-term peripheral venous access, widespread use was limited by its large size and cumbersome insertion technique.

The 1980s saw advances in technology and materials that led to a renewed interest in long-term peripheral venous access. New catheter materials and simplified insertion techniques increased the use of the peripheral vascular system for central venous access.

Current Status

Peripherally inserted central catheters (PICCs) are one of the most rapidly growing areas of vascular access devices. For many patients, they are the device of choice for vascular access. Presently, eight manufacturers offer more than 25 different products from which to choose (see Table 15–1). The PICC is used in inpatient and outpatient settings, and for home infusion therapy. In oncology, the PICC has many applications and fills the gap between the short-term peripheral I.V. device and the surgically placed long-term central venous catheter (CVC).

What Is a PICC?

The PICC line is a long catheter made of biocompatible material (medical grade silicon or polymer material). Sizes vary from 14–24 inches in length. Figure 15–1 shows a 4.0 FR catheter in relation to diameters of various veins. The catheter is inserted through an introducer (a needle or plastic cannula) into one of the veins in the antecubital region. The catheter then is advanced into the central venous system or to some predetermined location in one of the large vessels of the chest. Unlike a long-term CVC, the PICC is not tunneled subcutaneously and has no Dacron cuff. The PICC may be sutured in place or, more commonly, held stationary by a dressing placed on the catheter.

Indications for a PICC

Indications for a PICC line include:

A. **Poor venous access.** A patient who requires multiple attempts at venipuncture to gain venous access is a suitable candidate for a PICC. The clinician can spare the patient the pain, stress, and trauma that accompany repeated attempts at venipuncture by placing a more reliable venous access device at the beginning of therapy.

B. **Irritating/vesicant drug therapy.** The infiltration and extravasation that occur with short-term peripheral venous access rarely occur with the PICC line. The more reliable nature of the device greatly reduces the risk of injury to the patient.

C. **Hyperosmolar solutions.** Catheter tip placement in larger veins allows the administration of total parenteral nutrition (TPN) via the peripheral route. The greater hemodilution found in these larger vessels reduces the risk of vein irritation and thrombus formation.

D. **Lengthy treatment protocols.** The PICC line is an appropriate choice for the patient receiving infusion therapy for more than 4 to 5 days. Based on current standards of practice, the PICC line has no scheduled change or recommended length of dwell in the vein (Intravenous Nursing Society, 1990). PICCs usually remain in place between 1 week and 6 months. The length of time will vary with the device, type of therapy, and individual patient criteria. Average dwell time is 12 to 15 days in the acute care setting, and 45 to 50 days in the home care setting. In a few rare instances, PICC lines have remained in use for as long as 18 to 24 months; however, the appropriateness of such cases must be examined carefully. The responsible practitioner must choose a point in time when the question is asked: "Is this the most appropriate device for this patient?" Length of treatment is just one of the considerations when choosing a vascular access device.

E. **Patient preference.** As patients become more sophisticated about their health care, they look to the clinician to provide them with all the options in their course of treatment. Not every patient needs or wants a surgically placed central line. The patient can make an informed decision after being given the information about options by members of the health care team.

F. **Geographic location.** When treating patients in the outpatient or home care setting, reliable vascular access is important for a smooth course of therapy.

Advantages of the PICC Line

Advantages of the PICC line include:

1. **Fewer insertion-related complications.**
   a. The PICC line virtually eliminates all complications associated with the chest approach to central venous cannulization, including:
      (1) Pneumothorax.
      (2) Hemothorax.
      (3) Hydrothorax.
         (a) Proper placement further reduces the risks of cardiac arrhythmias.
   b. Reduction of:
      (1) Pain, stress, and trauma of repeated venipunctures.
      (2) Infiltration.
      (3) Extravasation associated with peripheral vascular access devices (Rountree, 1991; Markel and Reynen, 1990; Pauley et al., 1993).
2. **Decreased cost of therapy.**
   a. A PICC provides reliable central venous access at approximately one fifth the cost of surgically placed CVCs (Rountree, 1991).
   b. Length of hospital stay is reduced.
   c. Home care costs are lower because fewer visits are needed at home and in outpatient settings.
   d. Agency liability is reduced by the use of a more reliable vascular access device.

Table 15–1 PICC Product Comparison

DESCRIPTION	PER-Q-CATH (GESCO)	V-CATH (HDC)	C-PIC (COOK)	L-CATH (LUTHER)	LIFEVAC (VYGON)	GROSHONG (DAVOL)	CENTERMARK (MENLO CARE)
"Silastic" catheter	X						
Silicone catheter		X	X		X	X	
Polymer catheter				X			X
23 ga (2.0 FR) catheter	X	X		X	X		
Sheath		19 ga					
or needle	20 ga	19 ga		19 ga	19 ga		
20 ga (3.0 FR) catheter	X	X	X	X	X		X
Sheath		17 ga			17 ga		
or needle	19 ga	17 ga	17 ga	17 ga	17 ga		17 ga
18 ga (4.0 FR) catheter	X	X	X	X	X	X	X
Sheath		17 ga			17 ga		
or needle	17 ga	16 ga	15 ga	14 ga	17 ga	14 ga	15 ga
16 ga (5.0 FR) catheter	X		X	X			
Sheath							
or needle	15 ga		14 ga	14 ga			
Dual-lumen catheter	4 FR, 5 FR, 6 FR	5 FR only				5 FR only	
	$65 & $75					$104.50	

Feature	1	2	3	4	5	6	7
Breakaway needle				×	×		
Introducer sheath	×	×			×	×	×
Guidewire (spring)	×	×	×				
Guidewire (twisted)			×	×	×	×	
Insertion tray	× $40–$50	× $45–$56	× $47	× $50	× $58.50	× $71.50	× $58.00
Individual catheters	× $22	× $25–$32	× $36	× $18	× $25		
Individual needles				× $12	× $12		
Individual sheaths	× $12						
Reference marks	×	×				×	
Stainless steel instrmts.	×				×		
Repair kit	×	×			×	×	×
Dressing change tray	×				×		

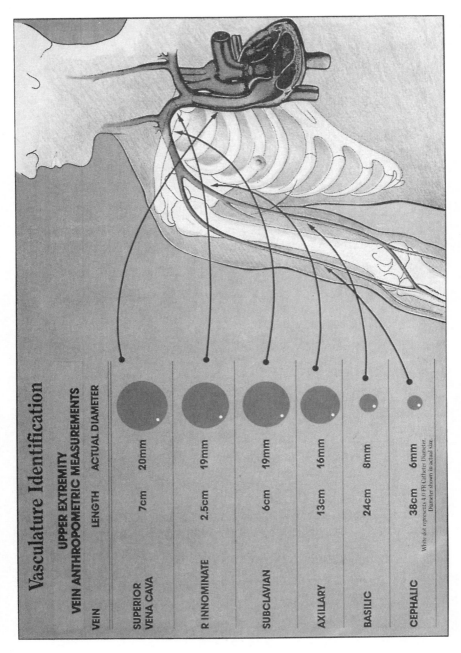

Figure 15–1. (Courtesy of Gesco International, Inc., San Antonio, TX.)

3. **Reliability.**
   a. More reliable than available short-term vascular access devices. Provides long-term vascular access equal to some of the more expensive, more invasive long-term devices with fewer risks (Hadaway, 1991).
   b. **Lower complication rates.**

Disadvantages of the PICC Line

The PICC line is not without problems or disadvantages. However, the advantages of the PICC line outweigh the few disadvantages that have been identified. Disadvantages include:

1. Training. The PICC line requires special training for placement. The Food and Drug Administration (FDA)-Central Venous Catheter Working Group strongly recommends that any clinician (physician or nurse) receive special training in the placement of central lines, including PICC lines (Hadaway, 1991). At least 48 states allow the placement of PICC lines by nurses and require that the nurse has special training, documents competency, and functions within the policy and procedures of the employing organization before independently placing a PICC line. A complete training program, derived from the recommendations of the FDA-Central Venous Catheter Working Group, should include:
   a. Indications and advantages of PICC lines.
   b. Anatomy review of the veins of the chest and upper extremities.
   c. PICC insertion techniques.
   d. Guidelines for verification of placement.
   e. Management of complications.
   f. Product review and evaluation.
   g. Legal issues.
   h. Demonstration of competency through supervised insertions.
   i. Ongoing quality assurance program.
2. Maintenance of skill levels. The number of clinicians placing PICC lines should be kept to a minimum to insure an adequate number of placements for each trained clinician. This will provide more accurate quality assurance data and allow for the maintenance of appropriate skill levels following training.
3. Patient selection. All patients are not suitable candidates for PICC line placement. The most frequent reasons are:
   a. Inadequate veins in the antecubital region.

    b. Inability to identify antecubital veins.

    c. Injury or trauma to the antecubital area.

    d. Pre-existing skin condition.

    e. Noncompliance with care and maintenance.

    These persons should be identified early in their course of therapy and referred for placement of a more appropriate vascular access device.

4. New problems. The PICC line will challenge the clinician with problems that are specific to the device. Complications that are not normally found with other types of CVCs or with short-term peripheral devices will present new challenges for creative catheter management.

Anatomy and the PICC Line

In adult and pediatric patients, the preferred placement sites are the superficial veins in the antecubital region of the upper extremity (Fig. 15–2). In infants and neonates, other veins, such as the scalp, temporal, and external jugular, are frequently used, but will not be discussed in this book.

The first choice for placement is the basilic venous system. This provides the straightest, most direct route from the superficial peripheral venous system into the central venous system. This system may be accessed by direct venipuncture into the basilic vein, or via the median antecubital basilic vein. The vein providing the largest and most superficial presentation would offer the least traumatic insertion.

A suitable second choice is the cephalic system. It is generally smaller than the basilic or median antecubital basilic, and travels a more tortuous route. These two factors may provide a slightly more difficult insertion when accessing the cephalic vein. The smaller size of this vein allows less blood flow around the catheter. This may increase the risk of mechanical phlebitis. Decreased hemodilution in this vein may result in a higher risk of chemical irritation.

Insertion Techniques

There are two insertion techniques that may be used for PICC line placement: the peel-away cannula technique, and the break-away needle technique.

The **peel-away** plastic cannula provides a simple and safe method of placement. It consists of a peel-away polymer cannula mounted over a needle (Fig. 15–3). The needle may have a flash chamber attached or

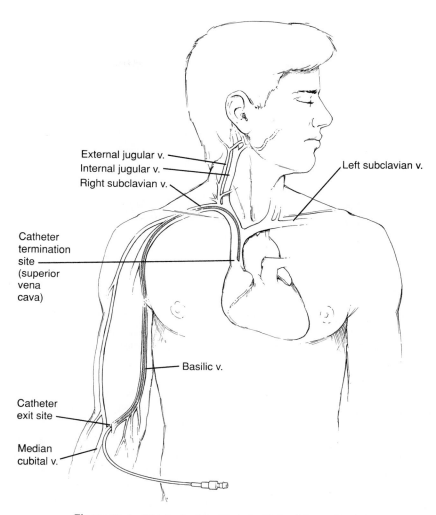

External jugular v.
Internal jugular v.
Right subclavian v.

Left subclavian v.

Catheter
termination
site
(superior
vena
cava)

Basilic v.

Catheter
exit site

Median
cubital v.

Figure 15–2. (Original art by Craig L. Kiefer, Naperville, IL.)

may allow the attachment of a syringe. The introducer unit (cannula and needle) resembles a short-term over-needle I.V. catheter. The insertion of the introducer unit is very similar also.

Venipuncture is performed using a very shallow angle (15° to 30°). When a blood return is noted in the flash chamber, advancement of the introducer is stopped. The peel-away cannula is pushed forward off the needle approximately ¼ to ½ inch. The needle is removed from the cannula and the catheter is threaded through the cannula.

This technique offers a simple, atraumatic placement procedure with

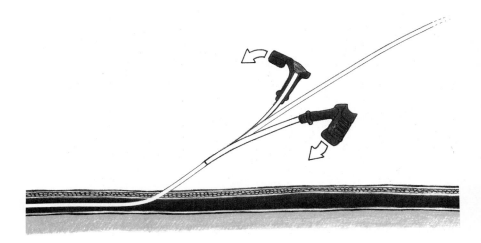

Figure 15–3. Peel-away plastic cannula. (Courtesy of Gesco International, Inc., San Antonio, TX.)

fewer complications than other methods. The possibility of damage to the catheter during the placement procedure is eliminated.

The **break-away** needle technique uses a stainless steel needle that can be split. The needle is designed to be split along its center axis (Fig. 15–4).

The venipuncture technique is similar to that used when obtaining a blood specimen. When a blood return is observed, the angle of the needle is made more parallel to the vein and the needle is advanced ¼ to ½ inch into the vein. The catheter then is advanced through the needle into the vein. The needle is removed from the vein and carefully pulled back along the catheter. The wings of the needle are separated, breaking the two halves of the needle from around the catheter. The clinician must take great care to assure that the catheter is not pulled back through the needle. Pulling the catheter back or pushing the needle forward over the catheter could cause catheter shearing.

Catheter Tip Location

Presently, there are two catheter tip locations in use throughout the United States. The first is a deep peripheral tip location. In this type, the catheter is threaded along a vein (preferably the basilic system) until the tip is located approximately 1 inch distal from the sternal head of the clavicle on the accessed side. This would position the catheter tip at the approximate junction of the axillary and subclavian veins. Since

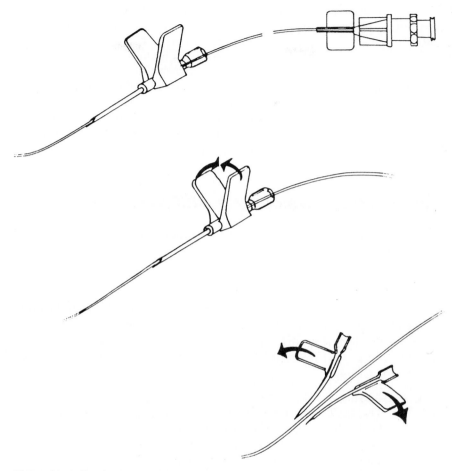

Figure 15–4. Break-away needle technique. (Courtesy of Gesco International, Inc., San Antonio, TX.)

the catheter is not within the confines of the thorax at this location, it could not be considered a central venous catheter. Although this catheter tip location is controversial, it is in popular use and, to date, has shown no higher incidence of complications than PICC lines placed with the tip in the superior vena cava. Due to the smaller size of the axillary-subclavian vein junction when compared to the superior vena cava (12 to 16 mm versus 19 to 21 mm), consideration should be given to the type of medications administered through a deep peripheral tip placement. Any drug that can be administered safely through a short-term peripheral intravenous catheter may be administered safely through a deep peripheral tip PICC. This guideline would limit the use of high concentration dextrose solutions, TPN, or vesicant/irritant chemotherapy infusions, or other drugs having unusual pH or osmolality.

The second choice for catheter tip location is the superior vena cava. The PICC line is threaded along the vein (preferably the basilic system) until the tip is in the upper half of the superior vena cava (Fig. 15–2). This assures tip location in a large central vein, with excellent blood flow and turbulence, and excellent hemodilution of infusates. A PICC line with a tip in the superior vena cava would have the same application and versatility as other types of central venous access devices.

Care and Maintenance of the PICC Line

The care of the PICC line is similar to that of other types of central venous access devices.

Dressing Changes

The sterile dressing performs two functions: it provides a sterile environment, and it prevents the catheter from migrating.

The PICC line dressing change should be a sterile procedure. Prepackaged kits used for other types of central line dressings work well for the PICC line.

1. **Guidelines for dressing changes.**
   a. The PICC line dressing should be changed at intervals similar to those of other central line dressings. Patients who are very active or who perspire profusely will need more frequent dressing changes.
   b. Transparent dressings were found to be safe and efficacious as a CVC site dressing for up to 7 days (Maki and Ringer, 1987).
   c. A transparent, permeable membrane dressing or a tape and gauze dressing may be used. The entire catheter hub and extension set union should be covered by the dressing.
   d. The use of a polymer skin coating will increase both patient comfort and dressing life.
   e. The initial dressing (first 24 hours) should have a gauze just above the insertion site to wick away any drainage. Subsequent dressings will not require a gauze unless drainage is excessive.
   f. If gauze is placed under a transparent, permeable dressing,

it must be changed according to standards for a tape and gauze dressing.

  g. To remove a transparent dressing, loosen at the distal end, anchoring the catheter hub with one hand, and peel the dressing toward the site and parallel to the skin.

  h. All dressings should be labeled clearly and positioned for easy site inspection.

2. **Flushing the PICC catheter.**

  a. The SASH method should always be used to eliminate problems with incompatible drugs. Final heparinization of the PICC line will require the proper amount, concentration, and interval.

  b. The amount of heparin required to flush the device should be equal to the system volume plus approximately 0.2 ml. Table 15–2 gives priming volumes for various catheters. A heparin concentration of 100 U/ml is popular in many areas and works well to maintain patency.

  c. Time intervals between flushes vary greatly. For smaller catheters (1.9 to 2.0 FR), a flush every 8 hours is adequate. Larger catheters, 2.8 FR and above, may be flushed daily or after each use.

  d. Extended flushing protocol (for patients who do not wish to perform daily maintenance):

   (1) Following treatment, flush the catheter with 1 ml of 5000 U/ml heparin every 2 to 3 weeks.

   (2) At the next treatment, remove the heparin and flush vigorously with 5 ml of normal saline solution.

3. **Declotting of PICC line.**

  a. The obstructed PICC may be cleared using urokinase (see Chapter 18). The small volume of the PICC line must be

Table 15–2 Priming Volumes for PICC Catheters

CATHETER SIZE (FR)	GAUGE (GA)/LENGTH (CM)	PRIMING VOLUME (ML)
2.0	23/38	0.06
3.0	20/60	0.20
4.0	16/60	0.30
5.0	16/60	0.40

Extension set volume varies from 0.2 to 0.6 ml.
Dual lumen capacity will vary with catheter size:
    Catheter set volume + Extension set volume = Priming volume.

taken into consideration, as well as catheter bursting strengths.

    b. Urokinase also may be used:

      (1) To restore flow rates to a catheter that has become sluggish after a lengthy dwell time.

      (2) In treatment of catheter sepsis not responsive to antibiotics, by destroying the fibrin matrix at the tip of the catheter, which may encapsulate or protect the bacteria.

4. **Use of pumps with PICC.**

    a. The PICC has been used successfully with all types of infusion pumps.

    b. The problems most often encountered are false occlusion alarms or inadequate flow rates.

    c. An improperly placed dressing may cause kinking of the catheter.

    d. Mini- or micro-tubing may cause high pressure readings by pump sensors.

5. **Blood sampling and administration.**

    a. For consistently good blood sampling, a larger catheter (4.0 FR) may be required.

    b. A gentle touch with a syringe rather than a vacutainer will yield a better blood sample.

    c. A 2-ml discard sample should clear the catheter and provide a reliable sample.

    d. The line should be flushed with at least 5 ml of normal saline solution following blood sampling to remove all blood within the device.

6. **Use of an extension set.**

    a. If a sterile extension set is attached to the sterile PICC line during the insertion procedure, it does not require change unless it becomes damaged, leaks, or if a precipitate is seen in the line.

    b. The volume of the extension set is important and will affect the flushing protocol.

Complications

PICC lines have demonstrated fewer complications than short-term peripheral devices or CVCs. Complications associated with neck and chest approaches to the central venous system may be eliminated by using a peripheral approach. Bleeding is more commonly seen with PICCs than with central lines and usually occurs in the first 24 hours following insertion. This may be caused by patient coagulopathies, anticoagulation therapy, vigorous physical activity, or traumatic insertion. More frequent dressing changes or a mild pressure dressing may prevent such problems. The most common complication is sterile mechanical phlebitis.

Controversial Issues

When any new product is introduced, controversy arises. Current controversial issues relating to PICC lines are:

A. Guidewire versus no guidewire.
B. Catheter tip placement—superior vena cava versus deep peripheral placement.
C. Radiographic verification of placement of device with tip in deep peripheral location.
D. Break-away needle versus peel-away cannula.
E. Training and education for the clinician placing PICC lines.
F. Certification versus qualification for placement of PICC lines.

Summary

Prior to the use of the PICC line, the oncology patient had the choice of a needle or intracath, or the surgically placed CVC. The PICC line has filled the gap between these two devices, and the oncology nurse has a new way of positively affecting patient care.

References

Hadaway, L.: State boards of nursing and advanced practice. J. Intravenous Nurs. *14*:274–279, 1991.
Intravenous Nursing Society: *Intravenous Nursing Society Standards of Practice, Standard III.* Philadelphia, J.B. Lippincott, 1990.
Maki, D.G., and Ringer, M.: Evaluations of dressing regimens for prevention of infection with peripheral intravenous catheters. JAMA *258*:2396–2403, 1987.
Markel, S., and Reynen, K.: Impact on patient care: 2652 PIC catheter days in the alternative setting. J. Intravenous Nurs. *13*:350, 1990.
Pauley, S., et al.: Catheter-related colonization associated with percutaneously placed central catheters. J. Intravenous Nurs. *16*:50–54, 1993.
Rountree, D.: The PIC catheter: A different approach. Am. J. Nurs. *91*(8):22–28, 1991.

Recommended Readings

Bagnall-Reeb, H.: Initial use of a peripherally inserted central venous access port: A review of the literature. J. Vasc. Access Nurs. 1(4):10–14, 1991.

Baranowski, L.: Central venous access devices: Current technologies, uses, and management strategies. J. Intraven. Nurs. 16(3):167–194, 1993.

Brown, J.M.: Peripherally inserted central catheters: Use in home care. J. Intravenous Nurs. 12:144–150, 1989.

Camp-Sorrell, D.: Advanced central venous access. J. Intravenous Nurs. 13:361–370, 1990.

Conohan, T.J., Schwartz, A.J., and Geer, R.T.: Percutaneous catheter introduction: The Seldinger Technique. JAMA 237:446–447, 1977.

Goodwin, M.L.: The Seldinger Method for PICC insertion. J. Intravenous Nurs. 12:238–243, 1989.

Goodwin, M.L., and Carlson, I.: The peripherally inserted central catheter: A retrospective look at 3 years of insertions. J. Intravenous Nurs. 16:92–103, 1993.

Giuffrida, D.J., et al.: Central vs. peripheral venous catheters in critically ill patients. Chest 90:806–809, 1986.

Guillatte, M.: Nursing management of external venous catheters. Adv. Clin. Care 5(4):12–17, 1990.

Hadaway, L.: An overview of vascular access devices inserted via the antecubital area. J. Intravenous Nurs. 13:297–300, 1990.

Hadaway, L.C.: Evaluation and use of advanced I.V. technology: Part I: Central venous access devices. J. Intravenous Nurs. 12:73–82, 1989.

Hedges, C., and Karas, B.S.: Peripherally inserted central catheters: Challenges for hospital management. Med. Surg. Nurs. 2(6):443–449, 1992.

Kyle, K.S., and Myers, J.S.: Peripherally inserted central catheters: Development of a hospital-based program. J. Intravenous Nurs. 13:287–290, 1990.

Loughran, S.C., Edwards, S., and McClure, S.: Peripherally inserted central catheters. J. Intravenous Nurs. 15:152–159, 1992.

Maki, D.G.: Infections associated with intravascular lines. In Swartz, M., and Remington, J. (eds.): *Current Topics in Clinical Infectious Diseases* (pp. 309–363). New York, McGraw-Hill, 1982.

Maki, D.G., and Ringer, M.: Evaluations of dressing regimens for prevention of infection with peripheral intravenous catheters. JAMA 24(258):2396–2403, 1987.

Masoorli, S., and Angeles, T.: PICC lines: The latest home care challenge. RN 53(1):44–51, 1990.

McKee, J.: Future dimensions in vascular access. J. Intravenous Nurs. 12:238–243, 1989.

Mears, C.: *Percutaneous Venous Catheter A.K.A. Peripherally Inserted Central (PIC) Line, Long Arm Catheter, Per-Q-Cath: Policy and Procedure.* Modesto, CA, California Cancer Center, 1989.

Mears, C.: P.I.C.C. and M.L.C. lines: Options worth exploring. Nursing 92 22(10):52–54, 1992.

Mirro, J., et al.: A prospective study of Hickman/Broviac catheters and implanted ports in pediatric oncology patients. J. Clin. Oncol. 213:222, 1989.

Morris, P., et al.: Instruments and methods: A peripherally implanted permanent central venous access device. Obstet. Gynecol. 78:1138–1142, 1991.

Pearl, J.M., Goldstein, L., and Ciresi, K.F.: Improved methods in long-term venous access using the P.A.S. port. Surg. Gynecol. Obstet. 173:313–315, 1991.

Prian, G.W., and Van Way, C.W.: The long arm silastic catheter: A critical look at complications. J. Intravenous Nurs. 13:297–305, 1988.

Rountree, D.: The PIC catheter: A different approach. Am. J. Nurs. 91(8):22–28, 1991.

Rutherford, C.: Insertion and care of multiple lumen peripherally-inserted central catheters. J. Intravenous Nurs. 2(1):16–19, 1988.

Rutherford, C.: A study of single lumen peripherally-inserted central line catheters. J. Intravenous Nurs. 2(3):169–173, 1988.

Weeks-Lozano, H.: Clinical evaluation of Per Q Cath for both pediatric and adult home infusion therapy. J. Intravenous Nurs. 14:249–256, 1991.

Whitlock, R., and Nickerson, B.: Percutaneously-inserted silastic catheters for prolonged intravenous therapy in pediatric patients. Bayviews 1:389–392, 1988.

Winters, V., et al.: A trial with a new peripheral implanted vascular access device. Oncol. Nurs. Forum 17:891–896, 1990.

Chapter 16

Implantable Ports

Linda Tenenbaum, R.N., M.S.N., O.C.N.
Dixie Brennan Scelsi, R.N., M.S., M.S.N.

Implanted infusion ports provide yet another mode of access to the vascular system. Like central venous catheters (CVCs) and peripherally inserted central catheters (PICCs), they have allowed for more chemotherapy administration in the outpatient or home setting. Implanted ports have several advantages over CVCs and PICCs. There is no exterior portion, thus decreasing the risk of infection. Flushing is necessary only after sampling blood or administering medication, or once monthly if the port is not in use.

From the patient's perspective, there are benefits of the implanted port as a vascular access device. A port has less effect on the client's body image than a CVC or PICC because it is completely implanted beneath the skin and has no visible external portion. Other advantages include that dressings and injection caps are not required, there is less interference with bathing and clothing changes, and there are fewer restrictions on activities. After incisions are healed, the client with a port may bathe, shower, or swim as usual.

Subcutaneous entrance for flushing or administering medication is relatively simple, and requires only a subcutaneous injection. Puncture of a port is often less painful than repeated venipuncture attempts. This may decrease pretreatment anxiety after insertion.

Description and Uses

An implantable port (Fig. 16–1) consists of a titanium or plastic chamber with a self-sealing septum, which is usually made of silicone rubber. The plastic material (most commonly polysulfone) is lightweight and durable. Many ports eliminate interference and distortion that may be caused by a metal port during magnetic resonance imaging (MRI) or computerized tomography (CT). A soft, radiopaque, biocompatible catheter (usually silicone or polyurethane) is attached to the port and terminates in the superior vena cava, approximately 2 cm above the right atrium. Other termination sites, illustrated in Figure 16–2, allow for regional delivery of medications into an artery or the peritoneal region. Another site not illustrated is the epidural region. Regional delivery allows for administration of a higher concentration of medication at a localized site with fewer systemic toxicities. In any location, the entire port and catheter system is implanted and secured with sutures during a relatively simple surgical procedure which is done on an inpatient or outpatient basis.

The port can be accessed to withdraw blood samples, or to administer intravenous (I.V.) fluids, medications, total parenteral nutrition (TPN), or blood products. Medication may be administered by bolus or continuous infusion. Dual lumen ports allow for the simultaneous administration of two solutions. Sample ports are shown in Figure 16–3. Component materials and features of each port are delineated in Table 16–1.

Commercially available ports include the following:

- A-Port
- Celsite port
- ChemoPort

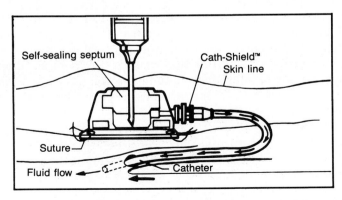

Figure 16–1. Sample vascular access port (Port-A-Cath). (Courtesy of Pharmacia Deltec, Inc., St. Paul, MN.)

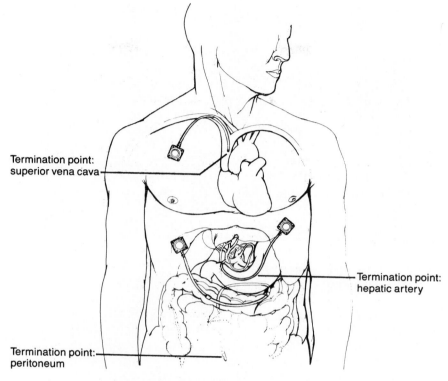

Figure 16–2. Termination sites for implanted infusion ports. (Courtesy of Pharmacia Deltec, Inc., St. Paul, MN.)

- Groshong port
- Hickman port
- Ideas'port
- IMPLANTOFIX-II
- ImPort
- Infuse-A-Port
- LifePort
- Norport
- OmegaPort
- Osteoport (investigational)
- P.A.S. Port
- Port-A-Cath
- Trim Port
- VasPort
- Vital Port

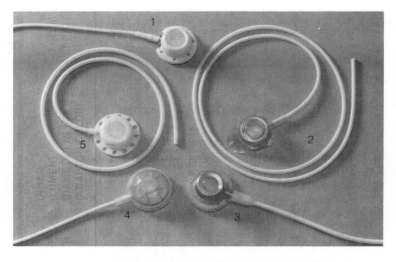

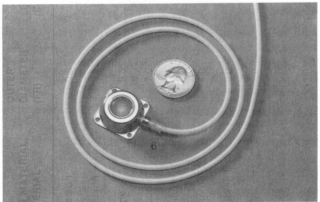

Figure 16–3. Vascular access ports. (1) ChemoPort Plastic. HDC Corporation, San Jose, CA. (2) Celsite Port. Courtesy of B. Braun Medical, Inc., Bethlehem, PA. (3) ChemoPort. Courtesy of HDC Corporation, San Jose, CA. (4) OmegaPort. Courtesy of Norfolk Medical Products, Inc., Skokie, IL. (5) VasPort. Courtesy of Gish Biomedical, Inc., Santa Ana, CA. (6) Port-A-Cath. Courtesy of Pharmacia Deltec, Inc., St. Paul, MN. (7) A^2-Port. (8) A-Port low profile port. (7) and (8) Courtesy of Therex Corp., Walpole, MA. (Photographs by Eric Schenk.)

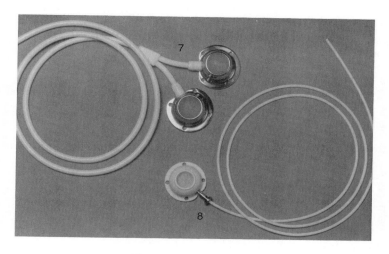

Figure 16–3. (Continued)

Two unique ports include the P.A.S. (Peripheral Access System) Port and the OsteoPort. The P.A.S.-Port (Fig. 16–4) is a small antecubital port connected to a PICC which has been placed under local anesthesia.

The Osteoport (Fig. 16–5), presently under investigation (Fiser, 1993; Kuhn, et al., 1993), allows repeated access to the vascular system via an intraosseus infusion directly into the bone marrow. The port is implanted subcutaneously like the other ports and screwed into a bone such as the iliac crest. Medications are administered as in any port, but are taken up by the venous sinusoids in the marrow cavity, and from there enter the peripheral circulation.

Implantation of Vascular Access Ports

The port to be implanted is selected considering such factors as one- or two-piece construction, single or double port, overall size, configuration, catheter size, and site of planned placement. In children or extremely thin adults, a smaller port is used to avoid extreme skin stretching, minimize the risk of skin breakdown, and provide maximum comfort to the patient.

In the female patient, a port should not be placed on the side of a previous mastectomy. The site selected should be free of pressure from bra straps. Placement near the midline provides a more stable base and less mobility than placement in the adipose tissue of the breast. This

(Text continued on page 455)

Table 16–1 Implantable Vascular Access Ports

NAME (COMPANY)	MATERIAL: PORT, CATHETER	TYPE	HEIGHT/BASE DIAMETER (MM)	WEIGHT (GM)	SEPTUM DIAMETER (MM)	NEEDLE PENETRATION DEPTH (MM)*	TYPE OF CATHETER	MAXIMUM RECOMMENDED PSI
A-Port (Therex)	Titanium, silicone	S	15.5 × 17.8	9.2	14.0	14.0	Att, det	40
A²-Port (Therex) (separate ports)	Titanium, silicone	D	15.5/28.6	18.4	14.0 each side	14.0	Att	40
A²-Port (Therex) (unified body)	Titanium silicone	D	15.5/28.6	16.0	14.0 each side	14.0	Att	40
A-Port low profile (Therex)	Plastic, silicone	S	10.0/25.0	3.6	10.0	8.38	Det	40
Celsite CVS-100 (B. Braun)	Epoxy-coated titanium, silicone	S	12/26	7.0	12.0	11.73	Det	40
Celsite CVS-150 (B. Braun)	Epoxy-coated titanium, silicone	S	9.2/36	4.0	9.0	9.3	Det	40
Celsite CAS-100 (B. Braun)	Cyrolite-coated titanium, silicone	S, A	12/26 × 32	7.0	12.0	11.73	Det	40
Chemo-Port (HDC)	Titanium, silicone	S	16.5/31.5	16.0	10.7	12.0	Att, det	40
Chemo-Port Low profile (HDC)	Titanium, silicone	S	12.0/27.8	9.0	9.1	9.0	Att, det	40
Chemo-Port (HDC)	Delrin plastic, silicone	S	13.5/29.8	7.4	5.5	10.0	Att, det	40
Hickman (Bard)	Titanium, silicone	S	14.0/31.7	16.0	12.7	12.8	Att, det	25
Hickman Lo Profile (Bard)	Titanium, silicone	S	9.4/24.8	7.7	9.0	7.9	Att	25
Hickman Dome (Bard)	Titanium, silicone	S	15.0/27.2	7.9	12.7	14.6	Det	25
Hickman MRI (Bard)	Delrin plastic, silicone	S	15.0/31.7	8.9	12.7	13.2	Att, det	25
Hickman MRI Dual (Bard)	Delrin plastic, silicone	D	14.0/35.5 × 53.6	14.0	12.7 each side	13.2 each side	Att	25
Ideas port (Ideas for Medicine)	Delrin plastic, silicone	S, D	13.8/30.9	8.3	12.7	11	Att, det	40/170
Ideas port (Ideas for Medicine)	Titanium, silicone	S, D	12.7/29.6	16.3	12.7	11	Att, det	40/170
Implantofix II (Braun)	Polysulfone/polyurethane	S, A	13.8/28.5	7.12	12.2	10.5	Att	120

452

ImPort (PS Medical)	Silicone/polymethylene, silicone	S	14.0/32	8.5	12.7	6.5	Att, det	30
Infus-A-Port MacroPort (Strato)	Silicone plastic, rubber	S, D	14.0/38	14.3	13.0		Att, det	40
Infus-A-Port Button port (Strato)	Polysulfone, polyurethane	S	11.0/24	4.4	9.0		Att	50
Infus-A-Port Micro Port (Strato)	Titanium, silicone	S, D, A,	14.0/30	10.6	8.0		Att	50
Infus-A-Port DualPort (Strato)	Titanium, silicone	D	13.0/46	17.9	13		Det	50
LifePort (Strato)	Titanium, silicone or Titanium, polyurethane	S	12.4/31.8	14.5	12.7		Att, det	40
LifePort (Strato)	Delrin, silicone	S	13.3/31.8	6.5	12.7		Att, det	40
LifePort dual port (Strato)	Titanium, silicone or Titanium, polyurethane	D, A	12.4/44.2 × 31.8	33.0	12.7		Att, det	40
LifePort dual port (Strato)	Delrin, silicone or Delrin, polyurethane	D	13.0/46.1 × 28.7	11.2	12.7		Det	40
LifePort low profile port (Strato)	Titanium, silicone	S	9.7/24.1	9.0	10.2		Att, det	40
LifePort Dual (Strato)	Delrin, polyurethane	D	13.0/46.1 × 28.7	11.2	12.7		Det	40
LifePort Dual (Strato)	Titanium, silicone	D	12.4/44.2 × 29.9	30.0	12.7		Att, det	40
LifePort Dual (Strato)	Titanium, silicone	D	12.4/44.2 × 31.8	38.0	12.7		Att, det	40
Norport (Norfolk)	Stainless steel or polysulfone, silicone	S, D	14/35	22.0	10.5	6.35	Att, det	40
Norport-SP (Norfolk)	Polysulfone, silicone	S, SE	15/38 × 38	9.0	12.0	12.0	Att	40
OmegaPort (Norfolk)	Titanium, silicone	S, D, multi-dimensional, domed	13/34	9.0	24.5	6.35	Att, det	40
Osteoport (Lifequest) (Investigational)	Stainless steel, silicone	S	7.5/21.5	7.7	12.7	8.0	†	45

(Continued)

453

Table 16–1 Implantable Vascular Access Ports (Continued)

NAME (COMPANY)	MATERIAL: PORT, CATHETER	TYPE	HEIGHT/BASE DIAMETER (MM)	WEIGHT (GM)	SEPTUM DIAMETER (MM)	NEEDLE PENETRATION DEPTH (MM)*	TYPE OF CATHETER	MAXIMUM RECOMMENDED PSI
P.A.S. Port (Pharmacia)	Titanium, polyurethane	S	10.0/27.7 × 16.5	5.6	6.6	5.6	Det	40
Port-A-Cath (Pharmacia)	Titanium, polyurethane	S, D	13.5/25	16.0	11.4	5.5	Att, det	40
Port-A-Cath (Pharmacia)	Titanium, silicone	S, D	13.5/25	16.0	11.4	5.5	Att, det	40
S.E.A.-Port (Harbor)	Titanium, silicone	D	12/40 × 33	17.0	19.1	5.1	Att, det	40
S.E.A.-Port (Harbor)	Titanium, silicone	S	14/32	15	19.1	5.1	Att	40
TrimPort (Gerard)	Titanium, silicone	S	14/32	15	16.0	12.0	Att, det	40
TrimPort (Gerard)	Delrin, silicone	S	14/32	8.0	16.0	12.0	Att, det	40
TrimPort (Gerard)	Titanium, silicone	D	14/45 × 23	13	16.0	12.0	Att, det	40
Vasport Low profile (Gish)	Fluoropolymer, silicone	S		7.0	12.4		Att, det	40
Vasport (Gish)	Fluoropolymer, silicone	S	14.0/31.7	9.7	12.4	6.7	Att, det	40
Vital Port (Cook)	Titanium, silicone	S	12.7/30.0	17.5	12.7	11.8	Att, det	40
Vital port (Cook)	Polysulfone, silicone	S	12.7/30	8.1	12.7	10.8	Att, det	40
Vital Port (Cook)	Titanium, silicone	D	12.7/49 × 29	47.0	12.7	11.8	Att, det	40
Vital Port (Cook)	Polysulfone, silicone	D	13.7/51 × 31	16.0	12.7	11.8	Att, det	40
Vital Port, Petite (Cook)	Titanium, silicone	S, P	9.7/24	9.0	10.2	9.1	Att, det	40
Vital Port, Mini (Cook)	Titanium, silicone	S, P	7.2/19	5.0	6.6	6.6	Att, det	40

S = single, D = dual, P = pediatric, SE = side entry, att = attached, det = detached.
*Needle penetration depth = distance from top of septum to floor of port chamber.
†Osteoport has no catheter; the outlet is a stainless steel shaft.

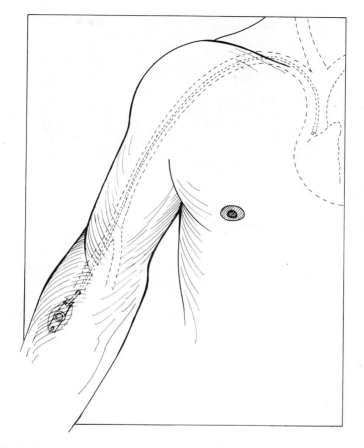

Figure 16–4. Anatomic location of P.A.S. Port. (Courtesy of Pharmacia Deltec, Inc., St. Paul, MN.)

location also facilitates self care. Ports placed in obese individuals may be more difficult to access.

The procedure for placement of the port with a detachable catheter is similar to that for placement of the long-term tunneled CVC. A small incision is made over the selected vein, a second incision is made lower on the anterior chest wall, and a pocket is created in the subcutaneous tissue. The catheter portion of the system is inserted into the vein and tunneled in the subcutaneous tissue toward the lower incision. The port is implanted into the subcutaneous pocket. After the position of the port and catheter is verified by fluoroscopy, the port is secured with sutures in the pocket and both incision sites are sutured.

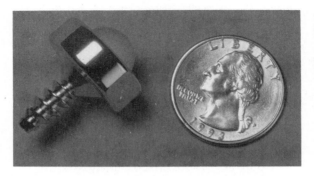

Figure 16–5. Osteoport. (Courtesy of LifeQuest Medical, Incorporated, San Antonio, TX.)

Nursing Care of the Client with an Implanted Port

Nursing care of the client with a vascular access port includes client assessment, patency maintenance, medication administration, and client education. The patient requires motivation to learn self care. He/she must also be taught and assisted to perform procedures required to maintain port patency and recognize problems that should be reported to the physician or nurse.

Nursing care includes:

- initial site care and dressing change
- accessing the port
- flushing the port
- heparinization
- obtaining a blood sample
- administering bolus medications
- administering continuous infusion therapy
- administering cyclic TPN or hyperalimentation (HAL)
- discontinuing infusion therapy
- troubleshooting problems

Further information on troubleshooting can be found in Chapter 18.

Initial Site Care and Dressing Change

Most clients have only steri-strips in place following port insertion. There may or may not be skin sutures in place. The site should be inspected for swelling, discoloration, redness, tenderness, or drainage. The patient must be assessed for temperature elevation; pain or swelling at the port site or in the shoulder, neck, or arm; or any other unusual finding. All findings should be documented and reported. Swelling that occurs more than 7 to 10 days after implantation may indicate migration of the catheter.

Accessing the Port

Noncoring needles with a deflected point, formerly known as "Huber point needles," must be used when accessing an implanted port. Puncture with other needles will damage the septum and shorten the lifespan of the port. Noncoring needles come in a variety of sizes and shapes; some are straight, others are angled. The straight noncoring needle is used for routine heparinization and administration of bolus injections, and may be used when accessing the Norport-SP or S.E.A.-Port. An angled noncoring needle or flexible port catheter should be used for the patient who is receiving a continuous infusion, for comfort and safety. Most noncoring port access needles used today for continuous infusions are part of a winged infusion set consisting of the needle and ½ to ⅝ inch of clear flexible tubing with a preattached flow control clamp (Fig. 16–6). The Surecath Port Access Catheter System allows for insertion of a flexible catheter into the port using a stylet that is contained within a disposable housing to avoid accidental needle sticks when accessing the port.

Additional caution should be taken when accessing a recently implanted port. Local tenderness, swelling, and discomfort or pain at the port site may be present for several days following insertion, making port access more difficult for the nurse and uncomfortable or painful for the patient. The port's septum is usually located close to the suture

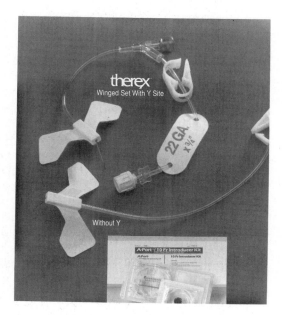

Figure 16–6. Winged infusion set with noncoring needle. (Courtesy of Therex Corporation, Walpole, MA.)

line, which may result in additional pain or discomfort when the port is accessed. After the site has healed, the client should experience only the minor discomfort associated with a subcutaneous injection each time the port is accessed.

The following general precautions should be noted:

1. Prevent rotation, rocking, tilting, or angling of the needle during and after insertion because this may cause damage to the port septum and skin.
2. Use a sturdy angled needle and avoid using too much force when accessing the port because this may bend the needle point. A bent needle point may cause septal damage upon removal.
3. For safety and patient comfort, a flexible port catheter (e.g., Surecath) may be used when accessing the port.
4. Flush the port or instill bolus medication with a 10- or 20-ml syringe, regardless of the amount of solution instilled. The smaller the syringe volume, the higher the pressure that can be generated. The maximum manufacturer-recommended pounds per square inch (PSI) of pressure for each port is indicated in Table 16–1.
5. Avoid excessive pressure on the syringe plunger when administering medication or flushing the port because this may result in catheter rupture or possible embolization of all or part of the catheter from the port body. High pressure may occur with clots in the catheter or administration of bolus injections while viscous solutions (TPN, lipids) are flowing.
6. Prevent air embolism by:
   a. Never leaving the noncoring needle open to the air.
   b. Using an extension set with a clamp or three-way stopcock.
   c. Instructing the client to perform the Valsalva maneuver when needles or tubings are changed or disconnected.
   d. Closing the clamp as the last 0.5 cc of solution is being injected from the syringe.
7. Flush with normal saline solution before, between, and following medication instillation or before heparinization to prevent drug incompatibilities and ensure patency.
8. Assess the patient carefully during administration of vesicant medications (see Chapter 2). If the patient feels or reports pain or an abnormal sensation at the injection site, this may indicate that the medication has extravasated. Should this occur, discontinue the medication, proceed with the extravasation protocol, and notify the physician immediately.

9. Blood or blood products must be administered via a large gauge (#19 or #20) needle. NOTE: DO NOT use a 19-gauge needle or infusion set when accessing the Infuse-A-Port Button Port, Therex Low Profile Port, or Vital-Port Petite Port because this will compromise septum integrity. Use only a 20- or 22-gauge noncoring needle. Use only the Port-A-Cath needle to access the P.A.S. Port system.
10. Use caution when removing the noncoring needle to prevent accidental needle sticks. The septum may "hug" the needle, resulting in sudden release.
11. Always use syringes, needles, and extension tubings with Luer-Lok connections and tighten all connections before injecting or withdrawing.

Equipment for All Port Procedures

Accessing, Flushing, Medication Administration, Blood Sampling

- Cleansing agent of choice (e.g., povidone-iodine swabsticks).
- Alcohol swabsticks.
- Clean gloves.
- Sterile noncoring needle and I.V. extension tubing with clamp or stopcock, or winged infusion set with noncoring needle.*,†
- A 10-ml syringe with 5 to 6 ml of normal saline for injection.
- A 10-ml syringe with 5 ml of heparinized saline for injection. (NOTE: This is usually 100 IU/ml, but may be as low as 10 IU/ml.)
- Syringe(s) with medication(s). The syringe should be 10 ml or larger, regardless of the volume of medication. If multiple medications are being administered in sequence, additional 10-ml syringes with 5 ml of saline will be required for flushing between medications.
- I.V. solution bag and tubing (for drip administration).
- Dressing (gauze and tape, or transparent film dressing).
- Disposal container for old dressing.
- Accessible disposal container for sharps.

---

*NOTE: A straight or angled noncoring needle may be used with the Norport-SP or S.E.A.-Port.

†NOTE: The smallest gauge needle possible should be used to minimize patient discomfort and prolong the life of the port.

Accessing and Flushing the Port

Procedure

1. Wash hands.
2. Explain procedure to patient.
3. Assemble equipment.
4. Don gloves.
5. Apply a local anesthetic agent (e.g., Lidocaine) to skin over septum to reduce discomfort if ordered or in protocol. NOTE: Emla, a topical anesthetic, may be applied approximately 1 hour prior to port entrance.
6. Draw up 6 to 10 ml of saline in one 10-ml syringe and the designated amount of heparinized saline in the other.
7. Attach a noncoring (Huber point) needle to the syringe containing normal saline and purge air from the needle.
8. Locate the port by palpation of the outer perimeter.
9. Prepare the site with cleansing agent(s) of choice.
   a. Swab skin in a circular pattern, and extend area prepped beyond periphery of the port.
   b. Allow at least 1 to 2 minutes for povidone-iodine to air dry before accessing the port. This activates its bacteriocidal, fungicidal, and sporicidal properties.
   c. Place a sterile drape over the port site if required by agency policy.
10. Stabilize the port using spread fingers or thumb and finger.
11. Push the noncoring needle firmly through the skin and port septum perpendicular to the port. The needle is in place when the tip touches the back of the port chamber. To prevent damage to the skin and septum, avoid angling or rotating the needle in the port septum by exerting firm pressure on the right angle of the needle.
12. Aspirate and observe for blood return to verify placement, then flush with normal saline to ensure patency.
13. Leave needle in place and disconnect empty syringe.
14. Connect needle to syringe with heparinized saline and flush. Stabilize port with fingers while injecting (Fig. 16–7).
15. Stabilize port with fingers and remove needle.
16. Maintain positive pressure on the syringe plunger when removing the needle from the port to avoid reflux of blood into the catheter.
17. Dispose of sharps and other equipment per hospital or agency policy.
18. Reposition patient for comfort if necessary.
19. Document procedure according to agency policy.

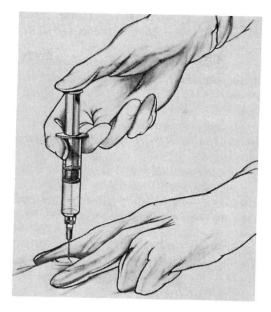

Figure 16–7. Administration of bolus medication into a vascular access port. The port is stabilized with the second and third fingers of one hand while the syringe is held in the other hand. (Courtesy of Pharmacia Deltec, Inc., St. Paul, MN.)

Administering I.V. Solution or Medication(s) via the Port

Procedure

1. Wash hands.
2. Explain procedure to patient.
3. Assemble equipment.
4. Don gloves.
5. Prepare solution or medication and prime tubing. Check medication compatibilities for simultaneously infusing solutions.
6. Follow instructions for accessing the port using a 19- to 22-gauge angled noncoring needle. NOTE: DO NOT use a 19-gauge needle or infusion set when accessing the Infuse-A-Port Button Port because this will compromise septum integrity. Use only a 20- or 22-gauge Port-A-Cath needle to access the P.A.S. Port system.
7. Prepare and purge air from a winged noncoring needle with pre-attached extension set and clamp tubing.
8. If additional access will be needed during infusion, prepare an extension set with a Y-site.

9. Draw up 6 to 10 ml normal saline solution in a 10-ml syringe and the designated amount of heparinized saline in a second 10-ml syringe.
10. Locate, access, and insert angled noncoring needle into the port following steps 8 through 12 for accessing and flushing the port.
11. Cushion the skin from the needle hub using a folded 2" × 2" qauze pad or other appropriate material.
12. Apply transparent dressing over access needle and proximal portion of extension.
13. Flush with 6 to 10 ml of normal saline solution.
14. Leave needle with extension tubing in place, disconnect empty syringe, and connect I.V. tubing (for continuous administration) or syringe with medication (for "bolus" administration).
15. Administer medication(s) or solution(s) as ordered. Follow manufacturer's directions for infusion pumps. NOTE: If the patient feels or reports pain or abnormal sensation at the injection site when receiving a vesicant medication, this may indicate that the medication has extravasated. Should this occur, discontinue medication, proceed with extravasation protocol, and notify physician immediately.
16. Flush between medications and after final medication or solution with 6 to 10 ml normal saline solution.
17. After final saline instillation, flush port with heparinized saline.
18. Stabilize port with fingers and remove needle, *or* (if subsequent medication or solution is to be administered)
19. Leave needle in place with the extension set capped and secured.

Obtaining a Blood Specimen

Procedure

1. Explain procedure to patient.
2. Assemble equipment.
3. Access port (see procedure for accessing and flushing port).
4. Withdraw and discard at least 2 to 3 ml of blood.
5. Connect a 10- to 20-ml syringe to noncoring needle.
6. Withdraw volume of blood necessary for laboratory tests.
7. Transfer specimen to appropriate tube(s).
8. Attach syringe and flush port with 10 to 20 ml of normal saline solution.
9. Attach syringe and flush port with 5 to 6 ml of heparinized saline solution or as specified in agency protocol.

10. Dispose of sharps and other equipment per hospital or agency policy.
11. Reposition patient for comfort if necessary.
12. Reinstate continuous infusion if in progress prior to blood withdrawal.
13. Document procedure according to agency policy.

Clearing the Blocked Port

See the procedure for clearing the occluded CVC in Chapter 14 and the procedure for clearing the blocked PICC in Chapter 15.

Troubleshooting Problems with Vascular Access Ports

See Chapter 18.

References

Fiser, D.H.: Intraosseous infusion. N. Engl. J. Med. 322:1579–1581, 1993.
Kuhn, J., et al.: Initial experience with a new intraosseous infusion device: The Osteoport. Proc. Am. Soc. Clin. Oncol. 12:439, 1993.

Recommended Readings

Bagnall-Reeb, H.: Initial use of a peripherally inserted central venous access port: A review of the literature. J. Vasc. Access Network 1(4):10–14, 1991.
Barrios, C.H., et al.: Evaluation of an implantable venous access system in a general oncology population. Oncology 49:474–478, 1992.
Beckton, D., et al.: An experience with an implanted port system in 66 children with cancer. Cancer 61:376–378, 1989.
Camp-Sorrell, D.: Advanced central venous access: Selection, catheters, devices and nursing management. J. Intravenous Nurs. 13:361–363, 1990.
Camp-Sorrell, D.: Implantable ports: Everything you always wanted to know. J. Intravenous Nurs. 15:262–273, 1992.
Camp-Sorrell, D.: Magnetic resonance imaging and the implantable port. Oncol. Nurs. Forum 17:197–199, 1990.
Gyves, J.W., et al.: A totally implanted injection port system for blood sampling and chemotherapy administration. JAMA 251:2538–2541, 1984.
Hadaway, L.: Evaluation and use of advanced I.V. technology: Part I: Central venous access devices. J. Intravenous Nurs. 12(2):73–82, 1989.
Hagle, M.E.: Implantable access devices for chemotherapy access and delivery. Semin. Oncol. Nurs. 3(2):95–105, 1987.
Henderson, M.L.: How to access an implanted port. Nursing 93, 23(1):50–53, 1993.
Kilbride, S.S.: A patient's guide to the implanted port. Oncol. Nurs. Forum 13(2):83–85, 1986.

Kwan, J.W.: Drug delivery technology. Cancer Bull. 42:383–390, 1990.

Kwan, J.W.: High-technology I.V. infusion devices. Am. J. Hosp. Pharm. 46:320–335, 1989.

Long, C., and Ovaska, M.: A comparative study of nursing protocols for venous access ports. Cancer Nurs. 15(1):18–21, 1992.

Marcoux, A., Fisher, S., and Wong, D.: Central venous access devices in children. Pediatr. Nurs. 16(2):123–133, 1990.

McKee, J.: Future dimensions in vascular access. J. Intravenous Nurs. 14:387–393, 1991.

Moore, C.L., et al.: Nursing care and management of vascular access ports. Oncol. Nurs. Forum 13(3):35–39, 1986.

Newton, R., DeYoung, J.L., and Levin, H.J.: Volumes of implantable vascular access devices and heparin flush requirements. J. Intravenous Nurs. 8(2):137–140, 1985.

Pearl, J.M., et al.: Improved methods in long-term venous access using the P.A.S. Port. Surg Gynecol Obstet 173:313–315, 1991.

Reed, W.P., et al.: Drug extravasation as a complication of venous access ports. Ann. Intern. Med. 102:788–789, 1985.

Riser, S.A.: Patient care manual for implanted vascular access devices. J. Intravenous Nurs. 11(3):166–168, 1988.

Schulmeister, L.: A comparison of skin preparation procedures for accessing implanted ports. N.I.T.A. 10(1):45–47, 1987.

Strum, S., McDermed, J., Korn, A., and Joseph, C.: Improved methods for vascular access, The Port-A-Cath: A totally implanted catheter system. J. Clin. Oncol. 4(4):596–603, 1986.

Viall, C.D.: Daily access of implanted venous ports: Implications for patient education. J. Intravenous Nurs. 13(5):294–296, 1990.

Wickham, R.: Techniques for long-term venous access. Nursing Management of the Patient Receiving Chemotherapy. Atlanta, American Cancer Society, 1987.

Wickham, R.S.: Advances in venous access devices and nursing management strategies. Nurs. Clin. North Am. 25(2):345–364, 1990.

Chapter 17

Ambulatory Infusion Devices

Linda Tenenbaum, R.N., M.S.N., O.C.N.
Dixie Brennan Scelsi, R.N., M.S., M.S.N.

Many persons with cancer are being treated in the outpatient setting. Some receive periodic chemotherapy and/or biotherapy in the physician's office, while others are treated in the home setting under the supervision of the home health care nurse. The nurse may administer bolus medications or initiate continuous infusion. The latter has been made possible by recent technical advances and delivery devices described in this chapter.

Purposes of Ambulatory Infusion Devices

Ambulatory infusion pumps allow the slow, continuous, low-volume delivery of chemotherapeutic and other agents, including intravenous (I.V.) hydration solutions, total parenteral nutrition (TPN), antibiotics, or pain medications. This chapter will only discuss their use in the administration of chemotherapy.

Chemotherapy may be administered via an ambulatory infusion pump as a short-term infusion, over several hours to several days, or as a long-term infusion, over days, weeks, or months. The pump allows for the safe, effective administration of chemotherapy and gives the client maximum independence and participation in self care. A regional infusion can be administered, providing a higher concentration of medication at a localized site. Many clients may continue to work and participate in day-to-day activities with fewer restrictions while receiving a continuous infusion via the pump.

Pump Features

Most pumps contain a battery as the power source, and many can be adapted to function on AC electrical current as well. Other features common to most include a reservoir, a pump mechanism, a programmer, a prime mover, and a method of connecting the pump to the patient. Elastomeric pumps include a reservoir with pumping pressure and delivery tubing. Specifications for ambulatory infusion pumps are described in Table 17–1.

Table 17–1 Features Basic to All Pumps

FEATURE	PURPOSE	COMMENTS
Power source	Provide energy.	Can be gravity, gas, windup, spring, or battery(s).
Prime mover	Make energy work.	Can be a motor, or elastomeric balloon.
Drug/fluid reservoir	Hold infusate.	Usually a disposable bag.
Program mechanism	Communicate an infusion mode to the pump.	Most have on-board programming, using knobs or buttons (mechanical or electrical programming) or computer programming/chips.
Method to connect pump to patient	Provide a pathway for movement of fluid from pump to patient.	Usually micro or minimum volume 60 inch tubing with or without a cassette, and (for multiple channels) a manifold tubing to link all channels to tubing connecting to the patient's vascular access device.
Pump mechanism	Action that actually displaces fluid from the drug/fluid reservoir to the patient. This is the pump's most identifying feature.	May be one of three actions: • peristaltic • piston • elastomeric.

Reprinted with permission from Lawson, M.: Guidelines for selecting an ambulatory infusion pump for outpatient intravenous therapy. J. Vasc. Access Nurs. 1(1):12, 1990.

Types of Ambulatory Infusion Devices

The major types of ambulatory infusion devices are:

External systems
• Peristaltic pumps
• Elastomeric balloon pumps
Implantable systems

External Ambulatory Infusion Devices

These devices are used in conjunction with a vascular access device (e.g., central venous catheter, port, peripherally inserted central catheter (PICC) line, or epidural catheter).

Peristaltic Infusion Pumps. These pumps function by use of a peristaltic mechanism which compresses the administration tubing to force fluid at a predetermined rate through the delivery pathway. The flow is controlled and monitored by a computer microprocessor, and a variety of delivery rates and modes are available. Fluid flow can be regulated between 0.1 and 400 ml/hr (see Tables 17–2, 17–3, and 17–4). Medication can be delivered from an internal reservoir. Some models allow connection to a standard I.V. bag. The Walkmed 350 (Fig. 17–1) features a pulsed motor and delivers medications at rates ranging from 0.10 to 19.99 ml/hr. The Pancretec Provider (Fig. 17–2) uses rotary peristaltic motion. The tubing is wound around a rotary cam, which propels fluid as it rotates. Other types of peristaltic infusion pumps function using a linear peristaltic action in which mechanical, fingerlike projections massage the tubing and move fluid along. Power sources and battery types vary. Most peristaltic action pumps weigh between 9.7 and 16 oz and can be worn in a pouch by the ambulatory patient.

Elastomeric Reservoirs/Pumps. Elastomeric reservoirs are lightweight, nonelectronic, disposable units that come in a variety of shapes. Each unit contains an outer shell and an inner elastomeric "balloon" reservoir. The reservoir stores medication and provides the pumping pressure to force the solution through the delivery tubing. A flow restrictor keeps fluid flowing at a constant rate. It should be noted that flow rate accuracy is calculated for normal saline solution at room temperature. Increased environmental or body temperature or contact between the fluid flow tubing and the patient's skin may increase the flow rate. A more viscous solution (e.g., 5% dextrose in water) may flow at a slightly slower rate. Some models have options such as a filter or patient control module. Specifications of these devices are listed in Table

(Text continued on page 474)

Table 17-2 Computer-Programmed Peristaltic Infusion Pumps

PUMP NAME (DISTRIBUTOR)	WEIGHT (OZ, APPROXIMATE)	SIZE (IN.)	BATTERY TYPE	RESERVOIR TYPE AND CAPACITY	PUMPING MECHANISM AND TYPE, FLOW RATE (ACCURACY)	ALARMS AND ALERTS/ ADDITIONAL FEATURES
CADD-1 model 5100 HFX (Pharmacia/ Deltec)	15	6.4 × 3.5 × 1.1	9-volt alkaline or lithium or RBP	50 ml, 100 ml. Remote reservoir adaptor for volumes greater than 100 ml.	Linear peristaltic, 1–299 ml in 24 hr or 90 ml/hr in fixed high flow mode, C (±6%).	Pump in stop mode, low battery, depleted battery, low reservoir volume, programmed volume depleted, high pressure, system error.
CADD-Plus model 5400 (Pharmacia/ Deltec)	15	6.4 × 3.5 × 1.1	9-volt alkaline or lithium or RBP	50 ml, 100 ml. Remote reservoir adaptor for volumes greater than 100 ml.	Linear peristaltic, 0–75 ml/hr, C, I (±6%).	Pump in stop mode, low battery, depleted battery, low reserve volume, programmed volume depleted, high pressure, system error.
MedMate 1100 (Patient Solutions)	17	4.4 × 3.3 × 1.1	Two internal 9-volt alkaline or optional RBP	Internal or external fluid container.	Linear peristaltic, 0.1–500 ml/hr, C, I (±5%).	Air-in-line, occlusion, door open, dose end, low bag, bag end, low battery, change battery, callback alert, program limit exceeded, prime limit, system fault.
Provider One Plus (Abbott)	12	5.2 × 3.4 × 1.3	9-volt alkaline or 12-volt rechargeable nickel cadmium, AC adaptor	(None—must be attached to a nonvented, collapsible I.V. bag [any capacity].)	Rotary peristaltic, 1–400 ml/hr (±5%).	Occlusion, air in line, low reserve, end of infusion, check line, system problem, computer error, low battery. Taper up/down—ramping.

Provider 5500 (Abbott)	14	5.2 × 3.4 × 1.3	Two 9-volt alkaline	As above.	Rotary peristaltic, 0.1–250 ml/hr, C, I (±5%).	Air in line, check line, occlusion, end of infusion, low reserve, system problem, low battery.
Provider 6000 (Abbott)	31	6.8 × 4.7 × 2.2	Two 9-volt alkaline, RBP	As above.	Rotary peristaltic, 0.1–250 ml/hr per channel, C, I, CB (±5%).	Occlusion, air in line, low battery, low reserve, system empty, end of infusion, check line, limit exceeded, amount too small, internal malfunction, callback alert. Can deliver two simultaneous infusions.
Verifuse (Block Medical)	17	7.2 × 4.0 × 1.5	Two 9-volt alkaline, AC adaptor or nickel cadmium available	Reservoir, 120 ml or standard I.V. solution container.	Single channel linear peristaltic, 0.1–300 ml/hr, C, I, T (±6%).	Low battery, change battery, occlusion, air-in-line, low reservoir, door open, pumping complete, end of program, bar code fault, malfunction. Can program or obtain current infusion status via a hand-held programmer, or from a remote location via a modem.
VIVUS-4000, 4000-2 (I-Flow)	32 (2-channel) 37 (4-channel)	7.75 × 4.5 × 1.8	5 AA or 10 AA	(No reservoir— adaptable to any size I.V. bag.)	Linear peristaltic, 0.1–200 ml/hr per channel, C, I (±6%).	Occlusion, low/ dead battery, stop, door open, empty, malfunction. Can be programmed from a remote site via telephone and downloaded into the Infuser via a modem.

(Continued)

469

Table 17–2 Computer-Programmed Peristaltic Infusion Pumps (Continued)

PUMP NAME (DISTRIBUTOR)	WEIGHT (OZ, APPROXIMATE)	SIZE (IN.)	BATTERY TYPE	RESERVOIR TYPE AND CAPACITY	PUMPING MECHANISM AND TYPE, FLOW RATE (ACCURACY)	ALARMS AND ALERTS/ ADDITIONAL FEATURES
WalkMed 350 (Medex)	12.8 (with battery)	4.4 × 4.0 × 1.8	9-volt alkaline; 450 ml at 1 ml/hr; 650 ml at 10 ml/hr	Disposable, 65, 150, or 250 ml bag.	Linear peristaltic, 0.1–19.99 ml/hr, C (±5%).	Occlusion, system malfunction, low battery, depleted battery, under-delivery, over-delivery, delivering, pump left in program mode, prime, door open.
WalkMed 440-PIC (Medex)	12.8 (with battery)	4.4 × 4.0 × 1.8	9-volt alkaline; 450 ml at 1 ml/hr; 650 ml at 10 ml/hr	Linear peristaltic. Disposable, 65, 150, or 250 ml bag.	Linear pumping action, 0.1–19.99 ml/hr, C (±5%).	Near-end, volume limit, occlusion, system malfunction, low battery, under-delivery, over-delivery, depleted battery, under-delivery, over-delivery, bar open, program error, total volume delivered.

C = continuous, I = intermittent, B = bolus, CB = continuous with bolus, T = taper dose, RBP = rechargeable battery pack.

Table 17-3 Disposable Elastomeric or Spring-Operated Infusion Pumps

PUMP NAME (DISTRIBUTOR)	TYPE, SHAPE	WEIGHT (OZ, WHEN FILLED TO CAPACITY)	SIZE (IN.)	RESERVOIR TYPE AND CAPACITY	ACCURACY	COMMENTS
Homepump 2 (Block)	E, round	6–8	Height—3.75; circumference—8.5	3-layer elastomeric membrane, 125 ml.	2 ± 15%	Equipped with integrated 1.2-μ particulate filter and 0.22-μm air-eliminating filter, 10 PSI. Entire unit disposable upon completion of infusion.
Homepump 5 (Block)	E, round	6–8	As above	As above.	5 ± 15%	
Infusor, models 2C1071 and 2C1080 (Baxter Healthcare)	E, cylindrical	4 (when filled)	6½ (length)	Outer shell blended non-PVC synthetic materials, tubing PVC, 65 ml.	0.5 or 2 ± 10% (varies with model)	Lightweight, disposable, contains 7-μm filter.
7-day Infusor, model 2C1082 (Baxter Healthcare)	E, cylindrical	5 (when filled)	8 (length)	As above, 95 ml.	0.5 ± 10%*	Lightweight, disposable, contains 7-μm filter.
Infusor LVS 2, LVS 5 (Baxter Healthcare)	E, shape of a baby bottle	275 ml (6 oz when filled)	5 (height)	Outer shell nonlatex synthetic product, inner reservoir—275 ml.	2 or 5 ± 10%† (varies with model)	Lightweight, disposable, contains 5-μm filter.
Paragon (I-Flow)	S, cylindrical	13	4.0 (diameter); 2.3 (height).	PVC, 110 ml.	0.5, 1.0, 2.0, 4 ± 10%*	Reusable with disposable reservoir and tubing.
Sidekick (I-Flow)	S, cylindrical	13.5	4.0 (diameter); 2.0 (height).	PVC, 65 and 110 ml.	50, 100, 200 ± 15%	Reusable infuser delivers up to 70,000 doses. Equipped with 1.2-μm filter.

E = elastomeric, S = spring-operated.
*Based on normal saline at room temperature. Increased environmental or body temperature can increase the flow rate. A more viscous solution (e.g., 5% dextrose in water) may flow at a slightly slower rate.
†Based on 5% dextrose in water as the diluent and the one-piece Luer keeping in contact with the skin.

471

Table 17–4 Implantable Infusion Pumps

PUMP NAME (MANUFACTURER)	WEIGHT (G)	DIAMETER (IN) × HEIGHT (IN)	ENERGY SOURCE	USABLE VOLUME IN RESERVOIR (ML)	PUMPING MECHANISM	FLOW RATE RANGES/ COMMENTS
Infusaid model 400 (Infusaid)	208	87 × 28	2-phase charging fluid.	50	Metal bellows with charging fluid.	2–3 ml/d. Available with 1 or 2 side-ports.
SyncroMed 8610 (Medtronic)	175	70.4 × 27.5; with access port: 85.2 × 27.5	Lithium battery (life: rate dependent, typically 44.5 mo at 0.5 ml/d).	18.0	Battery-powered, noninvasive programmability.	0.096–0.9 ml/d. Can be programmed to deliver bolus, intermittent doses.
Therex 30 ml Constant Flow Implantable Pump (Therex)	136	3.05 (diameter); 1.25 (thickness)	2-phase charging fluid (Freon), activated by patient's body temperature.	30	Compression-expansion cycle of sealed freon chamber.	Preset—0.5–2 ml/d.

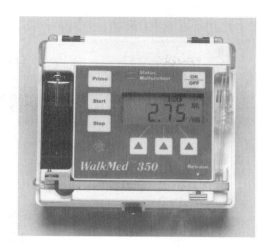

Figure 17–1. Computer-programmed pump (WalkMed 350 ambulatory infusion pump for continuous delivery). (Courtesy of Medex Ambulatory Infusion Systems, Broomfield, CO.)

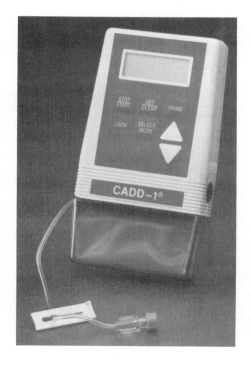

Figure 17–2. CADD-1 ambulatory infusion pump. (Courtesy of Pharmacia Deltec, Inc., St. Paul, MN.)

473

17–3. Sample elastomeric reservoirs/pumps are shown in Figures 17–3 and 17–4.

Implantable Infusion Systems

An implantable infusion system consists of a pump and an outlet catheter and has no external components. It is used for continuous regional infusion of chemotherapeutic agents or other medications (e.g., analgesics) into a localized space (e.g., intra-arterial, intrathecal, intraperitoneal). Regional infusion allows for a higher concentration of medication at the localized site. If a sideport is present on the pump, this allows for the bolus injection of chemotherapeutic agents and other medications if indicated. Two pumps currently in use, the Infusaid model 400 and the SynchroMed Infusion System, each function in a different manner. A third, the Therex pump, is in a clinical trial. Specifications for these devices are listed in Table 17–4.

Implantation Technique. The pump is surgically implanted in a subcutaneous pocket of tissue, most commonly located in the left lower quadrant of the abdomen. A silicone outlet catheter attached to the pump is tunneled to the desired infusion site. For an abdominally placed pump, this is usually the hepatic artery for treatment of primary or metastatic tumors of the liver. For further information on hepatic

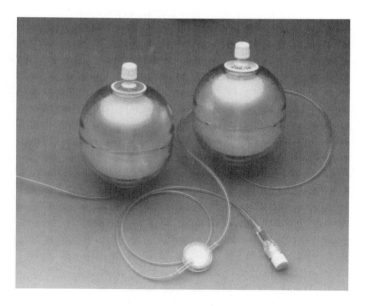

Figure 17–3. Homepump. (Courtesy of Block Medical, Inc., Carlsbad, CA.)

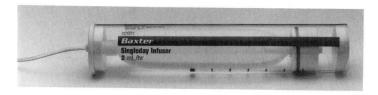

Figure 17–4. Infusor. (Courtesy of Baxter Healthcare Corp., I.V. Systems Division, Deerfield, IL.)

artery chemotherapy, see Chapter 2. The internal pump also may be placed in a pocket of tissue in the right or left subclavian fossa of the chest wall, with the termination site of the catheter in the superior vena cava for systemic intravenous infusion of chemotherapeutic agents.

The Infusaid model 400 (Fig. 17–5) is a totally implantable pump consisting of two chambers separated by flexible metal bellows (Fig. 17–6). The lower chamber contains a charging fluid (liquid Freon) in a completely sealed environment; the upper (medication) chamber contains the chemotherapeutic agent. As the pump is refilled, the bellows expand and exert pressure on the lower chamber, causing the vapor to condense to a liquid state. At body temperature the Freon vaporizes, exerting a constant pressure on the drug chamber. This pressure forces medication out of the chamber through an outlet filter and flow restrictor into the catheter for delivery to the selected body site.

The Synchromed Infusion System consists of a surgically implanted pump made of titanium, a silicone rubber catheter, and connecting tubings. The pump chamber can hold up to 50 ml of solution and can be programmed externally through a radiotelemetry link. Delivery time for medication varies from 0.025 to 0.9 ml/hr. Unlike other pump systems, flow rate is not affected by medication viscosity, atmospheric pressure, or temperature alterations. The pump is refilled by a sterile technique using a noncoring needle. Medication is added via the self-sealing septum (inlet septum) in the top center of the pump. The reservoir volume is 50 ml. Bolus medications may be administered via a sideport.

Excess pressure may result in dislodgement of the sideport septum. To prevent this, the following principles must be observed when administering sideport injections or clearing catheter occlusions via the sideport:

1. Sideport injections must be administered through a 10-ml or larger syringe, regardless of the amount of the bolus.
2. Injection rates must not exceed 10 ml/min.

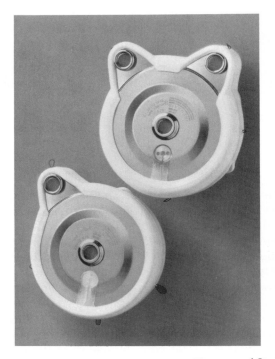

Figure 17–5. Infusaid model 400 implantable pump. (Courtesy of Strato Infusaid, Inc., Norwood, MA.)

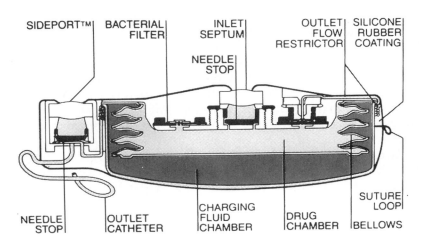

Figure 17–6. Infusaid model 400 implantable pump—internal view. (Courtesy of Strato Infusaid, Inc., Norwood, MA.)

Client Selection and Education for External Ambulatory Infusion Pumps

Clients with ambulatory continuous infusion pumps must be able to operate the pump, handle related equipment, monitor for side effects, and troubleshoot problems that may occur. Criteria for selection include:

1. Patient ability and desire to learn.
2. Adequate support (family and/or professional) at home.
3. An organized teaching program.
4. Follow-up by nurses with specific expertise to assure client compliance.
5. Reliable vascular access via catheter, port, or reservoir.
6. Drugs that are stable for several days at room temperature.
7. Patient desire for ambulatory or outpatient therapy.

General Instructions for Connecting Tubing of an External Pump to a Port or Catheter

1. Clamp silastic catheter or extension set on port.
2. Remove cap on end of pump tubing.
3. Remove cap from end of silastic catheter or extension set on port.
4. Attach a 10-ml syringe with 5 to 10 ml of sterile normal saline solution to the silastic catheter or extension set.
5. Open clamp on catheter or extension set and irrigate catheter or port.
6. Close clamp.
7. Connect end of pump tubing to silastic catheter or extension set.
8. Open clamps on pump tubing and silastic catheter or extension set.
9. Turn pump on.
10. Follow manufacturer's directions for regulation of specific pump and observance of pump alarms.

Nursing Care of the Client with an External Ambulatory Infusion Pump

Nursing care of the client with an ambulatory infusion pump includes client assessment and education regarding medications and equipment used. Clients selected to participate in a regimen of chemotherapy delivered via an ambulatory infusion pump should be able and motivated to learn and must have reliable manual dexterity, attention span, and memory. Good coping mechanisms and a support system are important as well. The client/significant other must be able to perform the following:

1. Flush the catheter.
2. Change I.V. bags or medication cassettes.
3. Understand basic operation of the pump (e.g., function of switches, alarms, lights).
4. Monitor pump settings.
5. Inspect extension sets and equipment.
6. Troubleshoot vascular access devices (e.g., change position, check all connections and clamps).
7. Recognize side effects of medications.
8. Recognize mechanical functioning.
9. Notify nurse or physician when indicated.

Nursing Care of the Client with an Implanted Infusion Pump

The nurse caring for the client with an implanted infusion pump should be familiar with the instruction manual for the pump. Institutions may permit only nurses who have been properly educated in this technology (e.g., filling, refilling pump). Written policies and procedures incorporating the manufacturers' recommendations for use should be available to the nursing staff responsible for care of these clients.

Most clients with an implanted pump are treated on an outpatient basis; thus, education for the clients and (when indicated) the significant others is essential. Teaching should include:

1. General information about the pump and its function.
2. Review of the patient teaching brochure or audiovisual material prepared by the manufacturer.
3. Treatment regimen.
4. Procedure for refilling the pump, including teaching, demonstration, and return demonstration.
5. Factors that alter the pump's infusion rate, such as changes in temperature, pressure, and altitude, and measures that should be taken if these alterations occur.
6. Side effects of medications administered via the pump and specific instructions about when to notify the physician or nurse should be provided in verbal and written form.
7. Troubleshooting measures.
8. Opportunity for questions and answers.

Referral to the home health care nurse should be made for follow-up care after the client leaves the hospital or clinic.

Recommended Readings

Catania, P.N., et al.: Ambulatory infusion devices for home chemotherapy. U.S. Pharmacist 14(11):94–100, 1989.

Hartsell, M.B.: Home infusion pumps. J. Pediatr. Oncol. Nurs. 6:134–136, 1991.

Kwan, J.W.: Drug delivery technology. Cancer Bull. 42:383–392, 1990.

Lawson, M.: Guidelines for selecting an ambulatory infusion pump for outpatient intravenous therapy. J. Vasc. Access Network 1(1):12–16, 1990.

Nadau, N.: Maintenance and care of patients with drug delivery systems. Rec. Results Cancer Res. 121:205–207, 1991.

Pasut, B.: Home administration of medications in pediatric oncology patients: Use of the Travenol infusor. J. Pediatr. Oncol. Nurs. 6(4):139–142, 1989.

Pharmacy Practice News: Pharmacy Practice News: 8th Annual Buyer's Guide to Pumps and Controllers. Pharm. Pract. News 19(7):13–19, 1992.

Schulmeister, L.: An overview of continuous infusion chemotherapy. J. Intravenous Nurs. 15:315–322, 1992.

Chapter 18

Management of Complications Associated with the Use of Venous Access Devices

Joseph Brown, R.N., B.S.N., C.R.N.I.
Dixie Brennan Scelsi, R.N., M.S., M.S.N.

The venous access device (VAD) is a catheter, or port with catheter attached, made of a foreign material that is surgically placed in the client's body. As with any mechanical and foreign material, the VAD may cause complications. The nurse must be aware of potential problems associated with VADs and should initiate appropriate measures to prevent their occurrence whenever possible. Problems include phlebitis, infection, catheter or port occlusion, catheter thrombosis, venous thrombosis, and extravasation of infusate. Ongoing nursing assessment is necessary to identify early evidence of complications and initiate appropriate interventions in a timely manner.

Phlebitis

The most common complication associated with short-term peripheral catheters, nontunneled central venous catheters, peripherally inserted central catheters (PICCs), and the P.A.S. (Peripheral Access System) Port is sterile mechanical phlebitis. It is not an infectious process but represents the body's response to a foreign material within the blood vessel. Criteria for infusion phlebitis can be used as a guide in assessing phlebitis (Box 18–1).

Box 18–1

Criteria for Infusion Phlebitis

Severity	Criteria
0	No pain, erythema, swelling, induration, or palpable venous cord at or around I.V. site.
1+	Pain at I.V. site, no erythema, swelling, induration, or palpable venous cord.
2+	Some erythema and/or swelling at site. No induration or palpable venous cord.
3+	Erythema and swelling at site. Induration or palpable venous cord <3 inches above site.
4+	Erythema and swelling at site. Induration or palpable venous cord >3 inches above site.

Sterile mechanical phlebitis more commonly occurs:

- in the first 48 to 72 hours after insertion,
- in women,
- with devices made of polymer materials,
- with left-sided insertions, and
- with large gauge catheters.

If phlebitis occurs and remains 3+ or less, the catheter may be left in place and treatment measures begun. Nursing interventions including application of warm, moist compresses, elevation of the extremity, and mild exercise have been effective in resolving or controlling the phlebitis.

The catheter must be re-evaluated and the possibility of removal contemplated when any of the following develop: phlebitis progressed beyond 3+; increased severity of pain and discomfort; temperature elevation; or drainage at the catheter insertion site.

Infection

Catheters and ports are associated with increased risk for infection because an invasive procedure is required for insertion. Catheter infections were documented in 12.7% of 55 patients with Groshong catheters and 11.3% of 53 patients with Hickman catheters (Pasquale et al., 1992).

The insertion and/or exit sites may be an entry portal for microorganisms. Microorganisms can migrate along the catheter or port tunnel, or be introduced through the catheter hub or port chamber, and result in septicemia. Infections associated with ports may also occur in the port pocket and may be related to sepsis or thrombus (Camp-Sorrell, 1992; Ross et al., 1988). Clients who are receiving total parenteral nutrition (TPN) or those who experience thrombus formation are more prone to the development of systemic infections. Infections are potentially life threatening in patients with neutropenia (neutrophil count <500 cells/mm^3) (Hughes et al., 1990).

The client with catheter sepsis typically has a fever, positive blood cultures, and/or hypotension. Increased vascular permeability and vasodilation may result in tissue ischemia, multisystem failure, shock, and, if left untreated, death. Systemic support and treatment with antibiotics should be accompanied by careful assessment and monitoring of the client's general status. Controversy exists regarding management of a central venous catheter in the presence of catheter-related sepsis. Antibiotics may be used in an attempt to save the catheter and a new line placed after the infection is resolved, or the VAD may be removed.

Occlusion

A VAD may be occluded as the result of mechanical obstruction (e.g., kinked or malpositioned tubing, closed clamps, clogged intravenous [I.V.] filter, pressure against body structure, obstruction in the portal reservoir), thrombotic occlusion (e.g., blood clot, fibrin sleeve, fibrin tail, mural thrombosis), or medication precipitates.

A **fibrin sheath** or **fibrin tail** may occur as the result of platelet aggregation and fibrin deposit. A fibrin sheath originates at the point of venous entry, and may occur as soon as 48 hours or as long as several months after placement (Wickham et al., 1992; Williams, 1990). The fibrin deposit may progress until it completely encases the surface of the catheter and causes retrograde flow of infusate up the length of the catheter (Bagnall-Reeb et al., 1992). Progressive difficulty in drawing blood may be noted. Should this occur, blood sampling may be facilitated by postural changes and/or by having the patient perform the Valsalva maneuver. Occasionally, the occlusion may be the result of a clot that is drawn into the catheter during attempts at blood sampling.

A fibrin tail is located at or extends off the catheter tip. This may not interfere with infusion, but may produce a "ball-valve" effect when attempting to aspirate a blood sample (Bagnall-Reeb et al., 1992; Lawson, 1991).

Thrombus formation at the catheter tip may not allow forward infusion of solutions or medications. However, if solutions are given at pressures exceeding venous flow, retrograde flow of infusate along the catheter may cause leakage from the vein into the surrounding tissues. The risk of this complication is increased in percutaneously placed catheters (Gemlo et al., 1988).

Venous Thrombosis

Damage to the vessel intima by the catheter may result in the formation of thrombi, which adhere to the vessel wall and sometimes extend onto the surface of the right atrium or tricuspid valve. This may develop secondary to the slow administration rate, the viscosity of the blood or blood products, or the back up of blood into the catheter (Holcombe et al., 1992). Damage to the venous intima is more common with stiff catheters (i.e., polyvinyl chloride), larger bore catheters, and catheterization from the left side; however, it may also occur with polyurethane and silicone catheters (Wickham et al., 1992). Signs and symptoms of venous thrombosis include difficulty maintaining fluid flow via a VAD, or inability to do so at all; pain in the chest wall or in the neck associated with fluid administration or flushing; or engorgement of the veins of the chest wall. Infusional difficulties, facial swelling, and neck vein distention are indicative of complete occlusion.

Other Causes of Catheter Occlusion

In addition to blood clots, VAD occlusion may occur as the result of drug precipitates that collect within the catheter lumen or port reservoir. Diazepam and phenytoin are two medications that have been reported to precipitate if a line has not been cleared thoroughly (Wachs, 1990). Factors that contribute to VAD occlusion include improper or inadequate flushing technique, pH of medications and I.V. diluent solutions, electrolyte ratios, and flow rates (Bagnall-Reeb et al., 1992).

VAD occlusion caused by drug precipitation may be evidenced by difficulty initiating or maintaining fluid flow, obstruction or resistance following infusion of incompatible medications, client discomfort during flushing, and/or inability to withdraw blood from a VAD. Drug precipitation should be suspected after inability to clear the catheter with urokinase (Bagnall-Reeb et al., 1992). Drug precipitates are difficult to clear and often cannot be cleared.

Lipids may be another cause of VAD occlusion. A waxy material ("lipid sludge") may form in the port or catheter of the patient who is receiving lipids piggybacked onto a dextrose/amino acid solution, and could cause progressive catheter occlusion over several days. This may be noted by increasing resistance each time the catheter is flushed (Holcombe et al., 1992). Attempts to clear the lipid sludge with urokinase may result in complete catheter obstruction (Pennington 1990; Pennington and Pithie, 1987).

Extravasation

Administration of vesicant medications via a VAD will not ensure that extravasation will be prevented. The client may complain of mild, temporary discomfort or more severe pain if extravasation occurs.

Factors that contribute to extravasation with VADs include incorrect catheter placement in small veins, disconnection of the catheter from the port, displacement or migration of the central venous catheter or port catheter tip into the jugular or smaller veins, incorrect port needle placement, or dislodgement of the port needle.

Displacement of a port catheter may occur by inadvertent traction on the catheter, or by manipulation of the catheter by the patient. This is known as "Twiddler's syndrome," and occurs most frequently in children (Gebarski and Gebarski, 1984; Servetar, 1992).

Extravasation may also occur with incorrect port needle placement or with dislodgement of the needle used for port infusions. Anatomic placement of the portal body may increase the risk of needle dislodgement (Camp-Sorrell, 1992). The ideal location for port placement is below the clavicle and above the breast, medial to the midclavicular line, where it is on a firm bony surface (Lambert et al., 1987; Mirro et al., 1990). Less optimal sites include the area over the pectoral muscle near the axilla or in the groin, deep in the subcutaneous tissue, under the breast tissue, or within excessive adipose tissue (Camp-Sorrell, 1992; Mirro et al., 1990).

Nonsiliconized needles should be used to access ports because siliconized needles can slip out of the port more readily. A deeper, more dense septum may decrease the chance of needle dislodgement (Strum et al., 1986).

If the needle dislodges from the port without exiting from the skin, it may appear as if the needle is still in place on inspection of the site. Verification of a blood return before and periodically during I.V. infusion of a vesicant drug is extremely important, and will assure safer delivery of potentially dangerous agents.

The degree of damage will vary depending on the type and amount of solution extravasated. The most common reactions observed with vesicant extravasation from a port include intense inflammation, epidermal erythema, and ulceration and/or necrosis of subcutaneous tissue (Camp-Sorrell, 1992). Ulcers appear as punched out lesions approximately 1 to 2 weeks after vesicant extravasation, and usually require plastic surgery (Camp-Sorrell, 1992). For further information on extravasation, see Chapter 2.

Catheter Damage

This may occur at the time of placement, with improper flushing, or during incorrect locking of the two-piece port and catheter system. Arm and shoulder movement may produce friction on and possible damage to the catheter when the port has been placed medially between the clavicle and first rib. Intermittent difficulties in infusion requiring postural changes of the client may be indicative of catheter damage. Should the catheter break completely, resulting in catheter embolus, the patient will present with sudden onset chest pain.

Difficulty in Accessing the Port

Placement of the port in the breast tissue or in excessive adipose tissue may make it difficult to access the port.

Other complications of VADs include pneumothorax (which usually develops immediately after insertion), pulmonary embolus resulting from embolization of air introduced into the central venous system, and perforation of vessel walls by the catheter tip.

Problems with Removal

PICCs may at times resist removal as a result of vasospasm, vasoconstriction, valve inflammation, or thrombophlebitis. This phenomenon has occurred in less than ⅛ of 1% of PICC line placements, and most often in catheters that have been in place for less than 2 weeks. Treatment involves placing tension on the catheter, re-dressing the catheter, and reattempting removal in 24 hours. Excessive tension should not be applied because this may cause the catheter to break. Warm compresses may be helpful in distending the vein and releasing the catheter.

Troubleshooting VADs

General Considerations

The nurse must assess clients for complications and institute appropriate nursing interventions when problems evolve. Monitoring clients for long-term follow-up requires knowledge of and experience with VADs, chemotherapy, antibiotics, TPN, I.V. pain regimens, and ambulatory infusion pumps, in addition to knowledge of and experience with the management of cancer and its related problems.

Nurses must be available on a 24-hour basis to clients receiving outpatient chemotherapy, TPN, or other medications through a VAD. Precipitating events which require troubleshooting usually are one or a combination of the following:

1. Inability to start infusion or flush catheter.
2. Inability to access port.
3. Inability to maintain flow rate.
4. Inability to draw blood from the catheter or port.
5. Pain or discomfort at the catheter exit site, port site, arm, or shoulder along course of catheter.
6. Edema or erythema at the port site.
7. Drainage from exit or port sites.
8. Any abnormal sensation or observation reported by the client.
9. Infusion pump alarms.
10. Malfunctioning or nonfunctioning equipment.

Nursing Responsibilities

The nurse must be thoroughly familiar with the chemotherapeutic agents administered, the treatment regimen and medication and hydration schedules, the VADs and their management, and the troubleshooting strategies for infusion pumps. The nurse must also be able to accurately assess the client/significant other regarding ability to learn self care and to identify evidence of complications to be reported to the health care team. Frequently, problems are solved by telephone; consequently, the nurse must be able to envision the most frequently encountered client problems and anticipate any unusual circumstances which may occur (mechanical or human). Skillful interviewing techniques are necessary to elicit specific information from the client/significant other. Written client records should be available to the nurse in the on-call situation so that a full assessment can be made. Complete and accurate documentation should include client condition, response to therapy, and problems encountered. The nursing record should also contain actions taken to troubleshoot potential or existing problems and their outcomes.

The first step in troubleshooting is accurate observation and assessment. The client and, when necessary, the caregiver (rather than the VAD or the equipment) are the focus of care, and listening to their description of what is happening is essential. Careful questioning to follow up on the patient's described problems is the next step. Particular emphasis should be placed on follow-up when troubleshooting with clients experiencing problems related to outpatient chemotherapeutic regimens and/or VADs and related equipment. This includes:

1. Assessing the urgency of the problem.
2. Obtaining a complete description of the problem.
3. Obtaining a history of events preceding the problem from the client or significant other.
4. Assessing the compliance and abilities of the client or significant other if self care is being performed.
5. Assessing the ability of the client or significant other to follow instructions and provide further information.
6. Amending or reinforcing client instructions as indicated.
7. Providing more detailed information and/or demonstrating performing specific skills as indicated.

Parameters that should be immediately assessed by direct inspection or initial questioning by phone should begin with the client and extend to VADs, dressings, tubings, infusion solutions, and infusion pumps or other equipment being used. The following should be evaluated:

1. **VAD or site. Catheters** should be inspected for integrity, position, and general appearance. The catheter should be in proper position (external portion should be appropriate for the type of catheter and the previously documented position for this client). Short-term catheters may be sutured, and the integrity of sutures should be observed. Markings on catheters should be noted and compared to the previously documented position. The position of the central venous catheter tip should be verified by x-ray.

Port sites should be inspected for general appearance. The sites should be compared to previous observations when possible. The outline of the septum is usually visible beneath the skin, and can be felt on palpation. Knowledge of and familiarity with the type of port the client has allows the nurse to accurately assess position when troubleshooting.

2. **Skin and surrounding area.** The skin at the catheter exit site (for catheters) or over the port injection area (for ports) should be assessed for warmth, redness, presence of dilated veins, drainage, and pain or discomfort. Knowledge of the medication or solution being infused is essential for accurate assessment of extravasation.

Observe the head, neck, and thorax for signs and symptoms of superior vena cava syndrome or venous thrombosis (e.g., swelling of head, face, neck, and arms, and distended collateral circulation over chest).

3. **Integrity of equipment** (including extension sets, noncoring needles, dressings, I.V. tubing connections, and clamps). Catheters should not be kinked and should be secured so that no tension is applied. Dressings should cover the site, secure tubings without kinking, and secure the noncoring needle. All connections should be tight. Clamps should be open for infusion and closed if no infusion is in progress.

Injection ports should be tightly attached with Luer-Lok connections, and may be taped for further security.

Noncoring needles used to access ports should be secured to the skin by tape under the dressing. The tip of the needle should rest against the back of the port chamber. Caution should be taken not to force the needle, which may cause the tip to bend.

4. **Ability to draw blood.** Attempt to draw blood with the client in the sitting, lying, arm-raised, standing, and side-lying positions. Having the client deep breathe and cough may also aid when drawing blood through problem catheters.

5. **Inserting and removing needles from ports.** All nurses who insert and remove needles from ports must receive education about this procedure and be properly supervised during an orientation period.

Clearing the Blocked VAD Line

The first step in resolving any problem is assessment of the problem. What medication(s) are running, and at what rate? Is there evidence of precipitation and/or thrombus formation? Initial measures to assess and restore patency of central venous catheters can be found in Boxes 18–2 and 18–3.

Dissolution of Lipid Sludge

Patency can be reestablished by instillation of a lipid solvent, ethyl alcohol, administered into the central venous catheter via a 0.22-μ filter and allowed to dwell for 1 to 2 hours (Holcombe et al., 1992; Pennington, 1990).

Use of Thrombolytic Agents

VAD occlusion due to partial occlusion by blood clots or blood may be cleared mechanically or with a thrombolytic drug such as urokinase (Holcombe et al., 1992; Lawson et al., 1982; Lawson, 1991; Wachs, 1990). The procedure for use of urokinase can be found in Box 18–2. Prophylactic use of a fibrinolytic drug to periodically cleanse the central venous catheter, or "locking" the central venous catheter with a dilute solution of fibrinolytic agent (2 ml of urokinase, 5000 IU/ml) monthly or every 2 months has proven effective in maintaining patency of the central venous catheter (Lawson, 1991). Holcombe and colleagues recently reported the use of 1 ml of urokinase, 5000 IU/ml, injected slowly and allowed to dwell for 30 to 60 minutes to restore catheter patency. In another study with pediatric central venous catheters, 1 ml of urokinase, 5000 IU/ml, was instilled into each occluded lumen. Catheter patency was restored with a single instillation in 62% of the cases, with two

---

Box 18–2

Procedure for Flushing Occluded Central Venous Catheters

1. Wash hands.
2. Don gloves.
3. Cleanse catheter/cap junction with povidone-iodine solution, place on sterile gauze, and allow to dry.
4. Clamp catheter and remove cap.
5. Attach a 1-ml syringe containing 5 ml of 0.9% sodium chloride solution.
6. Unclamp catheter.
7. Attempt to irrigate catheter. If unsuccessful, attempt to aspirate.
8. If catheter aspirates, but will not irrigate:
   a. Reposition patient (opposite side, or from lying to sitting position).
   b. Aspirate with smaller syringe (5 ml, 3 ml).
   c. Change patient's intrathoracic pressure by having patient raise arms and wave side to side, cough, deep breathe with slow exhale, or perform Valsalva maneuver.
9. If blood can be aspirated, flush vigorously with 10 to 20 ml of 0.9% sodium chloride solution, and connect to IV administration set. If IV not in progress, cap and heparinize catheter.
10. If able to irrigate catheter, but all attempts to aspirate fail, proceed with appropriate procedure to restore catheter patency.
11. If unable to infuse or aspirate, attempt to determine cause of occlusion and proceed with appropriate procedure to restore catheter patency.

Reprinted with permission from Holcombe, B.J., Forloines-Lynn, S., and Garmhausen, L.W.: Restoring patency of long-term central venous access devices. J. Intravenous Nurs. 15:37, 1992.

---

instillations in 30%, and with three instillations in 4% (Wachs, 1990). Urokinase instilled prophylactically into ports at 3- to 4-week intervals was reported to be successful in keeping the port free of residual deposits (Fraschini, 1991). Urokinase has been used in the home setting as well (Bjeltich, 1987). Procedures for use of urokinase vary widely. Two sample procedures can be found in Boxes 18–3 and 18–4.

Other Measures

There are some reports in the literature of success in clearing drug precipitates by increasing the pH with sodium bicarbonate (Goodwin, 1991), or decreasing the pH with 1 ml of 0.2 to 1.0 ml of 0.1% hydrochloric acid (Duffy et al., 1989; Shulman et al., 1988; Testerman, 1991).

Table 18–1 summarizes the problems, their possible causes, and the nursing interventions for troubleshooting VADs. See specific guidelines and procedures in Chapters 14 (central venous catheters), 15 (PICCs), and 16 (implanted ports).

Box 18–3

Procedure for Clearing a Blocked Central Venous Catheter (CVC), Peripherally Inserted Central Catheter (PICC), or Port Using Urokinase

NOTE: This is a generalized instruction guide. Follow manufacturer's instructions for specific catheters, PICCs, or ports when available.

Urokinase (Abbokinase Open-Cath), a fibrinolytic agent, is most often instilled by the physician. Institutional policies should specify who is responsible for performing this procedure. Nurses who perform this procedure should receive education in techniques, major action and side effects, and precautions to be taken when injecting urokinase to clear a catheter or port.

Procedure

1. Check under and around dressing to be sure that catheter is not kinked.
2. Clamp catheter and disconnect I.V. tubing or syringe.
3. Attempt to irrigate with heparinized saline and aspirate clot from catheter, using a 10-ml syringe. Do not apply excessive pressure, as this may cause catheter rupture. (NOTE: A three-way stopcock may be used to reduce the risk of catheter rupture (see Box 18–4).) If step 4 is not successful in clearing line:
4. Prepare urokinase solution:
   a. Remove protective cap.
   b. Turn plunger-stopper one-quarter turn and press to force diluent into lower chamber.
   c. Roll and tilt vial to dissolve solution. Avoid vigorous shaking or agitation.
   d. Withdraw solution into 10-ml syringe.
5. Slowly inject a volume of urokinase equal to the internal volume of the catheter or port using a 10-ml syringe. (NOTE: See product manual or Nursing Guide for specific amounts.)
6. Use a gentle push-pull action on syringe plunger to maximize solution mixing.
7. Remove syringe and attach an empty 10-ml syringe to catheter.
8. Wait at least 10–15 minutes before attempting to aspirate drug and residual clot.
9. Repeat aspiration attempts every 5–10 minutes.
10. If catheter is not open within 30 minutes, cap the catheter and allow urokinase solution to remain for an additional 30–60 minutes, then reattempt aspiration.
11. A second instillation of urokinase may be necessary in resistant cases.
12. When patency is restored, aspirate 4–5 ml of blood to assure removal of all drug and residual clot.
13. Remove the blood-filled syringe and flush with at least 10 ml of normal saline solution.

From Lawson, M., Bottino, J.C., and Hurtubise, M.R.: The use of urokinase to restore the patency of occluded central venous catheters. Am. J. IV Ther. Clin. Nutr. 9:29–30, 32, 1982; *Groshong Catheter Nursing Procedure Manual* (pp. 17–19). Salt Lake City, UT, Bard Access Systems, 1992; *Clinical Information: Port-A-Cath and P.A.S. Port Implantable Access Systems.* St. Paul, MN, Pharmacia Deltec, Incorporated, 1990.

Box 18-4

Procedure for Declotting a Blocked Peripherally Inserted Central Catheter (PICC) Using Urokinase

NOTE: Manufacturer's directions for use of urokinase illustrate use of a 1-ml syringe. The use of smaller syringes exposes central catheters to potential rupture by exertion of pressure at 120–150 psi. The use of positive pressure may result in catheter rupture. This procedure, using a three-way stopcock, removes excess pressure from the catheter. Once negative pressure is applied, it creates a vacuum within the catheter. As the stopcock is turned to open the port with the syringe containing urokinase, the vacuum draws the medication into the catheter down to the location of the clot. At no time during this procedure is the catheter expanded beyond its normal size. In addition, only the amount of medication needed is administered because only the dead space created by the aspiration is filled.

Equipment
Urokinase
Sterile gloves and mask
Sterile CVC dressing kit including cleansing agent of choice (e.g., povidone iodine swabsticks)
2 10-ml syringes
1 sterile three-way stopcock
Disposal container for old dressing
Accessible disposal container for sharps

Procedure
1. Check under and around dressing to be sure that catheter is not kinked and clamp is open.
2. Remove dressing only enough to expose connection of catheter hub to extension set tubing.
3. Keeping the patient's arm below the level of the heart, remove extension and swab catheter hub with povidone iodine.
4. Make sure lever on three-way stopcock is in OFF position and attach to hub of PICC.
5. Swab one port of stopcock with povidone iodine solution and attach an empty 10-ml syringe.
6. Swab the remaining port of stopcock with povidone iodine solution and attach a 10-ml syringe containing urokinase.
6. Turn the stopcock OFF to syringe containing urokinase and open to the empty 10-ml syringe.
7. Gently aspirate the catheter until the syringe plunger is pulled back to the 8–9 ml mark; then turn the stopcock OFF to the aspirating syringe and ON to the syringe containing urokinase. (NOTE: At this point, the medication will be drawn into the PIC catheter.)
8. Turn the stopcock to the OFF position and allow urokinase to remain in the catheter 5–15 minutes or per manufacturer's recommendations.
9. Open the stopcock and aspirate the line to check for residual clot and blood return. If blood is noted:
   a. Aspirate and discard 3–5 ml waste.
   b. Flush the line with 20 ml of 0.9% sodium chloride for injection.
   c. Remove the three-way stopcock.
   d. Attach a new extension tubing primed with heparinized saline solution.
10. If there is no blood, return to step 9, repeat aspiration attempts every 5–10 minutes.
11. If catheter is not open within 30 minutes, cap the catheter and allow urokinase solution to remain for an additional 30–60 minutes, then reattempt aspiration.
12. A second instillation of urokinase may be necessary in resistant cases.

From Bonstell, R.P., and Brown, J.M.: Declotting peripherally inserted central catheters with a new technique using urokinase. J. Vasc. Access Nurs. 2(1):10–12, 1992. Reprinted with permission.

Table 18–1 Troubleshooting Vascular Access Devices

MANIFESTATION	POSSIBLE CAUSE	NURSING INTERVENTIONS
Erythema, pain, warmth which follows course of the vein with peripheral I.V., midline catheter (MLC), or PICC.	Sterile mechanical phlebitis.	1. Assess associated factors: vital signs (VS), general condition of client, solution or medication being administered. 2. Continue to monitor site (see Box 18–2). 3. Local treatment to site as indicated or prescribed. 4. If phlebitis beyond 3+, may need to remove catheter.
Erythema, pain, warmth at catheter insertion site (PICC), catheter exit site (short-term or tunneled central venous catheter [CVC]), or port pocket site.	Local infection, cellulitis.	1. Assess associated factors: VS, general condition of client, solution or medication being administered. 2. Continue to monitor site. 3. Daily site care using meticulous aseptic technique. 4. If port pocket infection suspected, do not cannulate port. If needle is already in place, leave in for possible administration of antibiotics.
Pain along catheter track during infusion.	Extravasation of vesicant or irritant medication.	1. Assess site. 2. Assess associated factors: solution, flow rate. 3. Slow infusion. 4. Assess for other signs and symptoms of extravasation if medication being administered is a vesicant agent (see Chapter 2). 5. Apply warm compress to site to induce hemodilution around catheter.

(Continued)

493

Table 18–1 Troubleshooting Vascular Access Devices (Continued)

MANIFESTATION	POSSIBLE CAUSE	NURSING INTERVENTIONS
Fever, hypotension, warm flushed skin, edema, respiratory distress, clotting abnormalities.	Catheter sepsis. May progress to septic shock.	1. Assess VS, skin condition, sensorium, laboratory data, cultures. 2. Use meticulous care when manipulating catheter or cannulating port. 3. Continue to reassess patient's condition, and report changes to physician.
Inability to flush catheter or port or infuse solution or medication. Difficulty maintaining IV flow rate.	Catheter occlusion due to: • fibrin sheath formation • mural thrombus • negative pressure when aspirating • drug precipitation • drug incompatibility • improper or inadequate flushing.	1. Gently aspirate and attempt to irrigate with 15 ml of saline in a 30-ml syringe. Repeat. 2. DO NOT use force because this may force clot through catheter. 3. If successful, aspirate clot then flush with 20 ml of saline. Following saline flush, administer medications, restart I.V., or heparinize catheter or port. 4. If not successful, inform physician and follow agency protocol for clearing the blocked catheter (see Boxes 18–2, 18–3, and 18–4).
Progressive difficulty maintaining infusion flow rate, chest pain, neck pain, engorgement of veins in chest wall.	Possible mural thrombosis.	1. Assess patient status, VS, sensorium, laboratory data. 2. Check all infusion sets, clamps, pumps, equipment. 3. Reposition client. 4. If problem continues, notify physician and prepare for treatment with heparin, urokinase, streptokinase, or tPA.

	Extravasation caused by catheter tip migration, catheter damage, or dislodged port needle.	1. Immediately assess and evaluate client's complaints about abnormal sensation or pain. 2. If vesicant is infusing, stop infusion immediately. 3. Verify patency and placement (assess blood return) before infusing medication or solution, especially vesicants. 4. If no blood return, have patient change position and cough and attempt to aspirate again. 5. Follow agency protocol for verification of placement prior to infusion of medications or solutions.
Minor discomfort, stinging, warmth (as perceived by patient), or other abnormal sensation along the course of the catheter or in chest wall, arm, shoulder.		
	Catheter slippage.	1. Verify position of catheter prior to initiating infusion. 2. Observe catheter site, noting markings on catheter. 3. Assess for client discomfort.
	Catheter breakage or damage.	1. Assess integrity of catheter prior to infusion. 2. Assess for client discomfort. 3. Observe client handling of catheter.

	Incorrect needle placement in port, or dislodgement of needle from port.	1. Assess port site prior to cannulation and compare to normal for client.
		2. Avoid use of siliconized needles.
		3. Carefully access port, stabilizing port and using firm pressure to puncture septum without bending needle.
		4. Use noncoring needle only.
		5. Aspirate for blood return. If none:
		  • check position of needle
		  • have patient change position or cough and reattempt aspiration.

References

Anderson, K.M., and Holland, J.S.: Maintaining the patency of peripherally inserted central catheters with 10 units/cc heparin. J. Intravenous Nurs. 15:84–88, 1992.

Bagnall-Reeb, H., Ryder, M., and Anglim, M.A.: *Venous Access Device Occlusions: Independent Study Module.* Abbott Park, IL, Abbott Laboratories, 1992.

Bjeltich, J.: Declotting central venous catheters with urokinase in the home by nurse clinicians. J. Natl Intravenous Ther. Assoc. 10:428–430, 1987.

Bonstell, R.P., and Brown, J.M.: Declotting peripherally inserted central catheters with a new technique using urokinase. J. Vasc. Ac. Nurs. 2(1):10–12, 1992.

Camp-Sorrell, D.: Implantable ports: Everything you always wanted to know. J. Intravenous Nurs. 15:262–273, 1992.

Duffy, L.D., et al.: Treatment of central venous catheter occlusions with hydrochloric acid. J. Pediatr. 114:1002–1004, 1989.

Fraschini, G.: Urokinase prophylaxis of central venous ports reduces infections and thrombotic complications. In *National Association of Vascular Access Nurses, Fifth Annual Conference Syllabus Abstract* (p. 33). Menlo Park, CA, National Association of Vascular Access Nurses, 1991.

Gebarski, S.S., and Gebarski, K.S.: Chemotherapy port "twiddler's syndrome": A need for preinjection radiography. Cancer 54:38–39, 1984.

Gemlo, B.T., et al.: Extravasation: A serious complication of the split-sheath introducer technique for venous access. Arch. Surg. 123:490–492, 1988.

Goodwin, M.L.: Using sodium bicarbonate to clear a medication precipitate from a central venous catheter. J. Vasc. Access Network 1(2):23, 1991.

Holcombe, B.J., Forloines-Lynn, S., and Garmhausen, L.W.: Restoring patency of long-term central venous access devices. J. Intravenous Nurs. 15:36–41, 1992.

Hughes, W.D., et al.: Guidelines for the use of antimicrobial agents in neutropenic patients with unexplained fever. J. Infect. Dis. 161:138–148, 1990.

Lambert, M.E., et al.: Experience with the Port-A-Cath. Hematol. Oncol. 6:57, 1987.

Mirro, J., et al.: A comparison of placement techniques and complications of externalized catheters and implantable port use in children with cancer. J. Pediatr. Surg. 25:120–124, 1990.

Pasquale, M.D., Campbell, J.M., and Magnant, C.M.: Groshong versus Hickman catheters. Surg. Gynecol. Obstet. 174:408–410, 1992.

Pennington, C.R.: Management of catheter occlusion. J. Parenter. Enteral Nutr. 14:551, 1990.

Pennington, C.R., and Pithie, A.D.: Ethanol lock in the management of catheter occlusion. J. Parenter. Enteral Nutr. 11:507–508, 1987.

Ross, M.N., et al.: Comparison of totally implanted reservoirs with external catheters as venous access devices in pediatric oncology patients. Surg. Gynecol. Obstet. 167:141–145, 1988.

Shulman, R.J., et al.: Use of hydrochloric acid to clear obstructed central venous catheters. J. Parenter. Enteral Nutr. 12:509–510, 1988.

Servetar, E.M.: A case report of Twiddler's syndrome in a pediatric patient. J. Pediatr. Oncol. Nurs. 9:25–28, 1992.

Strum, S., et al.: Improved methods for vascular access: The Port-A-Cath, a totally implanted catheter system. J. Clin. Oncol. 4:596–603, 1986.

Testerman, E.J.: Restoring patency of central venous catheters obstructed by mineral precipitation using hydrochloric acid. J. Vasc. Access Network 1(2):22–23, 1991.

Wachs, T.: Urokinase administration in pediatric patients with occluded central venous catheters. J. Intravenous Nurs. 13:100–102, 1990.

Wickham, R., Purl, S., and Welker, D.: Long-term central venous catheters: Issues for care. Semin. Oncol. Nurs. 8:133–147, 1992.

Williams, E.C.: Catheter-related thrombosis. Clin. Cardiol. 13:134–136, 1990.

Recommended Readings

Atkinson, J., Bagnall, H., and Gomperts, E.: Investigational use of tissue plasminogen activator (t-PA) for occluded central venous catheters. J. Parenter. Enteral Nutr. 14: 310–311, 1990.

Bagnall, H., Gomperts, E., and Atkinson, J.: Continuous infusion of low-dose urokinase in the treatment of central venous catheter thrombosis in infants and children. Pediatrics 83:953–966, 1989.

Bagnall-Reeb, H., and Ruccione, K.: Management of cutaneous reactions and mechanical complications of central venous access devices in pediatric patients with cancer: Algorithms for decision making. Oncol. Nurs. Forum 17:677–681, 1990.

Bern, M.M., et al.: Very low doses of warfarin can prevent thrombosis in central venous catheters. Ann. Intern. Med. 112:423–428, 1990.

Bonstell, R.P., and Brown, J.M.: *Declotting Peripherally Inserted Central Catheters with a New Technique Using Urokinase.* San Antonio, TX, Gesco, International.

Brown, L.H., Wantroba, I., and Simonson, G.: Reestablishing patency in an occluded central venous access device. Crit. Care Nurse 9:114–121, 1989.

Brown-Smith, J.K., et al.: Tunneled catheter thrombosis: Factors related to incidence. Oncol. Nurs. Forum 17:543–549, 1990.

Clarke, D.E., and Raffin, T.A.: Infectious complications of indwelling long term central venous catheters. Chest 97:966–972, 1990.

Corona, M., et al.: Infections related to central venous catheters. Mayo Clin. Proc. 65:979–987, 1990.

Crow, S.: Infection risk in I.V. therapy. J. Natl Intravenous Ther. Assoc. 10:101–105, 1987.

Cunliffe, M.T., and Polomano, R.C.: How to clear catheter clots with Urokinase. Nursing 16(12):40–43, 1986.

Dawson, S., et al.: Right atrial catheters in children with cancer: A decade of experience in the use of tunneled exteriorized devices at a single institution. Am. J. Pediatr. Hematol. Oncol. 13:126–129, 1991.

Duffy, L.F., et al.: Treatment of central venous catheter occlusion with hydrochloric acid. J. Pediatr. 114:1002–1004, 1989.

Goode, C.J.: A meta-analysis of effects of heparin flush and saline flush: Qualitative and cost implications. Nurs. Res. 40:324–330, 1991.

Goodwin, M.L.: Central venous catheter tip malposition following optimal placement in the superior vena cava. J. Vasc. Access Network 1:18–21, 1991.

Goodwin, M.L., and Carlson, I.: The peripherally inserted central catheter: A retrospective look at 3 years of insertions. J. Intravenous Nurs. 16:92–103, 1993.

Haire, D., et al.: Obstructed central venous catheters: Restoring function with a 12-hour infusion of low dose Urokinase. Cancer 66:2279–2285, 1990.

Hall, P., Cedermark, B., and Swedenborg, J.: Implantable catheter system for long-term intravenous chemotherapy. J. Surg. Oncol. 41:39–41, 1989.

Hamilton, R.A., et al.: Heparin sodium versus 0.9% sodium chloride injection for maintaining patency of indwelling intermittent infusion devices. Clin. Pharmacol. 7:439–443, 1988.

James, L., Blesdow, L., and Hadaway, L.: A retrospective look at tip location and complications of peripherally inserted central catheter lines. J. Intravenous Nurs. *16*:104–109, 1993.

Lawson, M.: Partial occlusion of indwelling central venous catheters. J. Intravenous Nurs. *14*:157–159, 1991.

Lawson, M., et al.: The use of urokinase to restore the patency of occluded central venous catheters. Am. J. Intravenous Nurs. Clin. Nutr. *9*:29–32, 1982.

Lum, P.S., and Soski, M.: Management of malpositioned central venous catheters. J. Intravenous Nurs. *12*:356–365, 1989.

Maki, D., et al.: Prospective randomised trial of povidone-iodine, alcohol, and chlorhexidine for prevention of infection associated with central venous arterial catheters. Lancet *338*(8763):339–343, 1991.

Maki, D.G., and Ringer, M.: Evaluations of dressing regimens for prevention of infection with peripheral intravenous catheters. JAMA *258*:2396–2403, 1987.

May, S., and Davis, C.: Percutaneous catheters and totally implanted access systems: A review of reported infection rates. J. Intravenous Nurs. *11*:97–103, 1988.

Monturo, C.A., Dickerson, R.N., and Mullen, J.L.: Efficacy of thrombolytic therapy for occlusion of long-term catheters. J. Parenter. Enteral Nutr. *14*:312–314, 1990.

Mukau, L., Talamini, M.A., and Sitzmann, J.V.: Risk factors for central venous catheter-related vascular erosions. J. Parenter. Enteral Nutr. *15*:513–516, 1991.

Plans, W.J.: Delayed pneumothorax after subclavian vein catheterization. J. Parenter. Enteral Nutr. *14*:444–445, 1990.

Prian, G.W., and Van Way, C.W.: The long arm silastic catheter: A critical look at complications. J. Intravenous Nurs. *11*(1):16–19, 1988.

Scott, W.: Complications associated with central venous catheters: A survey. Chest *94*: 1221–1224, 1988.

Schulmeister, L.: Needle dislodgement from implanted venous access devices: Inpatient and outpatient experiences. J. Intravenous Nurs. *12*:90–92, 1989.

Smith, J.M.: Occluded access devices: Nursing guidelines. Probl. Solv. Office Oncol. Nurs. *3*(3):1–3, 1989.

Smith, S., et al.: Maintenance of patency of indwelling central venous catheters: Is heparin necessary? Am. J. Pediatr. Hematol. Oncol. *13*:131–143, 1991.

Stokes, D.C., et al.: Early detection and simplified management of obstructed Hickman and Broviac catheters. J. Pediatr. Surg. *24*:257–262, 1989.

Stuart, R.K., Shikora, S.A., and Akerman, P.: Incidence of arrhythmia with central venous catheter insertion and exchange. J. Parenter. Enteral Nutr. *14*:152–155, 1990.

Thielen, J.B., and Nyquist, J.: Subclavian catheter removal: Nursing implications to prevent air emboli. J. Intravenous Nurs. *14*:114–118, 1991.

van Hoff, J., Berg, A.T., and Seashore, J.H.: The effect of right atrial catheters on infectious complications of chemotherapy in children. J. Clin. Oncol. *8*:1255–1262, 1990.

Weeks-Lozano, H.: Clinical evaluation of Per Q Cath for both pediatric and adult home infusion therapy. J. Intravenous Nurs. *14*:249–256, 1991.

Chapter 19

Client Education

Dixie Brennan Scelsi, R.N., M.S., M.S.N.

Current Trends

The past two decades have brought a great deal of progress in the management of cancer, and more clients with cancer are being treated on an outpatient basis. This is partially due to the development of long-term venous access devices (VADs) (described in Chapters 14 through 17), and is partially the result of current trends toward reduced length of hospital stays. Thus, more chemotherapy and biotherapy must be administered in the outpatient clinic, the physician's office, or the home. A benefit is that the client may remain in the home and work settings and can be as productive as possible while undergoing therapy for cancer. The trend toward early discharge and more home care has increased the patient's responsibility for his/her care. A well-planned client education program must assure that the client receives the knowledge and is assisted in developing skills necessary to maintain self-care. In many cases, family members participate in caring for the client or serve as backup caregivers. Self-care is used here to denote the emphasis on the client as the preferred caregiver.

Goals of Client Education

A program of client education must inform the client about the medications he/she is receiving, the anticipated side effects, and related precautions. The client and family must be taught procedures for medication administration and informed of expected toxicities of medications administered. The educational program may enhance the client's self confidence, allowing him/her to maintain maximal independence while receiving therapy. Client and family participation in the treatment regimen must be encouraged. Time must be allowed for questions, and answers must be presented in a manner that is understandable to the client.

Assessing and Planning

Client education ideally begins as soon as a diagnosis and treatment plan have been established. Today, with shorter hospital stays, less time is available for inpatient client education. This requires early assessment and initiation of client education in the hospital setting, with communication and coordination between the acute care setting and the home care or office nurse to assure continuity of client education.

As both lifespan and the number of successful cancer therapies increase, so does the number of older clients. This, along with the multicultural backgrounds of clients, provides additional challenges to the nurse. The older adult may learn at a slower pace and may have more difficulty remembering new information. He/she may need more repetition and reinforcement. Visual changes that accompany aging may impede the reading of printed material if the print size is too small.

Education must be carefully planned and personalized to each client, taking into consideration his/her age, cultural beliefs, and educational background. A variety of educational strategies and continuous reinforcement are necessary to assure compliance in self-administration of prescribed medications (Levine et al., 1987; Yarbro, 1992).

The Process of Client Education

Educating the client is an integral part of the nursing process, and caring allows the interactions between nurse and client and/or family that are necessary to facilitate learning to occur. Caring is the essence of nursing (Leininger, 1981). In the nurse–client relationship, caring has been defined as "the direct or indirect nurturant and skillful activities, processes, and decisions related to assisting people to achieve or maintain health" (Larson, 1984; Leininger, 1981; Mayer, 1986).

Client knowledge of and participation in the educational process are essential for the successful treatment regimen in outpatient chemotherapy. Learning is individual; possible for all age groups in the absence of dementing disease; patterned, active, purposeful, and creative; and involves transfer of understanding (Knowles, 1978).

The three domains of learning are cognitive, psychomotor, and affective. Cognitive learning involves intellectual activities geared toward understanding. Psychomotor learning results in client mastery of physical skills. Affective learning involves the client's feelings and attitudes. The client and/or family who will administer chemotherapy in the home setting must learn many "facts" about medications and equipment, techniques for handling equipment, and strategies for coping with side effects, body image alterations, and feelings and attitudes about cancer and the therapy.

Many medications can be taken orally, some require subcutaneous injection, and the majority require venous access, utilizing one of several types of devices. With proper education, many clients in the home setting are able to self-administer chemotherapy, biotherapy, and/or supportive regimens (e.g., antiemetics, antidiarrheals) and can properly identify significant side effects.

Client Selection

Candidates for self-care are those who have:

1. Ability to understand the purpose and recognize side effects of chemotherapy, biotherapy, and other medications administered.
2. Manual skills and dexterity necessary to self-administer the proper dose of parenteral chemotherapy, biotherapy, and/or supportive agents by self-injection or venous access device.
3. Manual skills and dexterity necessary to handle venous access equipment safely and properly.
4. Motivation to learn and care for self.
5. Emotional stability.
6. A support system (family or significant other).

Each plan for nursing care in this book includes a knowledge deficit and describes goals and standards of care or nursing interventions for alterations associated with antineoplastic agents. Specific nursing measures for individual medications are included in the "nursing interventions" columns of tables in Chapters 3 and 4.

Utilization of Client Education Materials

Chemotherapy and You (National Cancer Institute, 1991) and *Understanding Chemotherapy: A Guide to Treatment of Leukemia, Lymphoma and Multiple Myeloma for Patients and their Families* (Leukemia Society, 1990) contain information about medications, toxicities, and toxicity management. Instruction sheets for most chemotherapeutic agents are available from the National Cancer Institute in English or Spanish. A sample is included in Box 19–1. Patient information about specific biologic response modifiers and how to self-administer them is available from the distributors of these products and appears in the Leukemia Society booklet (see Boxes 19–2 and 19–3). Flip charts and videos are also available. Appendix E lists many patient teaching aids that can be utilized in the teaching–learning process.

Education of the Client with a Vascular Access Device

Many clients must maintain and manipulate a vascular access device for the administration of chemotherapy and/or biotherapy. Additional planning and teaching by the nurse is imperative for these individuals.

Ideally, client education about a vascular access device (central venous catheter, peripherally inserted central catheter, port, or pump) begins prior to insertion of the vascular access device. At this time, the nurse should acquaint the client and family members or significant other with the overall goals of the therapy program and equipment that will be utilized. The nurse should assess the client's ability to perform necessary procedures at this time. A brief explanation of the insertion techniques can prepare the client and family and reduce anxiety. Anatomic illustrations, brochures, and/or videos can be utilized to reinforce verbal discussion by the nurse. It is helpful for the client to discuss specific placement of implanted ports with the physician prior to insertion, and placement in relation to the usual clothing the client wears (e.g., the bra band and straps) should be taken into consideration. This prevents trauma to the port site and allows the client to continue wearing his/her usual clothing.

The educational process will vary depending on each client's knowledge base and learning needs. The nurse initiates a structured teaching program, incorporating information about specific medications and equipment for medication delivery. The first session with a client who has a vascular access device is devoted to explaining and demonstrating catheter (or port) care procedures, such as dressing, flushing, clamping, and capping. Demonstration materials are used to show step-by-step procedures to the client/family and are followed by a return demonstration and the opportunity for the client to receive answers to questions. The nurse should monitor return demonstrations of procedures by the patient and, when indicated, significant other including handwashing, changing dressings, drawing heparin, and (if indicated) using a Tubex device. Written instructions are given to the client at this time (see sample client instructions in Boxes 19–6 through 19–23).

Subsequent teaching sessions are utilized to reinforce all steps taught and demonstrated. Additional instructions include teaching about:

1. Clamping the catheter.
2. Flushing the catheter or port.
3. Changing tubing on the noncoring needle.
4. Changing the noncoring needle (if indicated).

Demonstration and nurse-supervised return demonstration should continue until the client is able to perform procedures in proper sequence and with proper technique.

When treatment is initiated in the hospital, office, clinic, or home, the client must be supervised. If teaching was initiated in a hospital or clinic, follow-up instruction is given in the home setting after discharge by the home health nurse. Follow-up visits in the home setting should continue until the client is performing the necessary procedures properly and independently.

The client who is treated in an ambulatory program is taught utilizing the established protocols of the home health care agency or institution providing the education. All protocols are based on specific medical orders, or standing orders of the physician or agency. The physician's orders for client education are required. For a successful home chemotherapy program, the patient must be able to call a "hot line" should problems arise. A nurse should be accessible to troubleshoot patient problems and provide advice 7 days a week, 24 hours a day.

Client education must be individualized to fit the client, equipment (pumps, ports, extension sets, syringes), and vascular access accessories (caps, dressings, bags, clamps, needles, irrigation solutions).

Sample client instructions for medications, toxicity management, and a variety of vascular access devices can be found in the following pages (see Boxes 19–1 through 19–23).

Box 19-1

Sample Client Instructions: Tamoxifen

Questions and Answers About Tamoxifen

1. What is tamoxifen?

Tamoxifen (trade name Nolvadex) is a drug in pill form, taken orally, that interferes with the activity of estrogen (a female hormone). It has been used for nearly 20 years to treat patients with advanced breast cancer. More recently, it also is being used as adjuvant, or additional, therapy following primary treatment for early stage breast cancer. Tamoxifen is also being studied to determine whether it is useful in the treatment of other types of cancer, such as melanoma, endometrial (uterine) cancer, and certain leukemias.

2. How does tamoxifen work on breast cancer?

Estrogen promotes the growth of breast cancer cells. Tamoxifen works against the effects of estrogen on these cells. It is often called an "antiestrogen." As a treatment for the disease, the drug slows or stops the growth of cancer cells that are already present in the body. As adjuvant therapy, tamoxifen has been shown to help prevent the original breast cancer from returning and also prevent the development of new cancers in the opposite breast.

3. Are there other beneficial effects of tamoxifen?

While tamoxifen acts against the effects of estrogen in breast tissue, it acts like estrogen in other body systems. This means that women who take tamoxifen may share many of the beneficial effects of menopausal estrogen replacement therapy, such as a lowering of blood cholesterol and a slowing of bone loss (osteoporosis).

4. Can tamoxifen prevent breast cancer?

Research has shown that when tamoxifen is used as adjuvant therapy for early stage breast cancer, it not only prevents the recurrence of the original cancer but also prevents the development of new cancers in the opposite breast. Based on these findings, the National Cancer Institute is sponsoring a large clinical trial to determine whether tamoxifen can prevent breast cancer in women who have an increased risk of developing the disease.

5. What are some of the more common side effects of taking tamoxifen?

In general, the side effects of tamoxifen are similar to some of the symptoms of menopause. Some women will experience hot flashes, irregular menstrual periods, vaginal discharge or bleeding, and irritation of the skin around the vagina. As is the case with menopause, not all women who take tamoxifen have these symptoms.

6. Does tamoxifen increase fertility?

Tamoxifen has been shown to increase fertility in premenopausal women. In some countries, the drug has been used to stimulate ovulation in women who have had difficulty becoming pregnant. Premenopausal women should use some type of birth control while taking tamoxifen. Oral contraceptives (birth control pills) should not be used because they may change the effects of tamoxifen.

Box 19–1

Sample Client Instructions: Tamoxifen (Continued)

7. Does tamoxifen cause a woman to begin menopause?

Tamoxifen does not cause a woman to begin menopause, although it can cause some symptoms that are similar to those that may occur during menopause. In most women taking tamoxifen, the ovaries continue to act normally and produce female hormones (estrogens) in the same or slightly increased amounts.

8. Does tamoxifen cause blood clots?

Data from large clinical trials suggest that there is a small increase in the number of blood clots in women taking tamoxifen, particularly in women who are receiving anticancer drugs (chemotherapy) along with tamoxifen. The total number of women who have experienced this side effect is small. The risk of having a blood clot due to tamoxifen is equal to the risk of blood clots for women on birth control pills or estrogen replacement therapy.

9. Does tamoxifen cause depression?

In one trial, depression was reported by about 1 percent of the postmenopausal women using tamoxifen as adjuvant therapy. No other trials have reported this side effect.

10. Does tamoxifen cause uterine cancer?

Results from several large clinical trials suggest that women taking the usual dose of tamoxifen (20 milligrams per day) have an increased risk of cancer of the lining of the uterus (endometrial cancer). The risk of endometrial cancer is almost doubled by tamoxifen, an increase similar to that associated with estrogen replacement therapy in postmenopausal women.

11. Does tamoxifen cause liver cancer?

There has also been some concern that tamoxifen may cause liver cancer. In one adjuvant trial, liver tumors were reported in 2 of 931 breast cancer patients receiving a high dose (40 milligrams per day) of tamoxifen. In these cases, it is not known whether the liver tumors were caused by the drug or were the result of breast cancer that had spread to the liver. In six other trials using 20 milligrams of tamoxifen daily as adjuvant therapy, no liver cancers have been reported.

The Cancer Information Service (CIS), a program of the National Cancer Institute, is a nationwide telephone service for cancer patients and their families, the public, and health care professionals. CIS information specialists have extensive training in providing up-to-date and understandable information about cancer. They can answer questions in English and Spanish and can send free printed material. In addition, CIS offices serve specific geographic areas and have information about cancer-related services and resources in their region. The toll-free number of the CIS is 1–800–4–CANCER (1–800–422–6237).

From "Cancer Facts," National Cancer Institute, Bethesda, MD, 1988.

Box 19–2

Client Instructions: Doxorubicin

Doxorubicin

Pronunciation:
Dox-oh-ROO-bi-sin

Brand names:
A commonly used brand name is Adriamycin®.

How given:
Doxorubicin is given by injection.

Special precautions: While you are taking doxorubicin, your doctor may want you to drink extra fluids so that you will pass more urine. This will help prevent kidney and bladder problems and keep your kidneys working well.

Doxorubicin causes the urine to turn reddish in color, which may stain clothes. This is not blood. It is perfectly normal and lasts for only 1 or 2 days after each dose is given.

Side effects needing immediate medical attention: Unusually fast or irregular heartbeat; pain at place of injection; shortness of breath; swelling of feet and lower legs; wheezing.

If doxorubicin accidently seeps out of the vein, it may damage some tissues and cause scarring. Tell the doctor or nurse right away if you notice redness, pain, or swelling at the I.V. site.

Other side effects needing medical attention as soon as possible: Fever, chills, or sore throat; sores in mouth and on lips; side or stomach pain; joint pain, unusual bleeding or bruising; skin rash or itching.

Side effects needing immediate attention after you stop using this medicine: Irregular heartbeat; shortness of breath; swelling of feet and lower legs.

Side effects that usually do not require medical attention: Loss of hair; nausea or vomiting (unless severe); reddish urine; darkening of soles, palms, or nails.

From the Leukemia Society of America: *Understanding Chemotherapy: A Guide to Treatment of Leukemia, Lymphoma, and Multiple Myeloma for Patients and Their Families* (pp. 17–18). New York, Leukemia Society of America, 1990. Reprinted with permission.

Box 19-3

Client Instructions: Interferon-Alpha Recombinant

Interferon-alpha recombinant

Pronunciation:
In-ter-FEAR-on

Brand names:
Commonly used brand names are Intron® or Roferon®.

How given:
Interferon is given by intramuscular or subcutaneous injection.

Special precautions: While you are using interferon, your doctor may want you to drink extra fluids.

Side effects needing immediate attention: Numbness or tingling in fingers, toes or face; rapid heartbeat with fever; rash.

Side effects needing medical attention as soon as possible: Dizziness; diarrhea; flu-like symptoms.

Side effects that usually do not require medical attention: Loss of appetite; change in taste; fatigue, headache; nausea and vomiting; weight loss.

From the Leukemia Society of America: *Understanding Chemotherapy: A Guide to Treatment of Leukemia, Lymphoma, and Multiple Myeloma for Patients and Their Families* (p. 25). New York, Leukemia Society of America, 1990. Reprinted with permission.

Box 19-4

Sample Client Education for the Person Taking High-Dose Methotrexate with Leucovorin Rescue

1. Take leucovorin tablets **exactly as prescribed by your physician. Every dose must be taken at the prescribed time around the clock, and none can be omitted or delayed.**
2. If there is a problem taking the medication or keeping it down, notify your physician **immediately.**
3. Practice good oral hygiene measures.
4. Drink 12 to 18 8-oz glasses of fluid daily for 3 days after taking your high-dose methotrexate. This will help to mobilize and eliminate the end products of the drug.
5. If you are taking the tablet form of leucovorin, keep an accurate record of doses taken.
6. Should vomiting occur when you are taking the tablet form and you have been given alternative instructions, follow these.
7. Report any signs of an allergic reaction (itching, hives, facial flushing).
8. Keep an identification card with you at all times indicating that you are taking leucovorin and that continuity of the medication should be maintained if an emergency occurs. Your physician's name and phone number should be on the card as well.

Box 19–5

Sample Client Instruction Sheet: Altretamine (Hexalen)

HEXALEN®(altretamine)

*h*ome administration

Instructions for_____
_____Patient name

Schedule

You will be taking HEXALEN for_____days in a 28-day cycle.
_____number

Start taking HEXALEN on _____
_____month/day

Your last day on HEXALEN will be _____
_____month/day

Month:

SUN	MON	TUE	WED	THU	FRI	SAT

Dosage

You will take_____HEXALEN capsules each day.
_____number

Take_____capsules after breakfast, _____after lunch,
____number_____number

_____after dinner, _____at bedtime.
____number_____number

Box 19–5

Sample Client Instruction Sheet: Altretamine (Hexalen) (Continued)

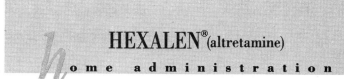

HEXALEN®(altretamine)

*h*ome   administration

Additional Information on HEXALEN Treatment

While most patients experience no nausea or vomiting while taking HEXALEN, some do. There are a number of steps you can take to help avoid this discomfort.

1. It is important to take your HEXALEN capsules on time.

2. Your doctor can prescribe medication that can help prevent nausea and vomiting. If you find it difficult to take oral medicine because of nausea, a suppository form can also be prescribed.

3. Good nutrition during therapy is important. It may help to eat a number of small, low-fat meals spaced throughout the day. Carbohydrates are easy to digest. Dry toast or crackers may help.

4. Drink plenty of clear liquids, but do not drink liquids with meals.

5. Sit up for at least one hour after eating.

Other Instructions

_____

_____

_____

If you are having any problems with your treatment, call your doctor.
Phone: _____

Box 19-6

Teaching Objectives for the Client with a Vascular Access Device

Upon the completion of instruction in the techniques of home chemotherapy, the client and/or family will be able to:

1. Identify the equipment and materials necessary for maintenance of the catheter or port.
2. Identify the equipment and materials necessary for the operation of the infusion pump.
3. List the steps for changing the dressing.
4. List the steps for irrigation of the catheter or port.
5. List the steps for pump setup (AutoSyringe, Cormed, Pancretec, Pharmacia).
6. Demonstrate all techniques listed above.
7. List signs and symptoms of side effects that should be reported to the physician.
8. Identify equipment problems.
9. Know the phone number of the home care nurse and have it available in the home.

Box 19-7

Sample of Client Education Material

General Information

The following information will help simplify the activities you will need to complete as you participate in your own therapy. In addition, you can help prevent some of the problems that can occur during therapy by your careful attention to detail.

Please store supplies in a clean area and keep them away from extreme heat or cold and moisture.

Follow the directions given to you, either orally or in writing, about storing any medications.

Keep your work area clean.

Always *wash your hands carefully* prior to handling any of the materials, medications, or equipment you will use in your therapy.

Your primary Registered Nurse will help you to develop a system for daily supply organization and usage, as well as a detailed step-by-step procedure for your particular therapy.

Should you have any questions, contact:

_____ , R.N.   Phone:_____

_____ , M.D.   Phone:_____

Box 19-8

Changing the Dressing on Your Vascular Access Catheter

1. Wash your hands carefully with iodine soap.
2. Assemble the supplies you will need:
   2" × 2" gauze pads
   Sterile package of iodine swabsticks
   Paper tape or transparent dressing
   Sterile alcohol wipes (to wipe catheter if needed)
   Open the packages, being careful not to touch the insides. *Use scissors to cut tape—before you handle the catheter.*
3. Remove old dressing and tape. Pick up dressing by corner and be careful not to touch the skin underneath. *Do not pull on the catheter.* At this time you should inspect the catheter site for swelling, redness, drainage, or pus. Call your doctor if any of these signs is present.
4. Clean the area around the catheter site, using the iodine swabsticks. Work in a circular motion from the catheter site to the edges. Clean a 2" circle around the catheter. Use each swabstick only once, then throw it away.
5. Place a sterile 2" × 2" gauze or transparent dressing over the catheter site. Use ointment only when prescribed by your doctor.
6. Tape all edges securely.
7. Tape a loop of catheter securely over the dressing (see illustration).

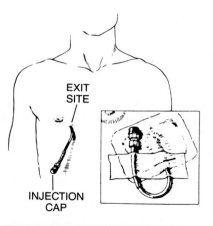

EXIT
SITE

INJECTION
CAP

Box 19–9

Filling Your Heparin or Saline Syringe

You will need the following for each irrigation (flush) of your central venous catheter:
10-ml syringe
Needle
Vial of heparin (100 units per ml) or saline
Alcohol swabs

Procedure
1. Attach needle to syringe.
2. Remove center metal disc from vial.
3. Swab rubber with alcohol.
4. Remove protective cap from needle and save.
5. Draw plunger of syringe back to _____.
6. Stick needle through rubber stopper into solution.
7. Push plunger in to 0 mark.
8. Turn hands so that vial is on top and syringe on bottom.
9. Allow plunger to return as far as it will, then pull it the remainder of the way to the _____ mark on syringe.
10. Take syringe and needle out of vial.
11. Replace protective cap until ready to use.

Precautions
Be careful not to touch the needle at any time. If you do touch it, or if it comes in contact with anything other than the rubber part of the vial, discard the needle and attach a new one. *Never* use a needle more than once, or near the central venous catheter—the catheter may be punctured.

Box 19–10

Irrigation of Your Central Venous Catheter or Peripherally Inserted Central Catheter

1. Prepare heparin or saline in syringe (see Box 19–9).
2. Clamp catheter.
3. Expel any air bubbles from syringe (hold syringe straight up, tap side of syringe to help air rise to top, and push plunger up).
4. Cleanse injection port with alcohol.
5. Insert needle carefully into center of injection port.
6. Unclamp catheter.
7. Gently push plunger of syringe to force fluid into catheter.
8. When syringe is almost empty (but while still pushing plunger), clamp catheter.
9. Disconnect syringe and needle and discard.

Points to Remember
You should experience very little resistance when pushing the fluid into the catheter.

Push gently in order not to damage the catheter.

Do not touch the end of the catheter or the syringe tip.

If the exterior of the catheter end is soiled, wipe with alcohol swab.

The catheter should never be left open to the air. Before you unclamp catheter, the cap or an I.V. or pump tubing must be connected to the catheter.

Box 19–11

Instructions for Emergency Interventions with Your Central Venous Catheter or Peripherally Inserted Central Catheter

If your neck or arm becomes swollen on the same side as the catheter, *notify your doctor immediately.*

Clotting

If your catheter has been allowed to remain unheparinized after a completed infusion, or if there has not been a constant flow of fluid (the bag has run dry and has gone unnoticed), there is a possibility that the blood will clot at some point along the catheter. If blockage or clotting should occur, the catheter should be irrigated with a heparin syringe (the same as for irrigation procedure). *If you meet firm resistance when irrigating, notify your doctor immediately and* **do not continue to try to irrigate.**

Breaking

Undue stress applied to the catheter while connecting and disconnecting the I.V., or while irrigating, can cause the catheter to break. If this should happen, *clamp the catheter immediately and notify your doctor.*

Blood Back-up

If a small amount of blood begins to back up and leak around the capped end of your catheter, the cap most likely has been attached improperly. *Clamp the catheter, remove the cap, irrigate the catheter with heparin, and replace the cap carefully.* Tape the cap/catheter connection and tape a loop in the catheter in the usual position.

Infection

You should observe for local or systemic symptoms of infection. Local symptoms include redness, swelling, tenderness, or drainage from around the catheter exit site. Some systemic symptoms include fever, chills, sweats, or lethargy. *You should call your doctor immediately if you have any of these symptoms.*

Chances of infection are minimal if procedures are followed carefully.

Air in the Catheter

Air may enter the catheter if any connection falls apart; if the cap, I.V. set, or syringe is removed without clamping; if the cap falls off the catheter; or if the I.V. set pulls out of the catheter.

The symptoms that would occur if air had entered the bloodstream include coughing, shortness of breath, and chest pain.

If you have these symptoms, *you should irrigate the catheter with heparin immediately, lie on your left side, and notify your physician.*

The symptoms should disappear within 20 minutes, but you still should notify your physician.

Carefully taping the cap/catheter connection should prevent air from entering. Always clamping the catheter when starting the infusion, stopping the infusion, and irrigating the catheter with heparin will also prevent air from entering.

Box 19-12

Avoiding Problems with Your Per-Q-Cath

The advantages of using a Per-Q-Cath are derived primarily from its small size. This allows the clinician to place the catheter thru a small needle and when in the vein, allows for a good flow around the catheter. The material that the Per-Q-Cath is made of is "Silastic", the most bio-compatible material available today.

Because of its small size, the clinician using a PICC line must take additional care in placing and maintaining it over what they may have been used to in the past with larger catheters or catheters made of less bio-compatible materials, that are much stiffer and tougher, e.g., plastics.

The fact that repair kits are provided by manufacturers of all central catheters tells us that problems can occur with PICC lines also. With this in mind we have compiled a list of possible problems that can be avoided and/or minimized with proper technique.

The four most common problems encountered with a PICC catheter and ideas for prevention and/or solutions to them are as follows:

Problem 1. Guidewire hard to remove.

Problem 2. Catheter breaks at or near hub.

Problem 3. Catheter develops a leak, after being used for a period of time.

Problem 4. Catheter develops a leak upon placement.

A new video has also been produced to provide the clinician with the most up-to-date procedures available. Following the steps in the video and the ideas presented herewith will avoid the most common problems encountered with PICC lines.

Reprinted with permission of Gesco International, San Antonio, TX.

Box 19-13

Avoiding Problems with Your Per-Q-Cath: Guidewire Hard to Remove

Problem 1: **Guidewire hard to remove.**

Cause: **Tortuous vessel path, bent and/or damaged guidewire occurring during procedure.**

Prevention:
1. Inspect wire upon removal from protector to make sure that the portion that will enter patient is straight.
2. Do not nick or cut guidewire when cutting catheter to length.
3. Select a vein with the least tortuous path, i.e., the basilic rather than the cephalic.

Box 19–13

Avoiding Problems with Your Per-Q-Cath: Guidewire Hard to Remove (Continued)

4. Slowly advance catheter and wire, approximately 1 inch at a time holding catheter gently with forceps. If resistance is met, the tip of the catheter is probably catching on a valve or in a turn in the vein. Re-distend the vessel and/or have patient rotate or raise arm. **Only if the introducer needle has been removed from the patient,** pull the catheter and wire back slightly in an attempt to free it from the obstruction. Do not force the catheter and wire as this can cause it to double over and bend the wire or damage the vein.

Removal:
1. If resistance is met when attempting to remove a guidewire from the catheter, the wire may be bent. This can be caused either by a sharp bend in the vessel where the catheter is being held very tightly against the wire, with no permanent damage to the wire, or by a bent or damaged wire. Do not force removal as this can damage the catheter.
2. Observe catheter to see if it is bunching (rippling) at the hub. If so, refrain from pulling on the guidewire allowing the catheter to relax to its normal shape and then apply light pressure with a 2×2 gauze pad over the catheter and insertion site. Then slowly resume removing the guidewire with a slight twisting motion. This should relieve the bunching and allow the wire to start being withdrawn.
3. If the wire does not begin to come out, slowly begin withdrawing both catheter and guidewire together, trying again as both exit the skin.
4. If a guidewire is forcefully removed when the catheter is bunched (rippled) at the hub, it will damage the catheter.

The Product: The guidewire in each Per-Q-Cath tray is made of a top grade stainless steel spring wire. It is then coated with Teflon to provide an ultra-smooth, durable, non-flaking surface. This coating is also designed to provide lubricity and resistance to abrasion while maintaining flexibility.

Each catheter is matched and assembled with a wire to insure that the wire can be removed with ease. The catheter and wire are also inspected for straightness prior to being placed in the protector.

If for any reason a bend is discovered in a wire prior to placement, return the product. GESCO will immediately replace the tray.

Reprinted with permission of Gesco International, San Antonio, TX.

Box 19–14

Avoiding Problems with Your Per-Q-Cath: Catheter Breaks at or near the Hub

Problem 2:   Catheter breaks at or near the hub.

Cause: Force causing the catheter to be stretched beyond its tensile strength.

Prevention: 1. Follow the taping and securing instructions and illustrations included in each Per-Q-Cath tray as follows:
   A. Leave about 1 inch of catheter, with a slight bend, between the entry sight and the hub of the catheter.
   B. Place one steri-strip over the wings of the catheter to stabilize the catheter. Do not place tape on catheter.
   C. Completely cover the catheter and wings with the non-occlusive dressing.
   D. Place a steri-strip under the hub and chevron over the wings and on top of the non-occlusive dressing. The chevron is the most important step in dressing the catheter as this takes all pressures off the catheter and distributes them over the surface of the non-occlusive dressing.

Summary: Following the above taping procedure provides maximum protection against breakage and leakage as the catheter is completely protected from any outside influence most of the time. If for some reason beyond control, a patient manages to break a catheter it may be repaired using a GESCO Repair Kit, a blunt needle, or the catheter portion of a standard I.V. placement unit, e.g., Angio-Cath. See instructions in each tray for sizes.

The Product: The Per-Q-Cath is manufactured from medical grade "Silastic" tubing, the most bio-compatible material on the market today. The tubing will stretch to 300% of its original size and withstand over 100 psi. During the manufacturing process each catheter is leak tested under 40 psi while being stretched approximately 25% of its original length to insure integrity of the catheter.

Reprinted with permission of Gesco International, San Antonio, TX.

Box 19–15

Avoiding Problems with Your Per-Q-Cath: Catheter Develops a Leak After Being Used for a Period of Time

Problem 3: Catheter develops a leak after being used for a period of time.

Probable Causes:
1. Clamping with instruments, i.e., hemostats. Never use any type of clamping device with the Per-Q-Cath. The catheter should be bent and held with the fingers when changing extension sets or heparin locks.
2. Accidental cut from sharp instrument during dressing change.
3. Improper dressing, leaving the catheter exposed rather than completely covered with the non-occlusive dressing will invariably lead to catheter damage.
4. Over-pressure "blow out" caused from a small bore syringe, normally occurring when the catheter becomes occluded.

   A 1cc or tuberculin syringe can generate in excess of 160 psi while a 3cc can generate over 100 psi using normal thumb pressure. A sudden thrust can exaggerate these pressures causing the catheter to rupture. By using the largest syringe that is practical, for the situation, and using gentle pressures on the plunger, this problem can be minimized or eliminated.
5. Using too much declotting agent when attempting to declot a catheter can cause the catheter to rupture. The priming volume for each catheter is shown in the instructions packaged in each tray, and range between .04 ml. and .34 ml. By using only the priming volume indicated and using gentle pressures with larger syringes, this problem can be eliminated.

The Product: The Silastic material, from which the Per-Q-Cath is made, is unaffected by chemicals and medications and, therefore, will not stiffen or embrittle but will remain soft and compliant throughout the life of treatment. If the catheter is patent upon placement, and has been functional for a period of time, the clinician should look to one of the above reasons if the catheter has developed a leak.

Reprinted with permission of Gesco International, San Antonio, TX.

Box 19–16

Avoiding Problems with Your Per-Q-Cath: Catheter Develops a Leak After Placement

Problem 4:   Catheter develops a leak after placement.

Probable Cause: 1. Guidewire becomes bent during catheter placement, is hard to remove and damages catheter when attempting withdrawal.

Prevention: Please refer to previous discussion on guidewire placement and removal.

Probable Cause: 2. Catheter is nicked by introducer needle during placement. This normally occurs during a difficult placement and is caused by withdrawing the catheter or guidewire while needle is in patient.

Prevention: After advancing the catheter a short distance into the vein (4 or 5 inches), completely withdraw the introducer needle, remove from catheter and discard. Continue to advance the catheter thru the skin. The needle is used only for access into the vein and once in the vessel, the catheter will thread very easily thru the skin.

                   Removing the needle early when placing the catheter will also eliminate the possibility of catheter emboli.

The Product: With the testing performed during the manufacturing process, as mentioned previously, it is improbable that the catheter could leak without having been damaged during the insertion process. Prior to placement, any Per-Q-Cath, with or without guidewire, may be flushed to check for patency. The end of the catheter can also be pinched off to verify that there are no leaks.

Reprinted with permission of Gesco International, San Antonio, TX.

Box 19–17

Guidelines for Home Flushing of the Port-a-Cath and P.A.S. Port Systems

If you or a family member has been instructed to flush the PORT-A-CATH or P.A.S. PORT system at home between treatments, remember these guidelines:

- *ALWAYS* follow the recommended procedure for cleansing the injection site.
- *ALWAYS* use a properly sterilized PORT-A-CATH needle (its specially shaped point does not damage the portal septum).
- *ALWAYS* insert the needle at a 90° angle to the skin.
- *ALWAYS* make sure the needle is inside the portal chamber and against the bottom before starting the injection.
- *NEVER* tilt or rock the needle once it is inside the portal chamber.
- *NEVER* leave the syringe or any attached tubing open to the air while the needle is inside the portal.
- *ALWAYS* stop the injection and call your physician at once if the heparin does not flow freely.
- *ALWAYS* call your physician if you have any questions or problems, or notice changes in the appearance of the area around the injection site.

Reprinted with permission of Pharmacia Deltec, Inc., St. Paul, MN.

Box 19–18

Caring for Your Implanted Port

Note: There are many brands of implanted ports. Consult manufacturer's product information for specifications and instructions.

The port is a totally implanted device used for intermittent infusion of chemotherapy, blood components, or I.V. solutions, and for drawing blood samples. It allows you to be active but provides easy access to the circulatory system when it is time to administer the chemotherapy that has been ordered by your doctor. When therapy is to be given, you will make an appointment with your doctor and be seen in the office. Notify the home care nurse to have the infusion pump available.

You and your family will be taught to care for the port. If an infusion pump is necessary, you will learn to use that as well.

Home care nurse: _____ , R.N.
Phone number: _____
Special instructions:
_____
_____
_____
_____

Box 19–19

Flushing Your Port

You will need:
   Betadine swabsticks
   Heparin solution (100 units per ml), _____ ml
   Noncoring needle
   Transparent dressing
   Sterile gloves

Procedure

1. Palpate edges of port.
2. Cleanse site with Betadine swabsticks.
3. Draw up 5 ml of heparin solution into syringe.
4. Open needle and put on sterile gloves. Attach noncoring needle to syringe. Push heparin through just until you see a drop at the end.
5. Hold two fingers of one hand on edges of port; stick needle into port at 90° angle. You will feel some resistance and will feel the needle reach the back of the port.
6. Slowly flush port.

(If needle is to be left in place):

7. Cover the needle with transparent dressing or occlusive dressing. Fold a 2″ × 2″ gauze pad and place under needle hub to prevent pressure on the skin.

The needle should be changed once weekly *or* when the skin around the needle site becomes reddened. A transparent dressing should be applied so that the hub of the needle can be easily accessed to administer chemotherapy or I.V. solutions.

Box 19–20

Removing a Noncoring Needle from an Implanted Port

You will be taught how to remove the needle from the implanted port when the infusion is finished. If you prefer, you may return to the physician's office to have the needle removed.

You will need:

Betadine swabsticks

Small dressing (BandAid or 2" × 2" gauze pad and tape)

For irrigation (the doctor will order):

Normal saline and/or heparin

Alcohol swabs

Syringe and needle

If you are told to irrigate the port prior to taking the needle out, refer to the instructions for drawing up the syringe.

Irrigate with _____ ml of _____.

Irrigate with _____ ml of _____.

Close slide clamp on extension set (if no extension set, hold your breath any time nothing is connected to the noncoring needle). To irrigate, remove the pump tubing from the noncoring needle and remove the needle from the syringe. Attach the syringe to the noncoring needle and slowly push the fluid in. Leave syringe attached and follow the instructions given below for removing the needle.

To Remove the Needle

1. Locate the edges of the port.
2. Place the fingers of one hand on either side of the port.
3. With other hand, firmly grasp needle and pull straight out.
4. Clean area with Betadine swabsticks.
5. Apply dry sterile dressing for 24 hours.
6. Leave open to air after dressing is removed.

Box 19–21

Instructions for an Ambulatory Infusion Pump with an Implanted Port

You will be seen in the doctor's office, where the nurse will puncture the port using sterile procedures; then the infusion will be started, using the special tubing attached to the ambulatory infusion pump.

You will be taught to observe for the following:

1. The digital display on the pump shows the amount of medication that has been given.
2. Your pump should read as follows during your therapy (read the display at the same time every day, 24 hours after the start of the infusion and every 24 hours thereafter):

Day 1 _____
Day 2 _____
Day 3 _____
Day 4 _____
Day 5 _____

3. If this number is off by _____, notify the nurse or physician.
4. Be sure the tubing is not kinked when you place the pump back into the zippered case after checking it.

Home care nurse: _____, R.N.
Phone number: _____
Special instructions:

_____

_____

Box 19–22

Sample Instructions for the Client with an Infusaid Pump

1. Avoid traumatic physical activity where the tissues adjoining the implant site may be damaged.
2. Consult your physician for dose rate changes before moving to a different altitude or embarking on long-distance air travel, since the flow rate of the pump will vary with altitude changes.
3. Avoid long, hot baths, extended exposure to saunas, or other activities that might alter pump temperature and, therefore, flow rate. Consult your physician if a febrile illness occurs.
4. Consult your physician for any unusual symptom or sign related to the specific drug you are receiving.
5. It is most important that fluid be maintained in the pump at all times. Refill appointments must be kept.
6. Notify your personal physician or consulting physician that you have an implanted pump so that appropriate precautions may be taken during a medical emergency.

Reprinted with permission of Strato Infusaid, Norwood, MA.

Box 19–23

Client Instructions: P.A.S. Port

What does a P.A.S. Port look like?
The P.A.S. Port (Fig. 1) consists of a portal (a small metal chamber), sealed at the top with a septum made of self-sealing silicone and the P.A.S. Port catheter (a thin, flexible tube). The unit is placed under your skin, with the portal near a vein in your arm. The tip of the catheter is advanced through the vein to a larger vein just above the heart.

How does the system work?
To access the system, a needle is inserted through the skin over the septum (Fig. 2). As the medicine is injected from the syringe into the port, it flows into the septum, up the thin tube in your vein, and is delivered into the bloodstream just above the heart. As your heart pumps, the medication is circulated to the areas where it is needed.

If you administer a bolus medication (all at one time), the needle is removed after the medication is given. If medication administered is from an I.V. bag over a period of time, the needle must remain in place until you have received all the medication or I.V. fluid.

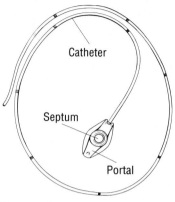

Figure 1. P.A.S. Port venous system

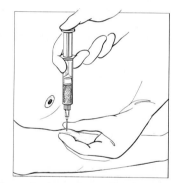

Figure 2. Accessing a P.A.S. Port venous system

(From *Patient Information: Port-A-Cath and P.A.S. Port Implantable Access Systems.* St. Paul, MN, Pharmacia Deltec, 1991. Illustrations reprinted with permission.)

References

Knowles, M.S.: *The Adult Learner: A Neglected Species.* Houston, Gulf Publishing, 1978.

Larson, P.J.: Important nurse caring behaviors perceived by patients with cancer. Oncol. Nurs. Forum 2(6):46–50, 1984.

Leininger, M.: *Caring: An Essential Human Need: Proceedings of Three National Caring Conferences.* Thorofare, NJ, Charles B. Slack, 1981.

Levine, A.M., et al.: Compliance with oral drug therapy in patients with hematologic malignancy. J. Clin. Oncol. 5:1469–1476, 1987.
Mayer, D.: Cancer patients' and families' perceptions of nurse caring behaviors. Top. Clin. Nurs. 8(2):63–69, 1986.
Yarbro, C.H.: Nursing implications in the administration of cancer chemotherapy. In Perry, M.C. (ed.): The Chemotherapy Source Book (pp. 873–883). Baltimore, Williams & Wilkins, 1992.

Recommended Readings

Brown, J.M.: Home care models for infusion therapy. Caring 9(5):24–26, 1990.
Coker, M., and Lampert, A.: Teaching checklist for home infusion therapy. Oncol. Nurs. Forum 17:923–926, 1990.
Demuth, J.S.: Patient teaching in the ambulatory care setting. Nurs. Clin. North Am. 24:645–654, 1989.
Dodd, M.J., Dibble, S.L., and Thomas, M.L.: Outpatient chemotherapy: Patients' and family members' concerns and coping strategies. Public Health Nurse 9:37–44, 1992.
Fernsler, J.I., and Cannon, C.A.: The whys of patient education. Semin. Oncol. Nurs. 7:79–86, 1991.
Goodman, M.: External venous catheters: Home management. Oncol. Nurs. Forum 15: 357–360, 1988.
Hiromoto, B.M., and Dungan, J.: Contract learning for self-care activities: A protocol among chemotherapy outpatients. Cancer Nurs. 14:148–154, 1991.
Howser, D.M., and Meade, C.D.: Hickman Broviac care: Developing organized teaching strategies. Cancer Nurs. 10:70–76, 1987.
Johnson, M.H., and Rhodes, V.A.: Patient education. In Perry, M.C. (ed.): The Chemotherapy Source Book (pp. 853–872). Baltimore, Williams & Wilkins, 1992.
Johnson, J.B., and Blumberg, B.D.: Teaching strategies: Patient education. In Groenwald, S.L., et al. (eds.): Cancer Nursing: Principles and Practice, 3rd ed. (pp. 1576–1586). Boston, Jones and Bartlett, 1993.
Lynch, M., and Yanes, L.: Flowsheet documentation of chemotherapy administration and patient teaching. Oncol. Nurs. Forum 18:777–783, 1991.
McCaffrey, D.: To teach or not to teach? Overcoming barriers to patient education in geriatric oncology. Oncol. Nurs. Forum 13(4):25–31, 1986.
Morra, M.E.: Developing strategies for patient education in cancer. In Baird, S.B., McCorkle, R., and Grant, M. (eds.): Cancer Nursing: A Comprehensive Textbook (pp. 944–956). Philadelphia, W.B. Saunders, 1991.
Nail, L.M., et al.: Use and perceived efficacy of self-care activities in patients receiving chemotherapy. Oncol. Nurs. Forum 18:883–887, 1991.
Nieweg, R., Greidanus, J., and de Vries, E.G.E.: A patient education program for a continuous infusion regimen on an outpatient basis. Cancer Nurs. 10:177–182, 1987.
Oncology Nursing Society: Outcome Standards for Cancer Patient Education. Pittsburgh, Oncology Nursing Society, 1982.
Reiger, P.T., and Rumsey, K.: Responding to the educational needs of patients receiving biotherapy. In The Biotherapy of Cancer-V: Proceedings of a Symposium (pp. 10–15). Pittsburgh: Oncology Nursing Press, 1992.
Reville, B., and Almadrones, L.: Continuous infusion chemotherapy in the ambulatory setting: The nurse's role in patient selection and education. Oncol. Nurs. Forum 16: 529–535, 1989.
Ruzicki, D.A.: Realistically meeting the educational needs of hospitalized acute and short-stay patients. Nurs. Clin. North Am. 23:629–637, 1989.

Somerville, E.T.: Knowledge deficit related to chemotherapy. In McNally, J.C., et al. (eds.): *Guidelines for Oncology Nursing Practice* (pp. 57–61). Philadelphia, W.B. Saunders, 1991.

Tripp-Reimer, T.: Cross-cultural perspectives on patient teaching. Nurs. Clin. North Am. 23:613–619, 1989.

Villejo, L., et al.: Strategies for cancer patient education: Overcoming barriers. Cancer Bull. 40:365–369, 1988.

Stevenson, E., and Crosson, K.: Patient education: History, development and future directions of the American Cancer Society and the National Cancer Institutes. Semin. Oncol. 7:134–142, 1992.

Welch-McCaffrey, D.: Evolving patient education needs in cancer. Oncol. Nurs. Forum 12(5):62–66, 1985.

Resources for the Nurse and Client

Chemotherapeutic Agents and Biologic Response Modifiers

GENERIC NAME	TRADE NAME	DISTRIBUTOR*
Aldesleukin	Proleukin	Cetus
Altretamine	Hexalen	U.S. Bioscience
Amsacrine	AMSA PD†	Parke-Davis
Aminoglutethimide	Cytadren	CIBA
Asparaginase	Elspar (U.S.)	Merck
	Kidrolase‡	Rhone-Poulenc Rorer
Bacillus Calmette-Guérin (BCG)	Theracys	Connaught
Bleomycin sulfate	Blenoxane	Bristol-Myers Squibb
Busulfan	Myleran	Burroughs Wellcome
Carboplatin	Paraplatin	Bristol-Myers Squibb
	Carboplatin	David Bull (Canada)
Carmustine (BCNU)	BiCNU	Bristol-Myers Squibb
Chlorambucil	Leukeran	Burroughs Wellcome
Cisplatin	Platinol	Bristol-Myers Squibb
	Platinol-AQ	Bristol-Myers Squibb
	Cisplatin	David Bull (Canada)
	Cisplatin	Frank W. Horner (Canada)
Cladribine	Leustatin	Ortho-Biotech
Conjugated estrogens	Premarin	Wyeth-Ayerst
Cyclophosphamide	Cytoxan	Bristol-Myers Squibb
	Neosar (U.S.)	Pharmacia Adria
	Procytox‡	Frank W. Horner (Canada)
Cyproterone acetate	Androcur†	Berlex (Canada)
Cytarabine (cytosine arabinoside)	Cytarabine	Chiron
	Cytarabine	David Bull (Canada)
	Cytarabine	Quad
	Cytosar-U	Upjohn
	Tarabine PFS	Pharmacia Adria

(Continued)

GENERIC NAME	TRADE NAME	DISTRIBUTOR*
Dacarbazine	DTIC-Dome (U.S.)	Miles
	DTIC (Canada)	Miles
Dactinomycin	Cosmegen	Merck
Daunorubicin	Cerubidine	Wyeth-Ayerst (U.S.)
	Cerubidine	Rhone-Poulenc Rorer (Canada)
Dexamethasone	Dalalone	Forest
	Decadron	Merck
	Dexamethasone	LyphoMed
	Hexadrol	Organon
Diethylstilbestrol diphosphate	Honvol‡	Frank W. Horner (Canada)
	Stilphostrol	Miles
Doxorubicin	Adriamycin PFS	Pharmacia Adria
	Adriamycin RDF	Pharmacia Adria
	Doxorubicin	Chiron
	Rubex	Immunex
Epoetin Alfa	Epogen	Amgen
	Procrit	Ortho-Biotec
Estramustine phosphate	Emcyt	Pharmacia Adria
Etoposide (VP-16)	VePesid	Bristol-Myers Squibb
Filgrastim, granulocyte-colony-stimulating factor (G-CSF)	Neupogen	Amgen
Floxuridine	FUDR	Roche
Fludarabine phosphate	Fludara	Berlex
5-Fluorouracil	Adrucil‡	Pharmacia Adria (Canada)
	Fluorouracil	Chiron
	Fluorouracil	David Bull (Canada)
	Fluorouracil	LyphoMed
	Fluorouracil	Roche
	Fluorouracil	Quad
Topical form:	Efudex	Roche Dermatologicals
	Fluoroplex	Allergan Herbert
Fluoxymesterone	Halotestin	Upjohn
Flutamide	Eulexin	Schering
Goserein acetate	Zoladex	Zeneca
Hydrocortisone	Hydrocortone	Merck
	Solu-Cortef	Upjohn
Hydroxyurea	Hydrea	Immunex
Idarubicin	Idamycin	Pharmacia Adria
Ifosfamide	Ifex	Bristol-Myers Squibb
Interferon alfa-2a, recombinant	Roferon-A	Roche

GENERIC NAME	TRADE NAME	DISTRIBUTOR*
Interferon alfa-2b, recombinant	Intron A	Schering
Leucovorin calcium for injection	Leucovorin Wellcovorin	Immunex Burroughs Wellcome
Leucovorin calcium tablets	Leucovorin Wellcovorin	Immunex Burroughs Wellcome
Leuprolide acetate	Lupron Injection Lupron Depot	TAP Pharmaceuticals TAP Pharmaceuticals
Levamisole	Ergamisol	Janssen Pharmaceutica
Lomustine (CCNU)	CeeNU	Bristol-Myers Squibb
Mechlorethamine, HN2, nitrogen mustard	Mustargen	Merck
Megestrol acetate	Megace	Bristol-Myers Squibb
Melphalan	Alkeran	Burroughs Wellcome
Mercaptopurine	Purinethol	Burroughs Wellcome
Mesna	Mesnex (U.S.) Uromitexan‡ (Canada)	Bristol-Myers Squibb Bristol-Myers Squibb
Methotrexate	Folex PFS Methotrexate Methotrexate Methotrexate Methotrexate LPF	Pharmacia Adria Chiron David Bull (Canada) Immunex Immunex
Methylprednisolone	Medrol Solu-Medrol	Upjohn Upjohn
Methyltestosterone	Oreton Methyl Testred	Schering ICN
Mitomycin-C	Mutamycin	Bristol-Myers Squibb
Mitotane	Lysodren	Bristol-Myers Squibb
Mitoxantrone	Novantone	Immunex
Paclitaxel	Taxol	Bristol-Myers Squibb
Pentostatin	Nipent	Parke-Davis
Plicamycin	Mithracin	Miles
Prednisolone	Delta-Cortef	Upjohn
Prednisone	Deltasone	Upjohn
Procarbazine	Matulane (U.S.) Natulan‡	Roche Hoffman–La Roche
Sargramostin (human recombinant GM-CSF)	Leukine Prokine	Immunex Hoechst

(Continued)

GENERIC NAME	TRADE NAME	DISTRIBUTOR*
Streptozocin	Zanosar	Upjohn
Tamoxifen citrate	Apo-Tamox‡	Apotex (Canada)
	Alpha-Tamoxifen‡	Genpharm (Canada)
	Nolvadex	Zeneca
	Nolvadex-D‡	Zeneca (Canada)
	Tamofen‡	Rhone-Poulenc Rorer (Canada)
	Tamone‡	Pharmacia Adria (Canada)
Teniposide	Vumon	Bristol-Myers Squibb
Testolactone	Teslac	Bristol-Myers Squibb
Testosterone cypionate	DepoTestosterone	Upjohn
	Virilon IM	Star
Thioguanine	Thioguanine (U.S.)	Burroughs Wellcome
	Lanvis‡	Burroughs Wellcome
Thiotepa	Thiotepa	Immunex
Vinblastine	Velban (U.S.)	Lilly
	Velbe‡	Lilly
	Vinblastine	Chiron
	Vinblastine	David Bull (Canada)
	Vinblastine	LyphoMed
Vincristine	Oncovin	Lilly
	Vincasar PFS	Pharmacia Adria
	Vincristine	David Bull (Canada)
	Vincristine	LyphoMed
Vindesine sulfate	Eldisine†	Lilly

*For distributors' addresses, see Appendix B.
†Available commercially in Canada; investigational in the United States.
‡Available in Canada only.

Manufacturers and Distributors of Chemotherapeutic Agents and Related Pharmaceuticals—United States and Canada

Author's note: Noncytotoxic agents used to treat symptoms in clients receiving chemotherapy and biotherapy are denoted by an asterisk. All medications are available in the United States and Canada unless indicated otherwise.

Allergan Herbert
Skin Care Division of Allergan, Inc.
2525 DuPont Drive
P.O. Box 19534
Irvine, CA 92713–9534
(714) 752–4500
(800) 347–4500
In Canada:
Allergan Canada
110 Cochrane Drive
Markham, Ont. L3R 951
(416) 940–7180
Fluoroplex topical solution and cream 1%* (fluorouracil)

Amgen, Incorporated
Amgen Center
Thousand Oaks, CA 91320–1789
(818) 499–5725
FAX: (818) 865–3707
(800) 888–7407
Epogen for injection (epoetin alpha)
Neupogen for injection (filgrastim)

Ayerst Laboratories
1025 Laurentian Boulevard
St. Laurent, QC H4R 1J6
Premarin (I.V., P.O.)—Canada

*NOTE: Used in treating *precancerous* lesions (actinic keratosis), not used for cancer therapy.

Berlex Laboratories, Inc.
15049 San Pablo Avenue
P.O. Box 4099
Richmond, CA 94804–0099
(800) 888–4112
In Canada:
2260 32 Avenue
Lachine, QC H8T 3H4
(514) 631–7400
FAX: (514) 636–9177
(800) 321–0288
    Fludara (fludarabine)

Bristol-Myers Oncology Division
A Bristol-Myers Squibb Company
P.O. Box 4500
Princeton, NJ 08543–4500
(609) 897–2126
FAX: (609) 897–6010
(800) 321–1335
In Canada:
Bristol-Myers Squibb of Canada
2365 Côte de Lisse Street
Montreal, QC H4N 2M7
(514) 333–3200
FAX: (514) 252–5855
(800) 267–1088
    BiCNU (carmustine)
    Blenoxane (bleomycin)
    CeeNU (lomustine)
    Cytoxan (cyclophosphamide)
        tablets
    Cytoxan (cyclophosphamide) for
        injection
    Ifex (ifosfamide)
    Lysodren (mitotane)
    Mesnex (mesna)*—U.S. only
    Paclitaxel (Taxol)
    Paraplatin (carboplatin)
    Platinol-AQ (cisplatin)
    Teslac (testolactone)—U.S. only
    Uromitexan (mesna)*—Canada
        only
    VePesid (etoposide) capsules
    VePesid (etoposide) for injection
    Vumon (teniposide)—Canada
        only

Burroughs Wellcome Company
Drug Information Department
3030 Cornwallis Road
Research Triangle Park, NC 27709
(919) 248–3000
(800) 443–6763

Burroughs Wellcome Inc.
16751 Transcanada Highway
Kirkland, QC H9H 4J4
(514) 630–7002
FAX: (514) 694–8201
    Alkeran (melphalan) tablets
    Alkeran (melphalan) for injection
    Lanvis (thioguanine)
    Leukeran (chlorambucil)
    Leucovorin for injection
    Leucovorin tablets
    Myleran (busulfan)
    Purinethol (6-mercaptopurine)
    Thioguanine
    Zyloprim (allopurinol)*

Chiron Therapeutics
4560 Horton Street
Emeryville, CA 94608–2997
FAX: (510) 420–4855
(800) 733–7025
    Doxorubicin
    Leucovorin calcium
    Metoclopramide*
    Methotrexate
    Proleukin (aldesleukin, human re-
        combinant interleukin-2)
    Vinblastine

CIBA Pharmaceutical Company
A Division of Ciba-Geigy Corpo-
    ration
555 Morris Avenue
Summit, NJ 07901
(201) 277–5000

CIBA Pharmaceuticals
A Division of Ciba-Geigy Canada
    Ltd.
6860 Century Avenue
Mississauga, Ont. L5N 2W5
(416) 821–4420
FAX: (416) 821–9815
    Cytadren (aminoglutethimide)

Connaught Laboratories, Inc.
Swiftwater, PA 18370
(717) 839–4235
1755 Steeles Avenue W.
Willowdale, Ont. L5N 2M6
(416) 667–2701
    TheraCys (BCG live-intravesical)

David Bull Laboratories (Canada), Inc.
334 Aimé-Vincent
Vaudreuil, QC J7V 5V5
(514) 424–0490
FAX: (514) 424–0490
(800) 567–2855
Carboplatin—Canada only
Cisplatin—Canada only
Cytarabine—Canada only
5-Fluorouracil—Canada only
Methotrexate—Canada only
Vinblastine sulfate—Canada only
Vincristine sulfate—Canada only

Fujisawa Pharmaceutical Corporation
3 Parkway North
Deerfield, IL 60015–2548
(800) 727–7003
Ganite injection (gallium nitrate injection)*
Pentam (pentamidine)

Hoffman–La Roche Limited
(In U.S., see Roche Laboratories)
2445 Meadowpine Boulevard
Mississauga, Ont. L5N 6L7
(905) 542–5555
FAX: (905) 542–5678
(800) 268–0440—except Newfoundland
Newfoundland: (800) 563–6037
Efudex cream (5-Fluorouracil)—Canada only
5-Fluorouracil—Canada only
Natulan (procarbazine)—Canada only
Roferon-A (interferon alfa-2a, recombinant)—Canada only
Versed (midazolam HCl)*—Canada only

Frank W. Horner, Inc.
5485 Ferrier Street
Ville-Mont-Royal, QC H4P 1M6
(514) 731–3931
FAX: (514) 738–4124
Honvol (diethylstilbestrol)—Canada only
Procytox (cyclophosphamide)—Canada only

ICI Pharma (see Zeneca Pharmaceuticals)

Immunex Corporation
51 University Street
Seattle, WA 98101
(206) 587–0430
FAX: (206) 223–5525
FAX: (800) 221–6820
(800) IMMUNEX (800–466–8639)
Hydrea (hydroxyurea)
Leucovorin (leucovorin calcium) for injection
Leukine (sargramostim, GM-CSF)
Methotrexate (methotrexate) tablets
Methotrexate (methotrexate sodium) parenteral
Methotrexate LFP (methotrexate LFP sodium) parenteral
Novantrone (mitoxantrone)
Rubex (doxorubicin)
Thiotepa (thiotepa)

Janssen Pharmaceutica, Inc.
1125 Trenton-Harbourton Road
P.O. Box 200
Titusville, NJ 08560–0200
(609) 730–2000
FAX: (609) 730–3044
(800) 253–3682
In Canada:
6705 Millcreek Drive Unit #1
Mississauga, Ont. L5N 5R9
(416) 567–2524
FAX: (416) 821–9427
Ergamisol (levamisol)
Inapsine (droperidol)*

Lederle Cyanamid Canada
88 McNabb Street
Markham, Ont. L3R 3E6
(416) 470–3600
Leucovorin (leucovorin calcium) for injection—Canada only
Methotrexate (methotrexate) tablets—Canada only
Methotrexate (methotrexate sodium) parenteral—Canada only
Methotrexate LFP (methotrexate LFP sodium) parenteral—Canada only
Novantrone (mitoxantrone)—Canada only
Thiotepa (thiotepa)—Canada only

Eli Lilly and Company
Lilly Corporate Center
Indianapolis, IN 46285
(317) 276–3714

Eli Lilly Canada, Inc.
3560 Danforth Avenue
Scarborough, Ont. M1N 2E8
(416) 694–3221
   Eldisine (vindesine sulfate)—
     Canada (investigational in
     U.S.)
   Oncovin (vincristine)
   Velban (vinblastine)—U.S. only
   Velbe (vinblastine)—Canada
     only

LyphoMed Division
Division of Fujisawa USA, Inc.
3 Parkway North Center
Deerfield, IL 60015–2548
(800) 727–7003
In Canada:
LyphoMed Canada
   Dacarbazine
   Dexamethasone
   Droperidol for injection*—U.S.
     only
   Fluorouracil
   Metoclopramide for injection*
   Nandrolone decanoate*
   Vinblastine
   Vincristine

Mead Johnson Pharmaceuticals
(same address and phone as Bristol-
  Meyers Squibb Company)
   Estrace (estradiol)

Merck and Company, Inc.
West Point, PA 19486–9989
(215) 652–7300
In Canada:
P.O. Box 1005
Pointe-Claire-Dorval, QC H9R 4P8
(514) 695–7920
FAX: (514) 630–2670
   Cortone sterile suspension,
     tablets
   Cosmegen (dactinomycin)
   Decadron (dexamethasone) tab-
     lets and injection
   Elspar (L-asparaginase)—U.S.
     only
   Mustargen (nitrogen mustard)

**Miles Inc., Pharmaceutical
Division**
400 Morgan Lane
West Haven, CT 06516
(203) 937–2000
(800) 468–0894

Miles Canada, Inc.
77 Belfield Road
Etobicoke, Ont. M9W 1G6
(416) 248–0771
(416) 248–9526
   DTIC-Dome (dacarbazine)
   Mithracin (plicamycin)
   Stilphostrol (diethylstilbestrol di-
     phosphate)

Organon Inc.
375 Mount Pleasant Avenue
West Orange, NJ 07052
(201) 325–4500
   BCG Vaccine Tice, USP

Ortho-Biotech
P.O. Box 300
Raritan, NJ 08869–0602
(800) 433–1015
   Leustatin (cladarabine)
   Procrit (epoetin alfa)

Parke-Davis
Division of Warner-Lambert
  Company
201 Tabor Road
Morris Plains, NJ 07950
(201) 540–2000
FAX: (201) 540–2248
(800) 223–0432
In Canada:
2300 Eglington East
Scarborough, Ont. M1L 2N2
(416) 288–2200
   AMSA-PD (Amsacrine)—Canada
     (investigational in U.S.)
   Nipent (pentostatin)

**Pharmacia Adria Laboratories
(formerly Adria Laboratories)**
Medical Services Department
P.O. Box 16529
Columbus, OH 43216–6529
(614) 764–8100
FAX: (614) 764–1802
(800) 729–2902

In Canada:
2280 Argentia Road
Mississauga, Ont. L5N 6H8
(416) 858–1144
  Adrucil (5-fluorouracil)—Canada
  Adriamycin PFS (doxorubicin)
  Adriamycin RDF (doxorubicin)
  Emcyt (estramustine phosphate
    sodium)
  Folex PFS (methotrexate)
  Idamycin (idarubicin)
  Neosar (cyclophosphamide)
  Tarabine PFS (cytarabine)

Roche Dermatologicals
Nutley, NJ 07110
(201) 812–2000
(800) 526–6367
  Efudex cream
  Efudex solutions

Roche Laboratories
Nutley, NJ 07110
(201) 235–5000
(800) 526–6367
  Fluorouracil injection
  Matulane (procarbazine)
  Roferon-A Injection (interferon
    alfa-2a, recombinant)

Schering Corporation
Galloping Hill Road
Kenilworth, NJ 07033
(908) 298–4000
(800) 526–4099

Schering Canada, Inc.
3535 Transcanada Highway
Pointe-Claire, QC H9R 1B4
(514) 426–7300
  Eulexin (flutamide)—U.S. only
  Euflex (flutamide)—Canada only
  Intron A (interferon alfa-2b, re-
    combinant)

TAP Pharmaceuticals
2355 Waukeegan Road
Deerfield, IL 60015
(800) 622–2011

In Canada:
6300 Côte de Lisse Road
Montreal, QC H4T 1Z1
(514) 340–7100
  Lupron (leuprolide acetate)
  Lupron Depot (leuprolide acetate
    depot suspension)

U.S. Bioscience Incorporated
One Tower Bridge
West Conshohocken, PA 19428
(215) 832–4504
FAX: (215) 832–4552
(800) 447–3969
  Hexalen (altretamine)

Wyeth-Ayerst Laboratories
P.O. Box 8299
Philadelphia, PA 19101
(215) 688–4400
  Ativan (lorazepam) for injection*
  Ativan (lorazepam) tablets*
  Benadryl (diphenhydramine hy-
    drochloride)*
  Cerubidine (daunorubicin)
  Phenergan (promethazine hydro-
    chloride)*
  Prochlorperazine*
  Premarin (conjugated estrogens)
    for injection
  Premarin (conjugated estrogens)
    tablets

Zeneca Pharmaceuticals
(formerly ICI Pharma)
Wilmington, DE 19897
(302) 886–2231
In Canada:
2505 Meadowvale Boulevard
Mississauga, Ont. L5N 5R7
(416) 821–8000
(800) 268–3992
  Nolvadex (tamoxifen citrate)
  Nolvadex-D (tamoxifen citrate)—
    Canada only
  Zoladex (goserlin acetate im-
    plant)

Comprehensive Cancer Centers

Alabama

Comprehensive Cancer Center
University of Alabama at
  Birmingham
University Station
1824 Sixth Avenue South
Birmingham, AL 35294–3300
(205) 934–5077

Arizona

Comprehensive Cancer Center
University of Arizona
1501 North Campbell Avenue
Tucson, AZ 85724
(602) 626–6372

California

Comprehensive Cancer Center
University of Southern California
P.O. Box 33804
1441 Eastlake Avenue
Los Angeles, CA 90033–0804
(213) 224–6416

Jonsson Comprehensive Cancer
  Center
UCLA Medical Center
100 UCLA Plaza, Suite 255
Los Angeles, CA 90024–1781
(800) 825–2631

Connecticut

Comprehensive Cancer Center
Yale University
205 William Wirt Winchester
P.O. Box 3333
New Haven, CT 06510–8028
(203) 785–4098

District of Columbia

Vincent T. Lombardi Cancer Research Center
Georgetown University Medical
  Center
3800 Reservoir Road N.W.
Washington, DC 20007–2197
(202) 687–2110

Howard University Cancer Research Center
2041 Georgia Avenue N.W.
Washington, DC 20060
(202) 636–7610 or 636–5665

Florida

Sylvester Comprehensive Cancer
  Center
University of Miami Medical Center
1475 N.W. 12th Avenue
Miami, FL 33136
(305) 545–1000

Maryland

Johns Hopkins Oncology Center
600 North Wolfe Street, Room 157
Baltimore, MD 21205
(301) 955–8638

Massachusetts

Dana Farber Cancer Institute
44 Binney Street
Boston, MA 02115
(617) 732–3323

Michigan

Meyer L. Prentis Comprehensive
   Cancer Center of Metropolitan
   Detroit
110 East Warren Avenue
Detroit, MI 48201
(313) 833–1088

Minnesota

Mayo Comprehensive Cancer
   Center
Mayo Clinic
200 First Street S.W.
Rochester, MN 55905
(507) 284–3413

New Hampshire

Norris Cotton Cancer Center
Dartmouth-Hitchcock Medical
   Center
2 Maynard Street
Hanover, NH 03756
(603) 646–5505

New York

Columbia University Cancer Center
College of Physicians and Surgeons
630 West 168th Street
New York, NY 10032
(212) 305–6730

Kaplan Cancer Center
New York University Medical
   Center
462 First Avenue
New York, NY 10016–9103
(212) 263–6485

Memorial Sloan-Kettering Cancer
   Center
1275 York Avenue
New York, NY 10021
(212) 794–7177
(800) 525–2225

Roswell Park Cancer Institute
Elm and Carlton Streets
Buffalo, NY 14263
(716) 845–2300
(800) ROSWELL (800–767–9355)

North Carolina

Duke University Comprehensive
   Cancer Center
P.O. Box 3843
Durham, NC 27710
(919) 684–6342 or 286–5515

UNC Lineberger Comprehensive
   Cancer Center
University of North Carolina School
   of Medicine
Chapel Hill, NC 27599
(919) 748–4354

Ohio

Ohio State University Comprehensive Cancer Center
Arthur C. James Cancer Hospital
410 West 10th Avenue
Columbus, OH 43210
(614) 293–8619
(800) 638–6966

Pennsylvania

Fox Chase Center
7701 Burholme Avenue
Philadelphia, PA 19111
(215) 728–6900

University of Pennsylvania Cancer
   Center
7 Silverstein Pavillion
3400 Spruce Street/HUP
Philadelphia, PA 19104–4283
(215) 662–3910

Pittsburgh Cancer Institute
200 Meyran Avenue
Pittsburgh, PA 15213–2592
(800) 537–4063

Texas

University of Texas M.D. Anderson
Cancer Center
1515 Holcombe Boulevard
Houston, TX 77030
(713) 792–6161

Vermont

Vermont Cancer Center
University of Vermont
1 South Prospect Street
Burlington, VT 05401
(802) 656–4580

Washington

Fred Hutchinson Cancer Research
Center
1124 Columbia Street
Seattle, WA 98104
(206) 467–4675

Wisconsin

University of Wisconsin Comprehensive Cancer Center
600 Highland Avenue
Madison, WI 53792
(608) 263–8090

Resources for Clients with Cancer

American Brain Tumor Association (ABTA)
2720 River Road
Suite 146
Des Plaines, IL 60018
(708) 827–9910
FAX: (708) 827–9918
Patient line: (800) 886–2282
A national organization providing free information for patients about brain tumors and their treatment. Services include patient education materials, listings of brain tumor support groups, referrals to support organizations, and information about treatment facilities. Their newsletter, *The Message Line*, published three times a year, describes research advances and publications.

American Cancer Society (ACS)
1599 Clifton Road, N.E.
Atlanta, GA 30329
In Atlanta, (404) 320–3333 (general information)
(404) 329–7616 (Department of Nursing)
From other regions, (800) ACS–2345 (227–2345)
Local branches—see the white pages of phone directory.
A voluntary organization offering information, counseling, guidance, sickroom supplies, and client transportation to hospital or treatment center for therapy. Offers professional education programs (local, regional, and national) and scholarships for Master's degree and doctoral students in Oncology Nursing. Support groups: CanSurmount, I Can Cope, International Association of Laryngectomees, and Reach to Recovery. Services may vary in specific region. Contact your local branch for further information.

American Foundation for Urologic Disease
300 West Pratt Street, Suite 401
Baltimore, MD 21201–2463
FAX: (410) 242–2383
(800) 828–7866
Provides educational materials for the public, patients, and professionals about all aspects of urologic diseases, including cancers. Services include patient education materials, the US TOO prostate cancer support groups, and the Bladder Health Council and Prostate Health Council. Quarterly publication: *Foundation Focus.*

Camps for Children with Cancer
Note: There are more than 60 summer camps in 36 states and Canada. Some are day camps; most offer 1- or 2-week overnight camp experiences. Many are free and are staffed by medical and/or nursing personnel; some administer chemotherapy if it is needed. For further information contact:
Children's Oncology Camps of America, Inc.
Children's Memorial Hospital
2300 Children's Plaza
Chicago, IL 60614
or the American Cancer Society at (800) ACS–2345

Canadian Cancer Society (CCS)
10 Alcorn Avenue
Suite 200
Toronto, Ont. MV4 3B1
(416) 961–7223
A lay organization offering information and counseling for persons with cancer and their families. May provide some financial assistance, sickroom supplies, and transportation for client and family to nearby hospital or cancer center. Plans professional conferences, awards fellowships for nurses and other health care personnel. Supports cancer research by diverting approximately half of total annual expenditure to the National Cancer Institute of Canada (NCIC). Sponsors support groups, including CanSurmount, Living with Cancer (Coping With Cancer in some divisions), and Reach to Recovery. Services may vary in 10 divisions (provinces). Contact your local branch for further information.

Canadian Palliative Care Association
c/o Manitoba Hospital Foundation
2109 Portage Avenue
Winnipeg, Manitoba R3J 0L3
(514) 843–1542
An independent national organization consisting of groups providing palliative care and others concerned with the care of terminally ill clients and their families or significant others.

Cancer Care, Inc.
1180 Avenue of the Americas
New York, NY 10036
(212) 221–3300
Contact: Priscilla Hartung, ACSW
Director of Social Services
(212) 302–2400

In New Jersey: 241 Milburn Avenue, Suite 241-C, Millburn, NJ 07041
(201) 379–7500, 141 Dayton Street, Ridgewood, NJ 07450 (201) 444–6630
On Long Island: 20 Crossways Park North, Suite 304, Woodbury, NY 11797
(516) 364–8130
Suffolk County office: 2855 Pond Road, Ronkonkoma, NY 11779
(516) 737–1836
In Connecticut: 120 East Avenue, Norwalk, CT 06851 (203) 854–9911
A nonprofit, nonsectarian social service agency founded in 1944 to help clients and their families and friends cope with the impact of cancer. Provides planning and counseling services for clients and families, psychosocial guidance, public education, social research, referral services, and work-site counseling and consultation services. Services are available free of charge to clients and their families at all stages of their illness.

Cancer Information Services (Canada)
Ontario region only: (800) 263–6750
Provides information about cancer, therapies, and resources for clients with cancer. In other provinces, contact the local branch of the Canadian Cancer Society (CCS).

Cancer Information Service (United States)
National Cancer Institute
Blair Building, Room 414
Bethesda, MD 20892–4200
(800) 4–CANCER (422–6237)
In Oahu, Hawaii, dial 524–1234 (from neighboring islands call collect)
Regional offices provide information about cancer, therapies, and sources of care for clients, families, professionals, and the general public. Trained staff and volunteers provide confidential answers to cancer-related questions. Will mail appropriate literature and answer questions. Spanish-speaking staff members are available in CA, FL, GA, IL, northern NJ, New York City, and TX.

The Candlelighters Childhood Cancer Foundation
7910 Woodmont Avenue
Suite 460
Bethesda, MD 20814
(301) 657–8401
(800) 366–2223
In Canada:
10 Alcorn Avenue
Suite 200
Toronto, Ont. M4V 3B1
(416) 926–1374
A nonprofit educational and support organization for families of children with cancer, survivors of childhood cancer, and professionals who work with them. The foundation maintains a network of over 400 peer support groups throughout the world; publishes newsletters and handbooks; answers requests for information through its Information Clearinghouse; and helps members experiencing discrimination in employment, education, or insurance. Local groups provide meetings at which parents (and, in many groups, children and teens) can exchange information and socialize. Groups also provide other services such as parent visitation, help with transportation, speakers, and conferences to educate the community. The Washington, DC, chapter is a registered lobbyist and monitors legislation and federal programs affecting members. Candlelighters' services are provided free of charge.

CanSurmount (contact via local ACS or CCS chapter)
A one-to-one limited-term visitation program for clients, family members, and significant others. Visitation is done by a trained volunteer who has had a personal experience with cancer and who is carefully selected, trained, and supervised by the American Cancer Society. Volunteer visitors provide emotional support and an outlet to voice fears and anxieties. Attempt is made to match client and visitor by age, sex, type and site of cancer, and other factors that might contribute to mutual understanding and ease of communication. Similar pairing is done when matching family members.

Children's Hospice International
901 Washington Street
Alexandria, VA 22314
(703) 684–0330
(800) 242–4453
A voluntary organization that acts as an international clearinghouse for information relating to care of the terminally ill child and his or her family. Provides lay information about terminal illness. Sponsors national, regional, and local seminars for health care professionals, volunteers, and families. Develops educational and training information for health care providers and assists in planning conferences, including provision of speakers. Serves as consultant for implementation of children's hospice programs. Publishes *Children's Hospice International Newsletter* quarterly. Membership open to terminally ill children and their families, health care professionals, and other interested persons; annual membership fee is $25.00.

Choice in Dying
200 Varick Street
New York, NY 10014–4810
(212) 366–5540
FAX: (212) 366–5337
(800) 989–WILL (989–9455)
A nonprofit educational organization that provides information about the "Living Will," advance planning for end-of-life care and death and dying. Advocates the recognition and protection of individual rights at the end of life. Provides guidance in completing advance directives and resolving conflicts over life-support decisions. Offers educational programs and materials, including a quarterly newsletter.

Compassionate Friends
P.O. Box 3696
Oak Brook, IL 60522–3696
(708) 990–0010
(708) 990–0246
In Canada:
Compassionate Friends, National Cancer Center of Canada
685 Williams Avenue
Winnipeg, Manitoba R3E OZ2
(204) 787–4896
A self-help organization incorporated in 1978 to offer friendship and understanding to bereaved parents and siblings. Provides support and aid to parents in the positive resolution of the grief experienced upon the death of their child; fosters the physical and emotional health of bereaved parents and siblings. National publications: *The Compassionate Friends Newsletter* (subscription is

$15.00/year) and *Sibling Newsletter* (subscription is $7.50/year) (both published quarterly). Membership by voluntary contribution. There are currently more than 665 local chapters. Aims of local chapters are to offer support and friendship to sorrowing parents; to listen with understanding; to provide "telephone friends"; to give cognitive information about the grieving process through programs and library; and to provide acquaintance with bereaved parents whose sorrow has softened and who have found fresh hope and strength for living. Local groups hold monthly meetings. Contact the national office for general and/or chapter information.

Corporate Angel Network, Inc. (CAN)
Westchester County Airport
Building 1
White Plains, NY 10604
(914) 328–1313
FAX: (800) 328–3938
    A nationwide program designed to give clients with cancer the use of available seats on corporate aircraft for travel to or from a recognized treatment center. Clients must be able to walk onto the plane and must be in stable condition. There is no cost to the patient, nor are there any financial need criteria. Requests for transportation should be made when a defined date for treatment or for discharge has been arranged. (*Note:* For Canada, see Mission Air.)

Hospice—for U.S., see National Hospice Organization; for Canada, see Canadian Palliative Care Association

I Can Cope (contact through local ACS chapter)
    A client and family education program offering information about cancer, its treatments, and modes of coping with the disease. Its goal is restoration of a sense of self-control through a greater understanding of cancer. Program consists of eight sessions (lectures, discussions, group, and individual activities) supervised by health care professionals.

International Association of Laryngectomees (IAL) see American Cancer Society for address. (Contact local chapter through local branch of the ACS or CCS.)
    A voluntary association that promotes and supports rehabilitation programs for persons who have had a laryngectomy. Provides educational programs, family education and information, support, and encouragement. Personal visits are made to clients in the hospital and/or home upon physician's request. Offers assistance with employment on an individual basis. Quarterly publication: *IAL News.*

International Myeloma Foundation
2120 Stanley Hills Drive
Los Angeles, CA 90046
(213) 654–3023
FAX: (213) 656–1182
(800) 452–CURE (452–2873)
    Promotes education about myeloma and research regarding prevention and treatment. Informs patients about available treatment options. Provides knowledge and support to community-based services and patient support groups. Quarterly publication: *Myeloma Today.*

International Ostomy Association, Inc. (IOA)
15 Station Road
Reading, Berkshire RG1 1LG
England
(714) 660–8624
A voluntary health organization dedicated to assisting people who have or will have intestinal or urinary tract diversions. Sponsors World Ostomy Congress and a World Ostomy Congress for Professionals. Publication: *Ostomy International* (a semi-annual publication).

Susan G. Komen Breast Cancer Foundation
5005 LBJ Freeway
Suite 370
Dallas, TX 75244
(800) I'M–AWARE (462–9273)
An organization dedicated to the eradication of breast cancer as a life-threatening disease by advancing research, education, screening, and treatment.

Leukemia Society of America, Inc.
600 Third Avenue
New York, NY 10016
(212) 573–8484
FAX: (212) 972–5776
(800) 955–4LSA (955–4572)
Offers financial assistance or referral to other means of support, educational materials, and consultation services for clients with leukemia and selected cancers (Hodgkin's disease, multiple myeloma).

Make-a-Wish Foundation of America
100 West Clarendon Street
Suite 2200
Phoenix, AZ 85013–3518
(602) 279–WISH (279–9474)
FAX: (602) 279–0855
(800) 722–WISH (722–9474)
The purpose of this foundation is to ensure that wishes are granted to children in the United States with a terminal illness or life-threatening medical condition creating the probability that the children will not survive beyond their eighteenth year. This is accomplished by chartering chapters and providing them with consistent policies, substantive resources, comprehensive training, and wholehearted support.

Make Today Count, Inc.
Mid America Cancer Center
1235 East Cherokee
Springfield, MO 65804–2263
(417) 885–2273
(800) 432–2273
An organization that brings together persons affected by life-threatening illnesses so that they may help one another learn to live in a positive and meaningful manner. Promotes openness and honesty in discussing and dealing with

cancer and other serious illnesses. Assists professionals in communicating with and meeting needs of client and family or significant others. Objectives are achieved by local meetings, including sharing of experiences, programs, and socialization.

Mission Air (Canada)
10 Alcorn Avenue
Toronto, Ont. M4V 3B1
(416) 924–9333
A nonprofit service organization providing transportation for patients with a life-threatening illness and their families when diagnosis or medical treatment is required outside of their own community. Patients fly free of charge through the use of donated empty seats on corporate, private, or government aircraft. Mission Air arranges for ground transportation at both ends of the flight. (For the U.S., see Corporate Angels Network.)

National Alliance of Breast Cancer Organizations (NABCO)
1180 Avenue of the Americas
Second Floor
New York, NY 10036
(212) 719–0154
FAX: (212) 768–8828
A not-for-profit central resource that provides individuals and health organizations with accurate, up-to-date information on all aspects of breast cancer, and promotes affordable detection and treatment. Active in efforts to influence public and private health policy on issues that directly pertain to breast cancer (e.g., reimbursement, legislation, funding policies). Publications: *NABCO News* (quarterly) and *NABCO Resource List* (updated annually). Membership: individual—$40.00/year; nonprofit organization—$75.00/year; business—$150.00/year.

National Cancer Institute (NCI)
Building 31, Room 11A52
Bethesda, MD 20892–4200
(301) 496–5615
(800) 422–6237 (4–CANCER)
A government agency that is part of the National Institutes of Health (NIH) of the Department of Health and Human Services (HHS). Conducts research and education relating to cancer. Activities include cancer drug development; research into causation, prevention, and treatment of cancer; programs on cancer control, prevention, and early detection; fellowships for education of professionals; and public and professional education (including Cancer Information Service). Clients who are receiving therapy as part of a clinical study may be housed free of charge at the hospital facilities of the NIH clinical center.

National Cancer Institute of Canada (NCIC)
77 Bloor Street West
Suite 1702
Toronto, Ont. M5S 3A1
(416) 961–7223
A volunteer scientific and professional agency that supports, coordinates, and conducts cancer research, training related to cancer research, and professional education.

National Coalition for Cancer Survivorship (NCCS)
1010 Wayne Avenue, 5th floor
Silver Spring, MD 20910
(301) 650–8868
Founded in 1986 with the purpose of developing the art and science of living after the diagnosis and treatment of cancer. Its mission is to promote a nationwide awareness of survivorship and to communicate that there can be vibrant, productive life following the diagnosis of cancer. Its objectives are to serve as a clearinghouse for information, publications, and programs for the many organizations working on the issue of survivorship; to provide a voice for many common and recurring issues of those organizations; to advocate the interests of cancer survivors in order to secure their rights and combat prejudice; and to promote study of the problems and potentials of survivorship. Membership available to organizations and individuals. Publications: *National Coalition for Cancer Survivorship (NCCS) Networker* (quarterly), *Charting the Journey* (an almanac of resources), *Facing Forward* (a guide for those finishing treatment), and *Teamwork: The Cancer Patient's Guide to Talking With Your Doctor.*

National Hospice Organization (NHO)
1901 North Moore Street
Suite 901
Arlington, VA 22209–1714
(703) 243–5900
FAX: (703) 525–5762
Hospice Helpline: (800) 658–8898
John J. Mahoney, President
An independent national organization whose membership consists of groups providing hospice care and other professionals concerned with care of terminally ill clients and their families. Addresses issues such as standards and criteria for care, research and evaluation, reimbursement and licensure, professional liaison, and ethics. Educates the public about hospice care through telephone, general information publications, workshops at regional and state levels, and an annual educational symposium.

National Kidney Cancer Association
1234 Sherman Avenue
Suite 200
Evanston, IL 60202–1375
(708) 332–1051
FAX: (708) 328–4425
E-Mail: (708) 322–1052 (see instructions below)
Basic purposes are to provide information to patients and physicians, sponsor research on kidney cancer, and act as an advocate on behalf of patients with the federal government, insurance companies, and employers. Provides physican referrals. Membership open to physicians, patients, and family members. Free information on kidney cancer; clinical trials by E-mail. Dues are $125.00/year and include a subscription to *Kidney Cancer News* (published quarterly). Other publications include *We Have Kidney Cancer* and a variety of public policy papers. To access E-mail: Dial (708) 332–1052, 1200–14, 400 baud, Full Duplex, 8 Data Bits, 1 Stop Vit, No Parity, No Echo.

Ronald McDonald House
One Kroc Drive
Oak Brook, IL 60521
(708) 575–7418
(*Note:* Same address and phone number for the U.S. and Canada.)
Serves as a "home away from home" for parents and families of children who are under treatment for serious illnesses (including cancer). Usually within walking distance of a treatment center. There are currently more than 150 houses open in the U.S. and nine other countries.

United Cancer Council, Inc.
Park Place Office Center
4010 W. 86th Street, Suite H
Indianapolis, IN 46268–1704
(317) 879–9900
A federation of independent voluntary cancer agencies whose mission is to promote, encourage, and assist in programs of service to cancer patients and public and professional education with regard to cancer and research. Offers a Cancer Patient Assistance Fund to provide direct financial assistance to qualified cancer patients for medical expenses. Affiliated member agencies also provide various reimbursement programs, educational programs, therapy and support groups, and research grants.

United Ostomy Association, Inc. (UOA)
36 Executive Park, Suite 120
Irvine, CA 92714–6744
(714) 660–8624
FAX: (714) 660–9262
(800) 826–0826
A nonprofit organization providing mutual aid, peer support (visit to hospital or home), and education. Holds local chapter meetings for education and support. Seeks to aid in development of better ostomy equipment and supplies. Sponsors educational conferences and encourages favorable legislation. Represents people with ostomies to allied agencies and manufacturers of ostomy products. Publication: *The Ostomy Quarterly*. Contact local chapters through the local ACS or CCS.

United Way
801 North Fairfax Avenue
Alexandria, VA 22314
(701) 836–7100
May provide financial assistance in certain situations. Eligibility and available resources vary.

US TOO International, Incorporated
Prostate Cancer Survivor Support Group
7501 Lemont Road, Suite 215
Woodridge, IL 60517
(708) 985–5255
FAX: (708) 985–0626
(800) 822–5277
An international support network devoted to helping survivors of prostate cancer and their families lead healthy and productive lives (physically, mentally,

and spiritually) by offering fellowship, shared counseling, and discussions pertaining to current medical options and a positive mental outlook. Provides a link between survivors and families, and the health care community. Currently, there are more than 180 US TOO groups in the U.S., Canada, and Istanbul, Turkey. Collaborates with the American Foundation for Urologic Disease to increase public awareness and education related to prostate cancer. Monthly publication: *US TOO Newsletter* (subscription fee: $24.00).

We Can Weekends
Nursing Director, Oncology
North Cancer Center
3300 Oakdale North
Robbinsdale, MN 55422
(612) 520–5155
   Weekend retreats for families dealing with cancer. Provides opportunity to focus on the problems and concerns that are encountered in living with cancer. Doctors, nurses, and therapists from medical and lay fields help families learn facts and fallacies about cancer, understand family dynamics, express feelings, learn problem-solving techniques, reduce stress, and utilize helpful resources. Interactions involve the whole family, and new friendships may develop for client and/or family. Cost for weekend is usually modest and scholarships are available. Designed for families with children. Baby-sitters available for infants and small children. Contact North Cancer Center to learn if there is a group in your region.

Y-ME Breast Cancer Support Program, Inc.
18220 Harwood Avenue
Homewood, IL 60430–2104
Hotline: (800) 221–2141
National office phone: (312) 799–8338
In Chicago: (312) 799–8228
Outside calling area: (800) 221–2141
   A nonprofit organization that provides information, hotline counseling, support, educational programs, and self-help meetings for patients with breast cancer and their families and friends. All trained volunteers have had breast cancer treatment. Activities include a telephone hotline manned by trained volunteers, who will answer questions and lend support; open-door educational meetings; a presurgical counseling and referral service, including reading materials, referral to physicians and clinics that specialize in breast cancer diagnosis and treatment, resource materials on options, and prostheses and wigs (when available); a speaker's bureau and workshop presentation to impress women about the importance of early detection, teach breast self-examination, and discuss alternative methods of diagnosis and treatment; training for hotline volunteers; and assistance in development of local groups. Publication: *Y-Me Hotline*. Membership fee on sliding scale.

Client Education
Materials

Note: For addresses, see Appendix F.

General Information

American Cancer Society: *Chemotherapy: What It Is, How It Helps.* Atlanta, American Cancer Society, 1990.

Dollinger, M., Rosenbaum, E., and Cable, G.: *Everyone's Guide to Cancer Therapy.* Toronto, Somerville House Books, Ltd., 1991.

Living with Cancer: A Guide to Self-Help. Coping with the Side Effects of Chemotherapy. Philadelphia, Wyeth-Ayerst Laboratories, 1991.

Understanding Chemotherapy. New York, Leukemia Society of America, 1992.

Adolescents

Help Yourself—Tips for Teenagers with Cancer. 40-page booklet and 45-minute cassette tape with user's guide. Pharmacia Adria Laboratories and National Cancer Institute, 1988. Available from Pharmacia Adria Laboratories or NCI.

Biotherapy

A Patient's Guide to Self-Injection. 20-minute video and accompanying pads of illustrated instruction sheets for subcutaneous injection. Seattle, WA, Immunex Corporation, 1991.

At Home With Roferon-A Therapy (audiocassette). Nutley, NJ, Roche Laboratories, 1990.

At Home With Roferon-A Therapy (videocassette). Nutley, NJ, Roche Laboratories, 1990.

A Patient Guide to Roferon-A Therapy. Nutley, NJ, Roche Laboratories, 1986.

A Guide for Patients Receiving Prokine (Sargramostim) (single sheet available on pads). Somerville, NJ, Hoechst-Roussel Pharmaceuticals, 1991.

Getting Ready for Epogen (flip chart). Thousand Oaks, CA, Amgen, Inc., 1990.

How to Give Yourself a Subcutaneous Injection (videocassette). Thousand Oaks, CA, Amgen, Inc., 1991.

Intron-A: Self-Administration Step by Step Subcutaneous Injection Technique (illustrated flip chart). Kenilworth, NJ, Schering Corporation, 1989. (Note: Fold-up illustrated instruction sheet available to accompany chart.)

Managing Interleukin Therapy. Bethesda, MD, National Cancer Institute.

Roferon-A Patient Administration Kit. Nutley, NJ, Roche Laboratories, 1990.

Roferon-A Subcutaneous Self-Administration Instruction Review (flip chart). Nutley, NJ, Roche Laboratories, 1990.

Roferon-A Administration Kit. Nutley, NJ, Roche Laboratories, 1990.

Self Administration of Intron-A. Kenilworth, NJ, Schering Corporation, 1990.

Self Injection of Intron-A (videocassette). Kenilworth, NJ, Schering Corporation, 1990.

Waldmann, T.A., and Schwartz, R.A.: *Understanding the Immune System.* Bethesda, MD, National Cancer Institute, 1991.

Bone Marrow Transplantation

Friends Helping Friends: Bone Marrow Transplant Resource Guide. 1992.

Bone Marrow Transplantation (BMT). New York, Leukemia Society of America, 1992.

Children's Books

Draw Me a Picture: A Coloring Book for Kids with Cancer (story/coloring book for children ages 3 to 6 years; includes guide book for adults). Research Triangle Park, NC, Glaxo Pharmaceuticals.

Parkinson, C.S.: *My Mommy Has Cancer* (storybook for children). Rochester, NY, Park Press, 1985. (Available from your Cerenex representative.)

Someone Likes You Beary Much (story/activity book). New York, Leukemia Society of America, 1990.

Clinical Trials

Cancer Treatments: Consider the Possibilities (pub. no. 89–3060). Bethesda, MD, National Cancer Institute.

Patient to Patient: Cancer Clinical Trials and You (15-minute videocassette and accompanying brochure). Bethesda, MD, National Cancer Institute, 1991.

What About Chemoprevention Trials? (pub. no. 93–3459). Bethesda, MD, National Cancer Institute, 1993.

What Are Clinical Trials All About? (pub. no. 90–2706). Bethesda, MD, National Cancer Institute, 1991.

Financial Issues

Cancer Treatments Your Insurance Should Cover: Information for Patients and Families. Rockville, MD, Association of Cancer Centers, 1991.

Genitourinary Cancers

Choices for the Prostate Cancer Patient (17-minute videocassette). Wilmington, DE, ICI Pharma, 1991.

Advanced Prostate Cancer: Treatment and Choices (videocassette). North Chicago, IL, TAP Pharmaceuticals, 1990.

Prostate Cancer: What It Is and How It Is Treated. Wilmington, DE, ICI Pharma, 1991.

Prostate Cancer: What Everyone Should Know. Deerfield, IL, TAP Pharmaceuticals, Inc., 1991.

Gynecological Disorders

Gynecologic Disorders Consultation Chart (flip chart for patient teaching). Princeton, NJ, Bristol-Myers Oncology Division, 1992.

Playing for Time: The Fight Against Ovarian Cancer. West Conshohocken, PA, U.S. Bioscience, 1992.

Hematologic Malignancies

Emotional Aspects of Childhood Leukemia: A Handbook for Parents. New York, Leukemia Society of America, 1993.

Hodgkin's Disease and the Non-Hodgkin's Lymphomas. New York, Leukemia Society of America, 1991.

Understanding Chemotherapy: A Guide to Treatment of Leukemia, Lymphoma and Multiple Myeloma for Patients and Their Families. New York, Leukemia Society of America, 1992.

Management of Side Effects (General)

Coping with the Side Effects of Chemotherapy. Philadelphia, PA, Wyeth-Ayerst Laboratories, 1991.

Living with Cancer: A Guide to Self-Help. Coping with the Side Effects of Chemotherapy. Philadelphia, Wyeth-Ayerst Laboratories, 1991.

Myelosuppression

Blood Counts and Infections: A Guide for Patients with Cancer. Columbus, OH, Pharmacia Adria Laboratories, 1993.

Nausea, Vomiting, Anorexia

Myths of Nausea and Vomiting: Ways to Manage Nausea and Vomiting During Cancer Treatment. Research Triangle Park, NC, Cerenex Laboratories, 1991.

New Horizons: Patient Intervention List and Patient Diary. Research Triangle Park, NC, Glaxo Pharmaceuticals, 1992.

Nutrition: An Ally in Cancer Therapy. Columbus, OH, Ross Laboratories, 1990 (available in English or Spanish).

Oncology Patient Care: Self-Help Tip Sheet: Managing Your Nausea and Vomiting. Philadelphia, Wyeth-Ayerst Laboratories, 1991.

Oral Hygiene

Beck, S.L., and Yasko, J.M.: *A Client's Guide to Oral Care.* Crystal Lake, IL, Sage Products, Inc., 1993.
Oral Care: Muco Care Products. *Treatment of Oral Complications of Cancer Therapy.* Buffalo Grove, IL, Unimed, Inc., 1993.
Your Oral Health: Improving or Maintaining a Healthy Mouth. Columbus, OH, Ross Laboratories, 1992.

Physical Appearance

Noyes, D.A., and Mellody, P.: *Beauty and Cancer: Looking and Feeling Your Best.* Dallas, Taylor Publishing Co. ($12.95 plus P&H).

Self-Administration of Medications

A Patient's Guide to Self-Injection (pads of illustrated instruction sheets for subcutaneous injection). Seattle, WA, Immunex Corporation, 1992.
The Challenge of Chemotherapy: Tolerance and Compliance. Oncology Patient Care, Wyeth-Ayerst Laboratories.
Toxic Reactions of Most Commonly Used Antineoplastics (laminated card). Columbus, OH, Pharmacia Adria Laboratories, 1992.

Vascular Access (General Information)

Curaflex Infusion Systems. Home Infusion Therapy: Resource Guide. Ontario, CA, Curaflex Infusion Systems, 1991.

Catheters

Bard Implanted Ports with Groshong Catheters: Use and Maintenance. Salt Lake City, UT, Bard Access Systems, 1992.
Care and Maintenance of Hickman, Broviac, and Leonard Vascular Access Catheters: Nursing Guide. Salt Lake City, UT, Bard Access Systems, 1992.
Care and Maintenance of Single and Multi-lumen Central Venous Catheters (C-VC-23) (18-minute videotape). Bloomington, IN, Cook Critical Care, 1991.
CathCap: Directions for Use. Irvine, CA, Gish Biomedical, Incorporated, 1991.
Groshong Catheter Nursing Procedure Manual. Salt Lake City, UT, Bard Access Systems, 1992.
Groshong Catheters and Bard Implanted Ports (wall chart). Salt Lake City, UT, Bard Access Systems, 1991.

Central Catheters

Diamond, E: *Managing Your Hickman Catheter.* Bethesda, MD, U.S. Department of Health and Human Services, 1990.
Groshong/Cath-tech CV Catheter: Patient's Information Manual. Salt Lake City, UT, Bard Access Systems, 1991.
Infuse-A-Cath Patient Manual. Beverly, MA, Strato Medical Corporation, 1992.

Patient Guide: How to Care for Your Hickman or Broviac Catheter at Home. Salt Lake City, UT, Bard Access Systems, 1988.

Peripherally Inserted Central Catheters (PICCs)

Avoiding Problems with Your Per-Q-Cath. San Antonio, TX, Gesco, International, 1991.
Clinical Information: Ventra Percutaneous Intravenous Catheters. St. Paul, MN, Pharmacia Deltec, Inc., 1993.

Ports

A Better Way: Patient Information for LifePort and Infuse-A-Port. Beverly, MA, Strato Medical Corporation, 1991.
A-Port: Instructions for Use. Walpole, MA, Therex Corporation, 1989.
About Your Trim-Port. Charlton, MA, Gerard Medical, Inc., 1993.
About Your Vital-Port. Leechburg, PA, CPC: A Cook Group Company, 1991.
Clinical Information: Port-A-Cath and P.A.S. Port Implantable Access Systems. St. Paul, MN, Pharmacia Deltec, Inc., 1990.
Implantofix Drug Delivery System: Patient Handbook. Bethlehem, PA, B. Braun Medical, Inc., 1990.
Implanted Ports with Hickman Catheter: Use and Maintenance. Salt Lake City, UT, Bard Access Systems, 1992.
Infuse-A-Port: Patient Manual. Norwood, MA, Infusaid, Incorporated, 1992.
Patient Choices for Vascular Access. St. Paul, MN, Pharmacia Deltec, Incorporated, 1990.
Patient Information: Port-A-Cath and P.A.S. Port. St. Paul, MN, Pharmacia Deltec, Incorporated, 1991.
Patient Manual: LifePort, Infuse-A-Port Implantable Port Systems. Beverly, MA, Strato Medical Corporation, 1993.
Patient to Patient: A Guide for Those Considering Tunneled Catheters and Implanted Ports (videocassette). Salt Lake City, UT, Bard Access Systems.

External Pumps

Baxter Infusor: Patient Instruction Guide. Round Lake, IL, Baxter Healthcare Corporation, I.V. Systems Division, 1991.
Homepump Patient Guide (pad containing 25 sheets). Carlsbad, CA, Block Medical, Inc. (cost: $2.00).
I-Flow Sidekick: The Patient's Guide (13-minute video). Irvine, CA, I-Flow Corporation.
Implantofix Drug Delivery System: Patient Handbook. Bethlehem, PA, B. Braun Medical, Inc., 1990.
Infusor Instruction Guide. Round Lake, IL, Baxter Healthcare Corporation, 1991.
Infusor: Question and Answer Reference Guide. Round Lake, IL, Baxter Healthcare Corporation, 1991.
LifeCare One Plus Inservice Videotape. North Chicago, IL, Abbott Laboratories, 1990.
LifeCare Provider 5500 System Inservice Videotape. North Chicago, IL, Abbott Laboratories, 1990.
Living with Your Provider 5500 Infusion System. North Chicago, IL, Abbott Laboratories, 1990.

Patient's Guide to the I-Flow Vivus 4000 Infusion System. Irvine, CA, I-Flow Corporation, 1991.

Provider 6000 Patient Guide. North Chicago, IL, Abbott Laboratories, 1990.

Verifuse Patient Inservice Video (12-minute videocassette). Carlsbad, CA, Block Medical, Inc., 1993 (cost: $50.00).

Implantable Pumps

Hoffmeister Stewart, J.: *Therex Implantable Pump: Patient Education Booklet.* Walpole, MA, Therex Corporation, 1991.

Infusaid Internal Pump: Patient's Manual. Norwood, MA, Infusaid, Inc., 1991.

Stewart, J.H.: *Therex Implantable Pump: Patient Education Booklet.* Walpole, MA, Therex Corporation, 1991.

Professional Education Materials

Biotherapy

Hernberman, R.B.: *Cetus ImmunoPrimer Slide/Lecture Guide.* Emeryville, CA, Cetus Oncology Division, 1991.

Intron-A: A Practical Guide for Nurses. Kenilworth, NJ, Schering Corporation, 1986.

Managing Your Patients on Roferon-A: Guidelines for the Health Care Professional. Nutley, NJ, Roche Laboratories, 1990.

Neupogen (Filgrastim) (pub. no. P40047). Thousand Oaks, CA, Amgen, Inc., 1992.

Neupogen (Filgrastim) Product Fact Card (laminated card). Thousand Oaks, CA, Amgen, Inc., 1993.

Patient Management Techniques for Interferon Therapy. Kenilworth, NJ, Schering Corporation, 1992.

The Interferons: Biology, Chemistry and Nomenclature (slides and commentary). Kenilworth, NJ, Schering Corporation, 1985.

The Management of Fatigue: An Overview for Nurses. Kenilworth, NJ, Schering Corporation, 1992.

The Right Start with Roferon-A Therapy: Managing Side Effects (videocassette). Nutley, NJ, Roche Laboratories, 1990.

Waldmann, T.A., and Schwartz, R.A.: *Understanding the Immune System.* Bethesda, MD, National Cancer Institute, 1991.

Chemotherapy Medications

Alberts, D.S., et al.: *Optimal Dosing of Carboplatin in Ovarian Cancer* (audiocassette and accompanying literature). Princeton, NJ, Bristol-Myers Oncology Products, 1991.

557

Alkeran (Melphalan Hydrochloride for Injection). Research Triangle Park, NC, Burroughs Wellcome Co., 1993.

An Introduction: Lupron Depot the Next Generation of GnRH Agonist Analogs. Deerfield, IL, TAP Pharmaceuticals, 1989.

Anticancer Drug Information Sheets (available in English and Spanish). Bethesda, MD, National Cancer Institute, 1991.

Birk, C., et al. *Administration of Paraplatin (Carboplatin for Injection): A Nursing Perspective* (audiocassette and accompanying brochure). Princeton, NJ, Bristol-Myers Squibb Company, 1993.

Bonami, P.D., et al.: *Community-Based Treatment of Lung Cancer: A Panel Discussion* (audiotapes and accompanying literature). Princeton, NJ, Bristol-Myers Oncology Products, 1990.

Cancer Chemotherapeutic Agents (wall chart). Atlanta, American Cancer Society, 1990.

Chemotherapy of Brain Tumors. Chicago, IL, American Brain Tumor Association (ABTA), 1989.

Dorr, R.T.: *Ifosfamide and Cyclophosphamide: Review and Appraisal*. Princeton, NJ, Bristol-Myers Oncology Products, 1992.

Garewal, H.S.: *Salvage Chemotherapy Regimens in Advanced Cancer*. Princeton, NJ, Bristol-Myers Oncology Products, 1988.

Geffner, E., and Best H. (eds.): *Handbook of Antineoplastic Agents*. Prepared by the editors of the compendium of Drug Therapy, 1990. Available from A.H. Robins Co.

Gregory, B., et al.: *1992/93 Guide for the Administration and Use of Cancer Chemotherapeutic Agents*. Philadelphia, Wyeth-Ayerst Laboratories, 1992.

Holmes, B.C., et al.: *Perspectives on the Use and Administration of Carboplatin: Nurse Panel Discussion* (audiotape and accompanying literature). Princeton, NJ, Bristol-Myers Oncology Division, 1991.

Kitrenos, J.G., and Santora, J.: *Guide for the Administration and Use of Cancer Chemotherapeutic Agents* (wall chart). Philadelphia, Wyeth-Ayerst Laboratories, 1988.

Lung Cancer Consultation Chart. Princeton, NJ, Bristol-Myers Oncology Division, 1991.

Nelson, M.C., and Turner, W.H.: *Leustatin (Cladribine) Injection: Guide to Continuous Infusion*. Raritan, NJ, Ortho Biotech, 1993.

Nurse Teaching Packet: Leucovorin. Wayne, NJ, Lederle Laboratories, 1992.

Pinkel, D., et al: *Burroughs Wellcome Oncology Products: Current Clinical Guide*, 2nd ed. Research Triangle Park, NC, Burroughs Wellcome, 1993.

Proceedings: New Survival Data in Ovarian Cancer: The Role of Hexalen (Altretamine, Hexamethylmelamine). West Conshohocken, PA, U.S. Bioscience, 1990.

Questions and Answers on Lupron Depot: The First Once-a-Month GnRH Agonist. Deerfield, IL, TAP Pharmaceuticals, 1990.

Quick Reference Guide for IV Alkeran (laminated card). Research Triangle Park, NC, Burroughs Wellcome Co., 1993.

Spain, R.C.: *Neoadjuvant Chemotherapy for Locally Advanced Non-Small Cell Lung Cancer*. Princeton, NJ, Bristol-Myers Oncology Division, 1988.

Zoladex: A Nurse's Guide. Wilmington, DE, Zeneca Pharmaceuticals, 1991.

Chemotherapeutic Protocols and Regimens (Combination Chemotherapy)

Bartel, S., Blanding, P., Harvey, C., et al.: *1992 Combination Cancer Chemotherapeutic Regimens* (wall chart). Thousand Oaks, CA, Amgen, 1992.

Dorr, R.T.: *Cancer Therapy Protocols: Drug Administration Regimens,* revised edition. Emeryville, CA, Cetus Oncology Corporation, 1992.
Non-Hodgkin's Lymphoma: Chemotherapy Dosing Guide for Aggressive Regimens. Princeton, NJ, Mead-Johnson Oncology Products, 1991.
Selecting Aggressive Therapy for Non-Hodgkin's Lymphoma Based on Patient Parameters. Princeton, NJ, Mead-Johnson Oncology Products, 1992.

Hypercalcemia

Hypercalcemia: Signs, Symptoms and Treatment. Deerfield, IL, Fujisawa Corporation, 1991.

Investigational Chemotherapy

Guidelines for the Clinical Evaluation of Antineoplastic Drugs. (HHS pub. no. [FDA] 81-3112). Rockville, MD, U.S. Department of Health and Human Services, 1981.

Preparation and Administration

A Guide to the Safe Handling of Antineoplastic Agents. Don Mills, Ontario, Health Care Occupational Health and Safety Administration, 1992.
ChemoCheck Training and Recertification Program (good for 12 C.E.U.s). Available from ChemoSafety Systems.
Chemoprotect Information Packet and Products Information, 1993. Available from Codan Medlon, Inc.
Chemotherapy Safety: Information Packet and Products Information. New Buffalo, MI, Healthcare Safety Systems.
National Institutes of Health: *Handling Chemotherapy Drugs Safely at Home.* Bethesda, MD, U.S. Department of Health and Human Services, 1990.
Safe Handling of Cytotoxic and Hazardous Drugs (laminated flip-chart). Emeryville, CA, Chiron Therapeutics, 1991.

Toxicities

Beck, S.L., and Yasko, J.M.: *Guidelines for Oral Care.* Crystal Lake, IL, Sage Products, Inc., 1993.
Calculating Absolute Neutrophil Count, and World Health Organization Neutropenia Grading System (laminated card). Thousand Oaks, CA, Amgen, Inc., 1993.
Cerenex Laboratories: *Zofran (Odansetron HCL Injection): Cancer Chemotherapy-Induced Emesis Series* (slides and commentary). Research Triangle Park, NC, Cerenex Laboratories, 1991.
Compazine Brand of Prochlorperazine: Questions and Answers. Philadelphia, SmithKline Beecham, 1990.
Gaddis, D., et al.: *New Horizons: Management of Chemotherapy-Induced Emesis* (20-minute videocassette). Research Triangle Park, NC, Cerenex Laboratories, 1992.
Gonzales, J.A., Hendrickson-Ferris, N., and Lee, P.: *Antiemetic Agents Used in Cancer Chemotherapy—1992* (wall poster). Research Triangle Park, NC, Cerenex Laboratories, 1992.
The Challenge of Chemotherapy: Tolerance and Compliance. Oncology Patient Care. Philadelphia, Wyeth-Ayerst Laboratories.
Toxic Reactions of Most Commonly Used Antineoplastics (laminated card). Columbus, OH, Pharmacia Adria Laboratories, 1992.

Vascular Access (General Information)

Curaflex Infusion Systems: *Home Infusion Therapy: Resource Guide.* Ontario, CA, Curaflex Infusion Systems, 1991.

Catheters

Bard Implanted Ports with Groshong Catheters: Use and Maintenance. Salt Lake City, UT, Bard Access Systems, 1992.
Care and Maintenance of Hickman, Broviac, and Leonard Vascular Access Catheters: Nursing Guide. Salt Lake City, UT, Bard Access Systems, 1992.
Care and Maintenance of Single and Multi-lumen Central Venous Catheters (C-VC-23) (18-minute videotape). Bloomington, IN, Cook Critical Care, 1991.
CathCap: Directions for Use. Irvine, CA, Gish Biomedical, Incorporated, 1991.
Groshong Catheter Nursing Procedure Manual. Salt Lake City, UT, Bard Access Systems, 1992.
Groshong Catheters and Bard Implanted Ports (wall chart). Salt Lake City, UT, Bard Access Systems, 1991.
Hemed Central Venous Access Catheters, Tunnelers, and Introducer Kit: Directions for Use. Irvine, CA, Gish Biomedical, Incorporated, 1993.
Hickman, Broviac, and Leonard Vascular Access Catheters (15-minute videocasette). Available in 3/4-in U-matic or 1/2-in VHS. Salt Lake City, UT, Bard Access Systems, 1992.
Implanted Ports with Hickman Catheter. Salt Lake City, UT, Bard Access Systems, 1992.
Ingle, R.J., and Nace, C.S.: *Venous Access Devices: Catheter Pinch-Off and Fracture.* Salt Lake City, UT, Bard Access Systems, 1993.
OmegaCath Long Term Vascular Access Catheter. Skokie, IL, Norfolk Medical Products, Inc., 1993.

Clearing the Blocked Catheter

Abbokinase Open-Cath (illustrated brochure). North Chicago, IL, Abbott Laboratories, 1993.
The Use of Urokinase to Restore the Patency of Venous Catheters (videocassette). North Chicago, IL, Abbott Laboratories, 1991.
Abbokinase Open-Cath (illustrated wall chart). North Chicago, IL, Abbott Laboratories, 1993.

Repairing the Damaged Catheter

Farish, J., and Bolton, D.: *Repair of Permanent Central Vascular Catheters* (C-VC-15) (15-minute videotape). Bloomington, IN, Cook Critical Care, 1987.
Hemed Central Venous Access Catheter Double Lumen Adhesive Repair Kit: Directions for Use. Irvine, CA, Gish Biomedical, Incorporated, 1991.
Hemed Central Venous Access Catheter Non-Adhesive Repair Kits. Irvine, CA, Gish Biomedical, Incorporated, 1991.
Hemed Central Venous Access Catheter Non-Adhesive Repair Kits (wall chart). Irvine, CA, Gish Biomedical, Incorporated, 1991.

Peripherally Inserted Central Catheters (PICCs)

Groshong PICC Insertion and Maintenance (video). Salt Lake City, UT, Bard Access Systems, 1987 (list price: $52.50).

Introduction to the Per-Q-Cath. San Antonio, TX, Gesco International, Inc., 1992.
Mears, C.: *Percutaneous Venous Catheter A.K.A. Peripherally Inserted Central (PIC) Line, Long Arm Catheter, Per-Q-Cath: Policy and Procedure*. Modesta, CA, California Cancer Center, 1992. (Available on request from Gesco International, Inc.)
Peripherally Inserted Central Venous Catheter Set with Peel-Away Introducer. Leechburg, PA, CPC: A Cook Group Company, 1990.

Ports

A-Port: Instructions for Use. Walpole, MA, Therex Corporation, 1989.
A²-Port Dual Lumen System: Instructions for Use. Walpole, MA, Therex Corporation, 1990.
Bard Implanted Ports with Groshong Catheters. Salt Lake City, UT, Bard Access Systems, 1992.
Celsite Drug Delivery System: Physician's Manual and Instructions for Use. Bethlehem, PA, B. Braun Medical, Inc., 1992.
Clinical Information: Port-A-Cath and P.A.S. Port Implantable Access Systems. St. Paul, MN, Pharmacia Deltec, Incorporated, 1993.
Groshong Catheters and Bard Implanted Ports (wall chart). Salt Lake City, UT, Bard Access Systems, 1991.
Groshong Venous Port: Nursing Manual. Salt Lake City, UT, Bard Access Systems, 1992.
Implantofix Drug Delivery System: Nursing Guide. Bethlehem, PA, B. Braun Medical, Inc., 1990.
Implanted Ports with Hickman Catheter: Use and Maintenance. Salt Lake City, UT, Bard Access Systems, 1992.
Infuse-A-Port: Care and Use of Venous Access Ports. Beverly, MA, Strato Medical Corp., 1992.
Infuse-A-Port: Care and Use of Venous Access Devices (12-minute videocassette). Includes objectives and post-test which can be returned for one C.E. contact hour. Beverly, MA, Strato Medical Corp., 1990.
Infuse-A-Port: Clinician's Manual. Norwood, MA, Infusaid, Inc., 1991.
LifePort Access and Maintenance Procedures (videocassette). Beverly, MA, Strato Medical Corporation, 1991.
LifePort, Infuse-A-Port: Quick Reference Guide (laminated wall chart). Beverly, MA, Strato Medical Corporation, 1991.
LifePort Vascular Access System: Instructions for Use. Beverly, MA, Strato Medical Corporation, 1991.
M.R.I. Dual Implanted Port with Septum Ridge Finder: Use and Maintenance. Salt Lake City, UT, Bard Access Systems, 1992.
Nursing Guidelines for Implantofix Drug Delivery System (9-minute video). Bethlehem, PA, B. Braun Medical, Inc., 1990.
OmegaPort: Guidelines for Standard Accessing (wall chart). Skokie, IL, Norfolk Medical Products, Inc., 1992.
OmegaPort Implantable Access System: Nursing Guidelines. Skokie, IL, Norfolk Medical Products, Inc., 1992.
OmegaPort Implantable Access System: User's Manual. Skokie, IL, Norfolk Medical Products, Inc., 1992.
OmegaPort Implantable Access System for All Therapies: Nursing Guidelines. Skokie, IL, Norfolk Medical Products, Inc., 1992.
Port-A-Cath "Body-in-a-Box" with Venous Demonstration Kit. St. Paul, MN, Pharmacia Deltec, Inc.

Port-A-Cath Implantable Access Systems (illustrated wall chart). St. Paul, MN, Pharmacia Deltec, Inc., 1989.

Port-A-Cath Nursing Inservice Video. St. Paul, MN, Pharmacia Deltec, Inc., 1989.

Port Access and Maintenance (laminated wall chart). Leechburg, PA, CPC: A Cook Group Company, 1992.

S.E.A.-Port Implantable Access System: Instruction Manual. Kenne, NH, Harbor Medical Devices (HMD, Inc.), 1992.

S.E.A.-Port TopSider Implantable Access System: Instruction Manual. Keene, NH, Harbor Medical Devices (HMD, Inc.), 1992.

SureCath Port Access Training Video. Broomfield, CO, Ivion Corporation, 1992.

The Care and Management of Implantable Vascular Access Ports. Norwood, MA, Infusaid, Inc., 1992. (Videotape and accompanying study packet.)

The Care and Use of Venous Access Ports. Beverly, MA, Strato Medical Corporation, 1990. (Presented as part of a series.)

Trim-Port Vascular Access System: Instructions for Use. Charlton, MA, Gerard Medical, Inc., 1993.

Vital-Port Dual Lumen Vascular Access System. Leechburg, PA, CPC: A Cook Group Company, 1992.

Vital-Port Mini Vascular Access System: Suggested Instructions for Use. Leechburg, PA, CPC: A Cook Group Company, 1993.

Vital-Port Petite Vascular Access System: Suggested Instructions for Use. Leechburg, PA, CPC: A Cook Group Company, 1992.

Vital-Port: Surgical Implantation with Access and Maintenance Suggestions (18-minute videocassette). Leechburg, PA, CPC: A Cook Group Company, 1992.

Vital-Port Vascular Access System: Suggested Instructions for Use. Leechburg, PA, CPC: A Cook Group Company, 1992.

Pumps

Baxter Infusor: Patient Instruction Guide. Round Lake, IL, Baxter Healthcare Corporation, I.V. Systems Division, 1991.

CADD-PLUS Pump: Operation Manual. St. Paul, MN, Pharmacia Deltec, Inc., 1992.

CADD-PLUS: Inservice Video. St. Paul, MN, Pharmacia Deltec, Inc., 1988.

CADD-PLUS: Operator Manual Model 5400. St. Paul, MN, Pharmacia Deltec, Inc., 1988.

I-Flow Paragon: User's Guide. Irvine, CA, I-Flow Corporation, 1993.

I-Flow Sidekick: Pharmacist's Guide (11-minute video). Irvine, CA, I-Flow Corporation.

Implantable Infusion Pump: Refill Procedure. Norwood, MA, Infusaid, Inc., 1992.

Infumed 400 Ambulatory Infusion Pump: Operations Manual. Broomfield, CO, Ivion Corporation, 1991.

LifeCare One Plus Inservice Videotape. San Diego, CA, Abbott Infusion Specialists, Inc., 1990.

Provider One Programming Guide. San Diego, CA, Abbott Infusion Specialists, Inc., 1992.

Provider 5500 Programming Guide. San Diego, CA, Abbott Infusion Specialists, Inc., 1992.

Provider 6000 Professional Field Reference. San Diego, CA, Abbott Infusion Specialists, Inc., 1992.

Therex Model 3000 Implantable Pump: Instructions for Use. Walpole, MA, Therex Corporation, 1991.

Verifuse Continuous Patient Therapy Guide (pad containing 25 sheets). Carlsbad, CA, Block Medical, Inc. (cost: $2.00).
Verifuse Intermittent Patient Therapy Guide (pad containing 25 sheets). Carlsbad, CA, Block Medical, Inc. (cost: $2.00).
Verifuse Nurse's Guide. Carlsbad, CA, Block Medical, Inc. (cost: $2.00).
Verifuse Pump (20-minute videocassette). Carlsbad, CA, Block Medical, Inc., 1993 (cost: $50.00).

Periodicals

Clinical Advances in Oncology Nursing. (Wyeth-Ayerst)
Innovations in Oncology. (Wyeth-Ayerst)
Innovations in Oncology Nursing. (Zeneca Pharmaceuticals)
Innovations in Urology Nursing. (Zeneca Pharmaceuticals)
Issues in Oncology. (A.H. Robins Company)
Newsaid. (Infusaid, Inc.)
Oncology Bulletin. (Cerenex Laboratories)
Oncology News/Update. (Miles Pharmaceuticals)
Oncology Patient Care. (Wyeth-Ayerst)
Oncology Update. (Boehringer Ingelheim Pharmaceuticals, Inc.)
Outpatient Chemotherapy. (Burroughs Wellcome)
Perspectives in Gynecologic Oncology. (U.S. Bioscience)
Roferon-A Highlights. (Roche Laboratories)
Updates. (Burroughs Wellcome)

Body Surface Area Slide Rules

Abbott Laboratories
Berlex Laboratories (includes Clinical Staging Systems for CLL and Fludara dose calculator)
Bristol-Myers Oncology Division (includes Creatinine Clearance Calculator and TNM Stager for Carcinoma of the Lung)
Immunex Corporation (includes Leukine Dosage Calculator)
A.H. Robins Company
Ortho Biotech (includes Procrit [epoetin alfa] dosage calculator)
Pharmacia Adria Laboratories
Roxane Laboratories
Upjohn (includes creatinine clearance calculator)
U.S. Bioscience (includes creatinine clearance calculator, and Ovarian Cancer Stager)

Breast Cancer: TNM Staging (Laminated Card)

Zeneca Pharmaceuticals

Patient Staging Scales—Karnofsky and ECOG

(laminated card): Emeryville, CA: Chiron Oncology

Wound Size Calipers

Berlex Laboratories

Addresses for Materials in Appendices E and F

Abbott Infusion Specialists, Inc.
15222-B Avenue of Science
San Diego, CA 92128
FAX: (619) 485–7709
(800) 338–7867

Abbott Laboratories
1 Abbott Park Road
North Chicago, IL 60064–3500
(708) 937–6100
(800) 633–9110
In Canada:
Abbott Laboratories Ltd.
6300 ch. Côte-de-Liesse
Montreal, QC H4T 1E3
P.O. Box CP 6150, Station A
Montreal, QC H3C 3K6
(514) 342–6244

**American Brain Tumor Association
(ABTA)**
2720 River Road
Des Plaines, IL 60018
(708) 827–9920
FAX: (708) 827–9918
Patient line: (800) 886–2282

American Cancer Society
(contact your local office to request
    information)
(800) ACS-2345
National Office:
1599 Clifton Road
Atlanta, GA 30329
In Georgia: (404) 320–4444
(800) ACS-2345
(800) 227–2345

Amgen, Incorporated
1840 Dehavilland Drive
Thousand Oaks, CA 91320–1789
(800) 77–AMGEN (772–6436)

Bard Access Systems
5425 West Amelia Earhart Drive
Salt Lake City, UT 84116
(801) 595–0700
FAX: (801) 595–4975
(800) 443–3385

Baxter Healthcare Corporation
I.V. Systems Division/Ambulatory
    Infusion Business (AIB)
Route 120 and Wilson Road
Round Lake, IL 60073–0490
(708) 270–4310
FAX: (708) 270–4320
(800) 285–2421

Berlex Laboratories, Incorporated
15049 San Pablo Avenue
P.O. Box 4099
Richmond, CA 94804–0099
(800) 888–4112
In Canada:
2260 32 Avenue
Lachine (PQ) H8T 3H4
(514) 631–7400
FAX: (514) 636–9177
(800) 321–0288

BioSafety Systems, Inc.
10225 Willow Creek Road
San Diego, CA 92131
In California: (619) 530–0400
FAX: (619) 530–2099
In Canada:
The Critical Asst. Group
31 Progress Court, Suite 11
Scarborough, Ontario M10 3Y5
(416) 289–7762
FAX: (416) 289–7765

Block Medical, Inc.
5957 Landau Court
Carlsbad, CA 92008
(619) 431–1501
FAX: (619) 431–1540
(800) 444–8681

**Boehringer Ingelheim
Pharmaceuticals, Inc.**
90 Eastridge
P.O. Box 368
Ridgefield, CT 06877
(203) 438–0311
In Canada:
977 Century Drive
Burlington, Ont. L7L 5J8
(416) 639–0333

B. Braun Medical, Inc.
824 Twelth Avenue
Bethlehem, PA 18018
(610) 691–5400
(610) 691–2202
(800) 523–9676

Breast Cancer Advisory Center
11426 Rockville Pike
Suite 406
Rockville, MD 20850

Bristol-Myers Squibb Company
Department of Medical Services
2402 W. Pennsylvania Street
Princeton, NJ 08543
(800) 321–1335
In Canada:
2625 Queensview Drive
P.O. Box 6313 Stn. J
Ottawa, Ont. K2A 3Y4
(613) 596–5850

Burroughs Wellcome Co.
3030 Cornwallis Rd.
Research Triangle Park, NC 27709
In North Carolina: (919) 248–3000
(800) 443–6763
In Canada:
Wellcome Medical Division
16751 Route Transcanadienne
Kirkland, QC H9H 4J4
(514) 694–8220

Cerenex Laboratories
A Division of Glaxo Pharmaceuticals, Incorporated
Five Moore Drive
Research Triangle Park, NC 27709
(919) 248–2100
(800) 545–2965

Chiron Therapeutics
4560 Horton Street
Emeryville, CA 94608–2997
(510) 601–3440
FAX: (510) 420–4855
Professional Services: (800) CHIRON-8; (800) 244–7668
Nurse Network: (800) IL2–NURS; (800) 452–6877

Clintec Nutrition Company
Three Parkway North
P.O. Box 760
Deerfield, Il 60015–0760
(708) 317–2800
FAX: (708) 317–3186
(800) 422–ASK2 (422–2752)

Codan Medlon, Inc.
3325 North Glenoaks Boulevard
Burbank, CA 91504
(818) 954–9541
FAX: (818) 848–7045
(800) 332–6326

Cook Critical Care
P.O. Box 489
925 South Curry Drive
Bloomington, IN 47402–0489
(812) 339–2235
FAX: (812) 339–5369
(800) 457–4500

CPC: A Cook Group Company
P.O. Box 529
Leechburg, PA 15656
(412) 845–8621
FAX: (412) 845–2848
(800) 245–4715

Cryogenic Laboratories, Inc.
2233 Hamline Avenue North
Roseville, MN 55113
(612) 636–3792
FAX: (612) 636–2199

Curaflex Infusion Systems
One Lakeshore Circle
3281 East Guasti Road, Suite 700
Ontario, CA 91761
(909) 460–2400
(800) 444–CURA (444–2872)

Fujisawa Pharmaceutical Corporation
Parkway North Center
Deerfield, IL 60015–2548
(800) 727–7003

Gerard Medical, Inc.
90 Worcester Road
Charlton, MA 01507
(508) 248–1562
FAX: (508) 248–1604

Germfree Laboratories
Department WC
7435 N.W. 41 Street
Miami, FL 33166
In Florida: (305) 592–1780
FAX: (305) 591–7280
(800) 922–1780, (800) 888–5357

Gesco International, Inc.
P.O. Box 690188
San Antonio, TX 78269
(210) 699–0444
FAX: (210) 699–8818
(800) 531–5814

Gish Biomedical, Incorporated
2681 Kelvin Avenue
Irvine, CA 92714–5821
(714) 756–5845
FAX: (714) 553–7392
(800) 938–0531

Harbor Medical Devices (HMD, Inc.)
160 E. Emerald Street
Keene, NH 03431
(603) 357–8322
(603) 358–6167
(800) 888–2408

Healthcare Safety Systems
Attn: Tom Roberts
P.O. Box 827
New Buffalo, MI 49117
(219) 293–0301
FAX: (219) 293–0202
(800) 727–3179

HDC Corporation
2109 O'Toole Avenue
San Jose, CA 95131
(408) 954–0340
FAX: (408) 954–1909
(800) 227–8162
In California: (800) 752–3999

I-Flow Corporation
2532 White Road
Irvine, CA 92714
FAX: (714) 553–8056
(800) 4IV-FLOW (448–3569)

Immunex Corporation
51 University Street
Seattle, WA 98101
(206) 587–0430
(800) 334–6273

Infusaid, Inc.
1400 Providence Highway
Norwood, MA 02062
(617) 769–8330
FAX: (617) 769–0072
(800) 451–1050

Ivion Corporation
Englewood, CO 80112
(800) 624–8466

Leukemia Society of America
600 Third Avenue
New York, NY 10016
(212) 573–8484
(800) 955–4LSA (955–4572)

LyphoMed, Inc.
10401 West Touhy Avenue
Rosemont, IL 60018
In Illinois: (312) 390–6500
(800) 621–3334
In Canada:
LyphoMed Canada, Inc.
6600 Goreway Dr.
Mississauga, Ont. L4V 1S6
In Ontario: (416) 673–1779
(800) 387–3986

Mead Johnson Nutritionals
2404 West Pennsylvania Street
Evansville, IL 47721
(800) 246–7893

Medex Ambulatory Infusion Systems
2400 Industrial Lane
Broomfield, CO 80020
(303) 465–6600
FAX: (303) 466–4955
(800) 543–7482

Medtronic, Inc.
800 53rd Avenue N.E.
Minneapolis, MN 55440–9087
(612) 572–5598
(800) 328–0810

Menlo Care
1350 Willow Road
Menlo Park, CA 94025
(415) 325–2500
(800) 752–8900

Miles Pharmaceuticals, Inc.
P.O. Box 340
Elkhart, IN 46515
(800) 468–0894

National Cancer Institute
Blair Building, Room 414
Bethesda, MD 20892–4200

National Cancer Institute
Office of Cancer Communications
Building 31, Room 10A–24
Bethesda, MD 20892

National Cancer Institute
International Cancer Information
Center
Building 82, Room 123
Bethesda, MD 20892

Norfolk Medical Products, Inc.
7307 North Ridgeway
Skokie, IL 60076
(708) 674–7075
FAX: (708) 674–7066
(800) 964–1544

NuAire Company
2100 North Fernbrook Lane
Plymouth, MN 55447
(612) 553–1270
FAX: (612) 553–0459
(800) 328–3352

Oncology Nursing Society
501 Holiday Drive
Pittsburgh, PA 15220–2749
(412) 921–7373
FAX: (412) 921–6525

Pharmacia Adria Laboratories
Medical Services Department
P.O. Box 16529
Columbus, OH 43216
FAX: (614) 764–1802
(800) 729–2902

In Canada:
2280 Argentia Road
Mississauga, Ont. L5N 6H8
(416) 858–1144

Pharmacia Deltec, Inc.
1265 Grey Fox Road
St. Paul, MN 55112
(612) 633–2556
FAX: (612) 639–2530
(800) 426–2448

A.H. Robins Company
Medical Department
1407 Cummings Drive
Richmond, VA 23220
(804) 257–2000
In Canada:
A.H. Robins Canada Inc.
2360 Southfield Rd.
Mississauga, Ont. L5N 3R6
(416) 821–8820

Roche Laboratories
340 Kingsland Street
Nutley, NJ 07110–1199
(800) 526–6367

Ross Laboratories
625 Cleveland Avenue
Columbus, OH 43216
(614) 624–ROSS (624–7677)
(800) 624–ROSS (624–7677)
or (800) 227–5767
In Canada:
5400 ch. Côte de Liesse
Montreal, QC H4P 1A5

Roxane Laboratories, Inc.
P.O. Box 16532
Columbus, OH 43216
In Ohio: (614) 276–4000
(800) 848–0120

Sage Products, Inc.
815 Tek Drive
P.O. Box 9693
Crystal Lake, IL 60014–9693
(815) 455–4700
FAX: (815) 455–5599
(800) 323–2220

Sandoz Nutritional Division
Route 10
East Hanover, NJ, 07936
(800) 333–3785

Schering Oncology/Biotech
Galloping Hill Road
Kenilworth, NJ 07033
(201) 298–4000
(800) 222–7579

SmithKline Beecham Laboratories
P.O. Box 7929
Philadelphia, PA 19101
(215) 751–4000
(800) 366–8900

Strato Medical Corporation
123 Brimbal Avenue
Beverly, MA 09105–1862
(508) 927–9419
FAX: (508) 927–7882
(800): 462–5005

TAP Pharmaceuticals
Medical Department
2355 Waukeegan Road
Deerfield, IL 60015
FAX: (708) 940–9801
(800) 622–2011

In Canada, see Abbott Laboratories
Ltd.

Taylor Publishing Company
1550 West Mockingbird Lane
Dallas, TX 75235
(800) 677–2800, ext. 8319

Therex Corporation
1600 Providence Highway
Walpole, MA 02081
(508) 660–1122
FAX: (508) 660–1819
(800) 322–1507

Unimed, Inc.
2150 East Lake Cook Road
Buffalo Grove, IL 60089
(800) 864–8330

U.S. Bioscience
One Tower Bridge
100 Front Street
West Conshohocken, PA 19428
(215) 832–4563
FAX: (215) 832–4552
(800) 447–3969

U.S. Clinical Products, Inc.
2552 Summit Avenue, Suite 406
P.O. Box 940129
Plaino, TX 75094–0129
(800) 527–4277
FAX: (214) 424–5845

U.S. Government Printing Office
Superintendent of Documents
Washington, DC 20402

Vygon Corporation
1 Madison Street
East Rutherford, NJ 07073
(201) 471–5200
FAX: (201) 471–5118
(800) 544–4907

Wyeth-Ayerst Laboratories
Drug Information Division
P.O. Box 8299
Philadelphia, PA 19101
(215) 688–4400
(800) 934–5556

In Canada:
Wyeth International
1120 Finch Avenue West
7th Floor, North York
Toronto, Ont. M3J 3H7
(416) 630–0280

Zeneca Pharmaceuticals
Wilmington, DE 19897
(302) 886–2231
In Canada:
2505 Meadowvale Boulevard
Mississauga, Ont. L5N 5R7
(416) 821–8000
(800) 268–3992

CALGB Expanded Common Toxicity Criteria

TOXICITY	GRADE				
	0	1	2	3	4
Hematologic					
WBC	≥4.0	3.0–3.9	2.0–2.9	1.0–1.9	<1.0
Platelets	WNL	75.0–normal	50.0–74.9	25.0–49.9	<25.0
Hemoglobin	WNL	10.0–normal	8.0–10.0	6.5–7.9	<6.5
Granulocytes/bands	≥2.0	1.5–1.9	1.0–1.4	0.5–0.9	<0.5
Lymphocytes	≥2.0	1.5–1.9	1.0–1.4	0.5–0.9	<0.5
Hematologic--other		Mild	Moderate	Severe	Life-threatening
Hemorrhage (clinical)	None	Mild, no transfusion	Gross, 1–2 units transfusion per episode	Gross, 3–4 units transfusion per episode	Massive, >4 units transfusion per episode
Infection	None	Mild; no active treatment (e.g., viral syndrome)	Moderate; requires outpatient P.O. antibiotic	Severe; requires I.V. antibiotic or antifungal or hospitalization	Life-threatening, e.g., septic shock
Gastrointestinal					
Nausea	None	Able to eat reasonable intake	Intake significantly decreased but can eat	No significant intake	

Vomiting	None	1 episode in 24 hr	2–5 episodes in 24 hr	6–10 episodes in 24 hr	>10 episodes in 24 hr or requiring parenteral support
Diarrhea	None	Increase of 2–3 stools/day over pre-Rx	Increase of 4–6 stools/day, or nocturnal stools, or moderate cramping	Increase of 7–9 stools/day, or incontinence, or severe cramping	Increase of ≥10 stools/day or grossly bloody diarrhea, or need for parenteral support
Stomatitis	None	Painless ulcers, erythema, or mild soreness	Painful erythema, edema, or ulcers, but can eat	Painful erythema, edema, or ulcers, and cannot eat	Requires parenteral or enteral support
Esophagitis/dysphagia	None	Painless ulcers, erythema, mild soreness or mild dysplasia	Painful erythema, edema, or ulcers or moderate dysphagia but can eat without narcotics	Cannot eat solids or requires narcotics to eat	Requires parenteral or enteral support or complete obstruction or perforation
Anorexia	None	Mild	Moderate	Severe	Life-threatening
Other GI					
Gastritis/ulcer	No	Antacid	Requires vigorous medical management or nonsurgical treatment	Uncontrolled by medical management; requires surgery for GI ulceration	Perforation or bleeding
Small bowel obstruction	No	—	Intermittent, no intervention	Requires intervention	Requires operation
Intestinal fistula	No	—	—	Yes	—
GI—other	—	Mild	Moderate	Severe	Life-threatening

(Continued)

TOXICITY	GRADE				
	0	1	2	3	4
Other Mucosal	None	Erythema, or mild pain not requiring treatment	Patchy and produces serosanguineous discharge or requires non-narcotic for pain	Confluent fibrinous mucositis or requires narcotic for pain or ulceration	Necrosis
Liver					
Bilirubin	WNL	—	$<1.5 \times N^*$	$1.5–3.0 \times N^*$	$>3.0 \times N^*$
Transaminase (SGOT, SGPT)	WNL	$\leq2.5 \times N^*$	$2.6–5.0 \times N^*$	$5.1–20.0 \times N^*$	$>20.0 \times N^*$
Alk Phos or 5' nucleotidase	WNL	$\leq2.5 \times N^*$	$2.6–5.0 \times N^*$	$5.1–20.0 \times N^*$	$>20.0 \times N^*$
Liver-clinical	No change from baseline	—	—	Precoma	Hepatic coma
Liver—other	—	Mild	Moderate	Severe	Life–threatening
Kidney, Bladder					
Creatinine	WNL	$<1.5 \times N^*$	$1.5–3.0 \times N^*$	$3.1–6.0 \times N^*$	$>6.0 \times N^*$
Proteinuria	No change	1+ or <0.3 g/100 ml or <3 g/l	2–3+ or 0.3–1.0 g/100 ml or 3–10 g/l	4+ or >1.0 g/100 ml or >10 g/l	Nephrotic syndrome
Hematuria	Neg	Micro only	Gross, no clots	Gross + clots	Requires transfusion

	WNL, <20	21–30	31–50	>50	
BUN mg%	WNL, <20	21–30	31–50	>50	—
Hemorrhagic cystitis	None	Blood on microscopic exam	Frank blood no treatment required	Bladder irrigation required	Requires cystectomy or transfusion
Renal failure	—	—	—	—	Dialysis required
Other Kidney/ Bladder					
Incontinence	Normal	With coughing, sneezing, etc.	Spontaneous some control	No control	—
Dysuria	None	Mild pain	Painful or burning urination, controlled by pyridium	Not controlled by pyridium	—
Urinary retention	None	Urinary residual >100 ml or occasionally requires catheter or difficulty initiating urinary stream	Self catheterization always required for voiding	Surgical procedure required (TUR or dilatation)	—
Increased frequency/urgency	No change	Increase in frequency or nocturia up to 2 × normal	Increased >2 × normal, but < hourly	With urgency and hourly or more or requires catheter	—
Bladder cramps	None	—	Yes		—
Ureteral obstruction	None	Unilateral, no surgery required	Bilateral, no surgery required	Not complete bilateral, but stents, nephrostomy tubes, or surgery required	Completed bilateral obstruction
GU Fistula	None	—	—	Yes	—
Kidney/Bladder—other	—	Mild	Moderate	Severe	Life-threatening

(Continued)

TOXICITY	GRADE				
	0	1	2	3	4
Alopecia	No loss	Mild hair loss	Pronounced or total hair loss	—	—
Pulmonary					
Dyspnea	None or no change	Asymptomatic, with abnormality in PFT's	Dyspnea or significant exertion	Dyspnea at normal level of activity	Dyspnea at rest
PO_2/PCO_2	No change or $PO_2 > 85$ and $PCO_2 \le 40$	$PO_2 > 70$ and $PCO_2 \le 50$, but not grade 0	$PO_2 > 60$ and $PCO_2 \le 60$, but not grade 0–1	$PO_2 > 50$ and $PCO_2 \le 70$ but not 0–2	$PO_2 \le 50$ or $PCO_2 > 70$
Carbon monoxide diffusion capacity (DLCO)	>90% of pretreatment value	Decrease to 76–90% of pretreatment	Decrease to 51–75% of pretreatment	Decrease to 26–50% pretreatment	Decrease to ≤25% of pretreatment
Pulmonary fibrosis	Normal	Radiographic changes, no symptoms	—	Changes with symptoms	—
Pulmonary edema	None	—	—	Radiographic changes and diuretics required	Requires intubation
Pneumonitis (noninfectious)	Normal	Radiographic changes, symptoms do not require steroids	Steroids required	Oxygen required	Requires assisted ventilation
Pleural effusion	None	Present	—	—	—

	None	Mild	Moderate	Severe	Life-threatening
Adult respiratory distress syndrome (ARDS)	None				Life-threatening
Other pulmonary:					
Cough	No change	Mild, relieved by OTC meds	Requires narcotic antitussive	Uncontrolled coughing spasms	—
Pulmonary—other	—	Mild	Moderate	Severe	Life-threatening
Heart					
Cardiac dysrhythmias	None	Asymptomatic, transient; requiring no therapy	Recurrent or persistent, no therapy required	Requires treatment	Requires monitoring; or hypotension, or ventricular tachycardia, or fibrillation
Cardiac function	None	Asymptomatic, decline of resting ejection fraction by less than 20% of baseline value	Asymptomatic, decline of resting ejection fraction by more than 20% of baseline value	Mild CHF, responsive to therapy	Severe or refractory CHF
Cardiac—ischemia	None	Nonspecific T-wave flattening	Asymptomatic, ST and T wave changes suggesting ischemia	Angina without evidence for infarction	Acute myocardial infarction
Cardiac—pericardial	None	Asymptomatic effusion, no intervention required	Pericarditis (rub, chest pain, ECG changes)	Symptomatic effusion: drainage required	Tamponade; drainage urgently required
Heart—other		Mild	Moderate	Severe	Life-threatening

(Continued)

TOXICITY	GRADE				
	0	1	2	3	4
Circulatory					
Hypertension	None or no change	Asymptomatic, transient increase by greater than 20 mm Hg (D) or to >150/100 if previously WNL. No treatment required	Recurrent or persistent increase by greater than 20 mm Hg (D) or to >150/100 if previously WNL. No treatment required	Requires therapy	Hypertensive crisis
Hypotension	None or no change	Changes requiring no therapy (including transient orthostatic hypotension)	Requires fluid replacement or other therapy but not hospitalization	Requires therapy and hospitalization; resolves within 48 hr of stopping the agent	Requires therapy and hospitalization for >48 hr after stopping the agent
Neurologic Other	—	Mild	Moderate	Severe	Life-threatening
Dermatologic					
Skin	None or no change	Scattered macular or papular eruption or erythema that is asymptomatic	Scattered macular or papular eruption or erythema with pruritus or other associated symptoms	Generalized symptomatic macular, papular, or vesicular eruption	Exfoliative dermatitis or ulcerating dermatitis

Local	None	Pain	Pain and swelling with inflammation or phlebitis	Ulceration	Plastic surgery indicated
Phlebitis/ thrombosis/ embolism	—	—	Superficial phlebitis (not local)	Deep vein thrombosis	Major event (cerebral/hepatic/ pulmonary/other infarction) or pulmonary embolism
Edema	None	1+ or dependent in evening only	2+ or dependent throughout day	3+	4+, generalized anasarca
Neurologic					
Neurosensory	None or no change	Mild paresthesias, loss of deep tendon reflexes	Mild or moderate objective sensory loss; moderate paresthesias	Severe objective, sensory loss or paresthesias that interfere with function	—
Neuromotor	None or no change	Subjective weakness; no objective findings	Mild objective weakness without significant impairment of function	Objective weakness with impairment of function	Paralysis
Neurocortical	None	Mild somnolence or agitation	Moderate somnolence or agitation	Severe: somnolence or agitation or confusion or disorientation, or hallucinations or aphasia, or severe difficulty communicating	Coma, seizures, toxic psychosis

*Upper limit of normal.

Adapted from Common Toxicity Criteria, SWOG Toxicity Criteria, CALGB Toxicity Grading. From Perry, M.C.: *The Chemotherapy Sourcebook* (pp. 1132–1140). Baltimore, Williams and Wilkins, 1992. Reprinted with permission.

Appendix *H*

Reimbursement/Patient Assistance Programs

COMPANY	PRODUCT(S) BRAND NAME (GENERIC NAME)	PHONE, FAX NUMBERS (TIME ZONE)
Adria Laboratories	(see Pharmacia Adria)	
Amgen, Inc.	Neupogen (filgrastim, GM-CSF)	(800) 272–9376 (EST) In Washington, DC: (202) 637–0376
Baxter Hyland Division	Gammaguard (Immune globulin)	(800) 548–IGIV (548–4448) (EST) In Washington, DC: (202) 637–0376
Berlex, Inc.	Fludara (fludarabine)	(800) 888–4112 (EST)
Bristol-Myers Oncology Division	All oncology medications (see Appendix B for list)	(800) 872–8718
Cerenex Pharmaceuticals	Zofran (ondansetron)	(800) 745–2967 (EST)
Chiron Therapeutics	Proleukin (aldesleukin, IL-2)	(800) 775–7533 (PST)
Fujisawa	Ganite (gallium nitrate)	(800) 366–6323 (EST)
Hoffman-La Roche, Inc.	Roferon-A (interferon alfa-2a)	(800) 443–6676 (EST)
Immunex Corporation	Leukine (sargramostim, GM-CSF)	(800) 321–4669 (EST)
Janssen Pharmaceutica	Ergamisol (levamisole HCl)	(800) 544–2987 (EST)
Organon	Tice-BCG	(800) 553–3851 (EST)
Ortho Biotech	Leustatin (cladribine) Procrit (epogen)	(800) 441–1366 (EST) FAX: (703) 648–1796
Parke-Davis	Nipent (pentamidine)	(800) 955–0120 (EST)
Pharmacia Adria	Adriamycin (doxorubicin)	(800) 729–2902 (EST)
Roche Cost Assistance Program	Roferon-A (Interferon alpha-2a)	(201) 235–5000 (EST)
Sandoz Pharmaceutical Corporation	Sandostatin (octreotide acetate)	(800) 447–6673 (EST)

COMPANY	PRODUCT(S) BRAND NAME (GENERIC NAME)	PHONE, FAX NUMBERS (TIME ZONE)
Schering-Plough Corporation	Intron-A (interferon alfa-2b)	(800) 521–7157 (EST)
TAP Pharmaceuticals	Lupron depot (leuprolide)	(800) 453–8438 (CST)
Zeneca Pharmaceuticals	Nolvadex (tamoxifen citrate) Zoladex (goserlin acetate)	(800) 767–4424 (EST)

INDEX

3
5-16

290
LBMT
P-21

CLE

ICI
INFORMATION
CONSERVATION, INC.

3 5282 00387 4669